D0337550

Diet, Nutrition, and Cancer

Committee on Diet, Nutrition, and Cancer
Assembly of Life Sciences
National Research Council

NATIONAL ACADEMY PRESS
Washington, D.C.   1982

NOTICE: The project that is the subject of this report was approved by the Governing Board of the National Research Council, whose members are drawn from the Councils of the National Academy of Sciences, the National Academy of Engineering, and the Institute of Medicine. The members of the committee responsible for the report were chosen for their special competences and with regard for appropriate balance.

This report has been reviewed by a group other than the authors according to procedures approved by a Report Review Committee consisting of members of the National Academy of Sciences, the National Academy of Engineering, and the Institute of Medicine.

The National Research Council was established by the National Academy of Sciences in 1916 to associate the broad community of science and technology with the Academy's purposes of furthering knowledge and of advising the federal government. The Council operates in accordance with general policies determined by the Academy under the authority of its Congressional charter of 1863, which establishes the Academy as a private, nonprofit, self-governing membership corporation. The Council has become the principal operating agency for both the National Academy of Sciences and the National Academy of Engineering in the conduct of their services to the government, the public, and the scientific and engineering communities. It is administered jointly by both Academies and the Institute of Medicine. The National Academy of Engineering and the Institute of Medicine were established in 1964 and 1970, respectively, under the charter of the National Academy of Sciences.

The work on which this publication is based was performed pursuant to Contract No. N01-CP-05603 with the National Cancer Institute.

Library of Congress Catalog Card Number 82-81777
International Standard Book Number 0-309-03280-6

Available from
NATIONAL ACADEMY PRESS
2101 Constitution Avenue, N.W.
Washington, D.C. 20418

Printed in the United States of America

First Printing, June 1982
Second Printing, September 1982
Third Printing, November 1982

Fourth Printing, May 1983
Fifth Printing, October 1984

Committee on Diet, Nutrition, and Cancer[1]

CLIFFORD GROBSTEIN, <u>Chairman</u>

JOHN CAIRNS, <u>Vice Chairman</u>

ROBERT BERLINER

SELWYN A. BROITMAN

T. COLIN CAMPBELL

JOAN D. GUSSOW

LAURENCE N. KOLONEL

DAVID KRITCHEVSKY

WALTER MERTZ

ANTHONY B. MILLER

MICHAEL J. PRIVAL

THOMAS SLAGA

LEE WATTENBERG

TAKASHI SUGIMURA, <u>Advisor</u>

<u>National Research Council Staff</u>:

SUSHMA PALMER, <u>Project Director</u>

KULBIR BAKSHI, <u>Staff Officer</u>

LESLIE J. GRAYBILL, <u>Research Associate</u>

ROBERT HILTON, <u>Research Associate</u>

FRANCES M. PETER, <u>Editor</u>

---

[1]See Appendix A for further information on committee members and staff.

Preface

Heightened interest in reducing the risk of three of the most dreaded diseases—heart disease, cancer, and stroke—has resulted in periodic efforts to "improve" food habits. These efforts attracted national attention during the last decade when a White House conference and congressional hearings explored the state of our knowledge concerning the status and health effects of nutrition in the United States. During the hearings there were inquiries about the relative emphasis placed on nutritional factors in the research strategy of the National Cancer Institute (NCI). The study described in this report is an outgrowth of these inquiries.

In June 1980, the NCI commissioned the National Research Council (NRC) to conduct a comprehensive study of the scientific information pertaining to the relationship of diet and nutrition to cancer. The NCI requested that the study committee (1) "review ... the state of knowledge and information pertinent to diet/nutrition and the incidence of cancer"; (2) "develop a series of recommendations related to dietary components (nutrients and toxic contaminants) and nutritional factors which can be communicated to the public"; and (3) "based on the above state-of-the-art appraisals and the identification of gap areas, develop a series of research recommendations related to dietary components and nutritional factors and the incidence of cancer." The agency also asked that two reports be prepared: the first to advise the NCI and the public whether evidence indicates that certain dietary habits may affect the risk of developing cancer and the second to inform NCI and the scientific community about useful directions research might take to increase our knowledge in this area. The first report is contained in this volume. It summarizes the most relevant scientific information on diet and cancer and recommends several interim dietary guidelines for dissemination to the public. In the second report, which is expected to be completed in approximately 1 year, the committee will consider potentially profitable areas for future research.

The NRC Governing Board assigned administrative responsibility for this project to the Executive Office of the Assembly of Life Sciences (ALS). Subsequently, a 13-member committee and one advisor were appointed to conduct the study. The diverse expertise represented on the committee includes such disciplines as biochemistry, microbiology, embryology, epidemiology, experimental oncology, internal medicine, microbial genetics, molecular biology, molecular genetics, nutrition, nutrition education, public health, and toxicology. Institutional affiliations and major research interests of the committee members and the staff are presented in Appendix A at the end of this report. This multidisciplinary composition has served to ensure comprehensive coverage of the scientific literature and to provide a broad perspective to the committee's conclusions. The work of the committee has been aided by extensive consultation with scientific colleagues, by specially arranged technical conferences on specific subjects, and by a public meeting to receive such additional information and advice as scientists and others wished to provide.

Food, nutrition, diet, and cancer are terms that encompass a very broad subject area, and the already vast accumulation of literature on the interrelationship of these factors is growing rapidly. Thus, the committee began its work by developing a preliminary map of its "territory." Having initially interpreted its charge to mean that no part should be arbitrarily excluded, the committee came to recognize that it would be wasteful to duplicate effort, especially when certain subjects have recently been evaluated in detailed reviews. After careful consideration, the decision was made to refer the reader to these comprehensive reviews and to concentrate in this report on the relationship between diet and its nutritional components and cancer in a narrower sense. Subjects not covered in detail include the health effects of nitrate, nitrite, and N-nitroso compounds, which have recently been studied by another ALS committee, and drinking water—a carrier of nutrients and potential toxic substances—also examined by an ALS committee. The Committee on Diet, Nutrition, and Cancer evaluated the evidence for selected contaminants and food additives, but did not discuss them in detail because the emphasis in this report is placed on the selection of particular foods or dietary regimens made by individuals or population groups, and the significance of these choices for cancer incidence.

During its preliminary mapping of territory, the committee recognized that its charge does not include the evaluation of diet and nutrition in relation to cancer therapy, but rather it stipulated that the committee's effort be directed toward the assessment of these factors in the etiology and prevention of cancer.

The committee is aware that several aspects of its charge are matters of controversy, either within the scientific and medical community or among the general population. Controversies are inevitable when data are neither clear-cut nor complete. Interpretations then depend on the criteria selected for evaluation and are influenced by individual or collective judgment. The committee has attempted to present the evidence as objectively as possible and to indicate the range of scientifically acceptable interpretation. It hopes that the results will be useful to all interested parties. The charge to the committee also included a request for dietary recommendations that could be used in the formulation of public policy. Although the committee decided that the data base is not yet adequate for firm recommendations to be made, it did conclude that there was sufficient justification for certain interim guidelines, which are presented in the Executive Summary (Chapter 1) of this report.

Scientifically valid data on diet and nutrition in relation to cancer are provided by three major sources: epidemiological studies on human populations; experimental studies on animals; and in vitro tests for genetic toxicity. All three types of studies provide useful information, especially when data derived from all sources point in the same direction. Accordingly, after a general introduction, this report presents the epidemiological and laboratory evidence for individual components of the diet, giving special attention to the degree of concordance between the epidemiological and experimental evidence. Nutrients are reviewed in Section A, and nonnutritive components are reviewed in Section B. Because of the great interest in the possible etiological and preventive roles of the dietary factors reviewed in Section B, a separate chapter is devoted to constituents that may act as inhibitors of carcinogenesis.

The trends in cancer incidence have been the subject of intense public interest and constant debate among scientists. Although this report does not purport to examine this issue in detail, Section C (Chapters 16 and 17) summarizes the current state of knowledge while focusing on the role that diet plays in the incidence of cancer at specific sites. Chapter 18 describes a framework for risk assessment with particular attention to the nuances that must be taken into account when quantifying the effects of so complex a mixture as diet.

In the Executive Summary (Chapter 1), the committee has assembled a general picture of the role of dietary and nutritional factors in the development and prevention of cancer from the detailed information presented in other chapters. The report concludes with a glossary of technical terms.

The committee particularly wishes to commend the able and devoted assistance of an NRC staff headed by Dr. Sushma Palmer, and consisting of Dr. Kulbir Bakshi, Mrs. Frances Peter, Mrs. Leslie Graybill, Mr. Robert Hilton, Mrs. Susan Barron, Mrs. Dena Banks, and Mrs. Eileen Brown.

The committee is also greatly indebted to Drs. Kenneth D. Fisher and Richard G. Allison from the Federation of American Societies for Experimental Biology; Dr. Michael Kazarinoff from Cornell University; Dr. Dietrich Knorr from the University of Delaware; Dr. Angela Little from the University of California at Berkeley; and Dr. Leonard Stoloff of the Food and Drug Administration, who served as consultants and in this capacity wrote manuscripts for the consideration and use of the committee, and extends thanks to those who gave testimony at the public meeting or, upon request, presented data and engaged in discussions during committee meetings, conferences, or workshops. Many others, especially Drs. Willard Visek, Kenneth Carroll, Morris Ross, Juanell Boyd, Joseph Rodricks, and Elizabeth Weisburger, also provided valuable advice to the committee from time to time.

Furthermore, the committee is grateful to Drs. Andrew Chiarodo and Diane Fink, the current and former project officers for this study at NCI, for their continuous interest and support; to Drs. Alvin G. Lazen and Robert Tardiff of the NRC staff; to members of the Board on Toxicology and Environmental Health Hazards for their advice in the planning of this study; to Ms. Barbara Jaffe, Miss Virginia White, and the staff of the Toxicology Information Center for their assistance and cooperation in supplying bibliographic material; to Ms. Estelle Miller and her coworkers at the NRC Manuscript Processing Unit; and to Mrs. Cecil Read, Mrs. Barbara Wensus, Mrs. Barbara Smith, and Mrs. Ute Hayman for their constant support in the preparation of the report.

CLIFFORD GROBSTEIN
Chairman
Committee on Diet, Nutrition, and Cancer

Contents

Diet, Nutrition, and Cancer

1 Executive Summary

Scientific pronouncements are usually viewed by the public as carrying a rather high level of certainty. Therefore, scientists must be especially careful in their choice of words whenever they are not totally confident about their conclusions. For example, it has become absolutely clear that cigarettes are the cause of approximately one-quarter of all the fatal cancers in the United States. If the population had been persuaded to stop smoking when the association with lung cancer was first reported, these cancer deaths would now not be occurring. Twenty years ago the "stop-smoking" message required some rather cautious wording. Today, the facts are clear, and the choice of words is not so important.

The public often demands certain kinds of information before such information can be provided with complete certainty. For example, weather forecasting is often not exact; nevertheless, the public asks that the effort be made, but has learned to accept the fact that the results are not always reliable.

The public is now asking about the causes of cancers that are not associated with smoking. What are these causes, and how can these cancers be avoided? Unfortunately, it is not yet possible to make firm scientific pronouncements about the association between diet and cancer. We are in an interim stage of knowledge similar to that for cigarettes 20 years ago. Therefore, in the judgment of the committee, it is now the time to offer some interim guidelines on diet and cancer.

Approximately 20% of all deaths in the United States are caused by cancer. Although the number of cancer cases is steadily increasing as the population grows, the age-adjusted total cancer incidence and mortality rates for sites other than the respiratory tract (cancers of which are primarily due to cigarette smoking) have as a whole remained stable during the last 30 to 40 years.

The search for the causes of cancer has been an important branch of cancer research. Considerable effort has been devoted to studying the influence of both environmental and genetic factors on the incidence of cancer. In the course of this research, it has become clear that most cancers have external causes and, in principle, should therefore be preventable. For example, blacks and Japanese residing in the United States develop the spectrum of cancers that is typical for the United States but different from that in Africa and Japan.

But what might these external causes be? Many factors in our environment are potential causes of cancer. They include substances in the air we breathe, the water we drink, the regions in which we work and

1

live, and the foods we eat. Our exposure to some of these factors varies in ways that can be precisely measured. For most factors, however, the measurement of the exposures and the assessment of their effects are neither precise nor straightforward. Among the factors whose precise effects are difficult to assess are the diets consumed by different groups of people. The measurements are difficult not only because it is hard to learn what people eat but also because the foods comprising their diets are so complex.

Studies of the association between diet and cancer have focused on cancers of the gastrointestinal tract, the breast and other tissues susceptible to hormonal influence, and, to a lesser extent, the respiratory tract and the urinary bladder. After assessing the resultant literature, the committee concluded that the differences in the rates at which various cancers occur in different human populations are often correlated with differences in diet. The likelihood that some of these correlations reflect causality is strengthened by laboratory evidence that similar dietary patterns and components of food also affect the incidence of certain cancers in animals.

Chapters 16 and 17 provide information about the trends in cancer incidence and the relationship between diet and the incidence of cancer at specific sites.

Epidemiologists have found it relatively easy to demonstrate a correlation between diets consumed in modern affluent societies and the incidence of cancers in such organs as the breast, colon, and uterus. But it has proved to be much more difficult to establish causal relationships and to determine which, if any, of the dietary components is responsible.

Similarly, difficulties are encountered in laboratory experiments. Like humans, most animals have a significant incidence of cancer in old age, and the rates of these cancers often tend to be affected by changes in diet. However, the influence of diet on spontaneous and experimentally induced cancers is not easily investigated because the underlying mechanisms and molecular biology of the cancers are still not fully understood. Indeed, the effects of diet were often regarded as a nuisance--i.e., yet another variable standing between the investigators and their measurement of carcinogenicity. As a consequence, researchers have only recently returned to the study of diet as a factor in carcinogenesis.

It is possible that research in progress will generate more definitive information that will be useful in formulating dietary recommendations to minimize the risk of cancer. In the meantime, the committee believes that the evidence at hand justifies certain interim guidelines. These guidelines appear at the end of this chapter following a summary of the committee's findings and the conclusions it believes can be drawn from the scientific evidence.

SUMMARY AND CONCLUSIONS

Dietary Patterns and Components of Food

Since the turn of the century, new methods of processing and storage have resulted in a proliferation of the kinds and numbers of food items available to the U.S. population. Unfortunately, little is known about the ways in which such innovations have altered the specific composition of the diet. The only components of food that have been monitored regularly are the nutrients. The dietary levels of most nutrients have changed relatively little over the past 80 years.

Attempting to determine which constituents of food might be associated with cancer, epidemiologists have studied population subgroups, including migrants to the United States, to examine the relationship between specific dietary patterns or the consumption of certain foods and the risk of developing particular cancers. In general, the evidence suggests that some types of diets and some dietary components (e.g., high fat diets or the frequent consumption of salt-cured, salt-pickled, and smoked foods) tend to increase the risk of cancer, whereas others (e.g., low fat diets or the frequent consumption of certain fruits and vegetables) tend to decrease it. The mechanisms responsible for these effects are not fully understood, partly because nutritive and non-nutritive components of foods may interact to exert effects on cancer incidence.

In the laboratory, investigators have attempted to shed light on the mechanisms by which diet may influence carcinogenesis. They have examined the ability of individual nutrients, food extracts, or non-nutritive components of food to enhance or inhibit carcinogenesis and mutagenesis, thereby providing epidemiologists with testable hypotheses regarding specific components of the diet. Because the data from both types of studies are generally grouped according to dietary constituents, the committee found it advantageous to organize its report in a similar fashion.

Total Caloric Intake

The committee reviewed many studies in which the variable examined was the total amount of food consumed by humans or animals, rather than the precise composition of the diet. This review is contained in Chapter 4, which is entitled "Total Caloric Intake," even though the studies did not indicate whether the observed effects resulted from the changes in the proportion of specific nutrients in the diet or from the modification of total caloric intake.

Since very few epidemiologists have been able to examine the effect of caloric intake per se on the risk of cancer, their reports have provided largely indirect evidence for such a relationship, and much of it is based on associations between body weight or obesity and cancer.

In laboratory experiments, the incidence of tumors is lower and the lifespan much longer for animals on restricted food intake than for animals fed ad libitum. However, because the intake of all nutrients was simultaneously depressed in these studies, the observed reduction in tumor incidence might have been due to the reduction of some specific nutrient, such as fat. It is also difficult to interpret experiments in which caloric intake has been modified by varying dietary fat or fiber, both of which may by themselves exert effects on tumorigenesis.

Thus, the committee concluded that neither the epidemiological studies nor the experiments in animals permit a clear interpretation of the specific effect of total caloric intake on the risk of cancer. Nonetheless, the studies conducted in animals show that a reduction in total food intake decreases the age-specific incidence of cancer. The evidence is less clear for human beings.

Lipids (Fats and Cholesterol)

Many epidemiological and laboratory studies have been conducted to examine the association between cancer and intake of lipids, i.e., total dietary fat, saturated fat, polyunsaturated fat, and cholesterol.

Fats. Epidemiological studies have repeatedly shown an association between dietary fat and the occurrence of cancer at several sites, especially the breast, prostate, and large bowel. In various populations, both the high incidence of and mortality from breast cancer have been shown to correlate strongly with higher per capita fat consumption; the few case-control studies conducted have also shown this association with dietary fat. Like breast cancer, increased risk of large bowel cancer has been associated with higher fat intake in both correlation and case-control studies. The data on prostate cancer are more limited, but they too suggest that an increased risk is related to high levels of dietary fat. In general, it is not possible to identify specific components of fat as being clearly responsible for the observed effects, although total fat and saturated fat have been associated most frequently.

The epidemiological data are not entirely consistent. For example, the magnitude of the association of fat with breast cancer appears greater in the correlation data than in the case-control data, and several reports on large bowel cancer fail to show an association with fat. Possible reasons for these discrepancies are apparent. These are discussed in Chapter 5 (see pages 5-5 and 5-18).

Like epidemiological studies, numerous experiments in animals have shown that dietary lipids influence tumorigenesis, especially in the breast and the colon. An increase in fat intake from 5% to 20% of the weight of the diet (i.e., approximately 10% to 40% of total calories) increases tumor incidence in various tissues; conversely, animals consuming low fat diets have a lower tumor incidence. When the intake of total fat is low, polyunsaturated fats appear to be more effective than saturated fats in enhancing tumorigenesis. However, this distinction becomes less prominent as total fat intake is increased.

Dietary fat appears to have a promoting effect on tumorigenesis. For example, some studies suggest that the development of colon cancer is enhanced by the increased secretion of certain bile steroids and bile acids that accompanies high levels of fat intake. Nonetheless, there is little or no knowledge concerning the specific mechanisms involved in tumor promotion. This lack of understanding contributes to our overall uncertainty about the mechanisms that underlie the effect of diet on carcinogenesis. Although most of the data ·suggest that dietary fat has promoting activity, there is not enough evidence to warrant the complete exclusion of an effect on initiation.

The committee concluded that of all the dietary components it studied, the combined epidemiological and experimental evidence is most suggestive for a causal relationship between fat intake and the occurrence of cancer. Both epidemiological studies and experiments in animals provide convincing evidence that increasing the intake of total fat increases the incidence of cancer at certain sites, particularly the breast and colon, and, conversely, that the risk is lower with lower intakes of fat. Data from studies in animals suggest that when fat intake is low, polyunsaturated fats are more effective than saturated fats in enhancing tumorigenesis, whereas the data on humans do not permit a clear distinction to be made between the effects of different components of fat. In general, however, the evidence from epidemiological and laboratory studies is consistent.

Cholesterol. The relationship between dietary cholesterol and cancer is not clear. Many studies of serum cholesterol levels and cancer mortality in human populations have demonstrated an inverse correlation with colon cancer among men, but the evidence is not conclusive. Data on cholesterol and cancer risk from studies in animals are too limited to permit any inferences to be drawn.

Chapter 5 contains a more detailed discussion of these studies.

Protein

The relationship between protein intake and carcinogenesis has been studied in human populations as well as in the laboratory. These studies are discussed in Chapter 6.

Results of epidemiological studies have suggested possible associations between high intake of dietary protein and increased risk for cancers at a number of different sites, although the literature on protein is much more limited than the literature concerning fats and cancer. In addition, because of the very high correlation between fat and protein in the diets of most Western countries, and the more consistent and often stronger association of these cancers with fat intake, it seems likely that dietary fat is the more active component. Nevertheless, the evidence does not completely preclude the existence of an independent effect of protein.

In most laboratory experiments, carcinogenesis is suppressed by diets containing levels of protein at or below the minimum required for optimal growth. Chemically induced carcinogenesis appears to be enhanced as protein intake is increased up to 2 or 3 times the normal requirement; however, higher levels of protein begin to inhibit carcinogenesis. There is some evidence to suggest that protein may affect the initiation phase of carcinogenesis and the subsequent growth and development of the tumor.

Thus, in the judgment of the committee, evidence from both epidemiological and laboratory studies suggests that high protein intake may be associated with an increased risk of cancers at certain sites. Because of the relative paucity of data on protein compared to fat, and the strong correlation between the intakes of fat and protein in the U.S. diet, the committee is unable to arrive at a firm conclusion about an independent effect of protein.

Carbohydrates

As discussed in Chapter 7, information concerning the role of carbohydrates in the development of cancer in humans is extremely limited. Although some studies suggest that a high intake of refined sugar or starch increases the risk of cancer at certain sites, the results are insufficient to permit any firm conclusions to be drawn.

The data obtained from studies in animals are equally limited, providing too little evidence to suggest that carbohydrates (possibly excluding fiber) play a direct role in experimentally induced carcinogenesis. However, excessive carbohydrate consumption contributes to caloric excess, and this in turn has been implicated as a modifier of carcinogenesis.

Dietary Fiber

Considerable effort has been devoted to studying the effects of dietary fiber and fiber-containing foods (such as certain vegetables, fruits, and whole grain cereals) on the occurrence of cancer (see Chapter 8).

Most epidemiological studies on fiber have examined the hypothesis that high fiber diets protect against colorectal cancer. Results of correlation and case-control studies of dietary fiber have sometimes supported and sometimes contradicted this hypothesis. In both types of studies, correlations have been based primarily on estimates of fiber intake obtained by grouping foods according to their fiber content. In the only case-control study and the only correlation study in which total fiber consumption was quantified rather than estimated from the consumption of high fiber foods, no association was found between high fiber intake and a lower risk of colon cancer. However, the correlation study indicated that the incidence of colon cancer was inversely related to the intake of one fiber component--the pentosan fraction, which is found in whole wheat products and other food items.

Laboratory experiments also have indicated that the consumption of some high fiber ingredients (e.g., cellulose and bran) inhibits the induction of colon cancer by certain chemical carcinogens. However, the results are inconsistent. Moreover, they are difficult to equate with the results of epidemiological studies because most laboratory investigations have focused on specific fibers or their individual components, whereas most epidemiological studies have been concerned with fiber-containing foods whose exact composition has not been determined.

Thus, the committee found no conclusive evidence to indicate that dietary fiber (such as that present in certain fruits, vegetables, grains, and cereals) exerts a protective effect against colorectal cancer in humans. Both epidemiological and laboratory reports suggest that if there is such an effect, specific components of fiber, rather than total fiber, are more likely to be responsible.

Vitamins

In recent years, there has been considerable interest in the role of vitamins A, C, and E in the genesis and prevention of cancer. In contrast, less attention has been paid to the B vitamins and others such as vitamin K. Chapter 9 contains more detailed information on the evidence summarized below.

Vitamin A. A growing accumulation of epidemiological evidence indicates that there is an inverse relationship between the risk of cancer and the consumption of foods that contain vitamin A (e.g., liver) or its precursors (e.g., the carotenoids in green and yellow vegetables). Most of the data do not show whether the effects are due to carotenoids, to vitamin A itself, or to some other constituent of these foods. In these studies, investigators found an inverse association between estimates of "vitamin A" intake and carcinoma at several sites, e.g., the lung, the urinary bladder, and the larynx.

Studies in laboratory animals indicate that vitamin A deficiency generally increases susceptibility to chemically induced neoplasia and that an increased intake of the vitamin appears to protect against carcinogenesis in most, but not all cases. Because high doses of vitamin A are toxic, many of these studies have been conducted with its synthetic analogues (retinoids), which lack some of the toxic effects of the vitamin. Retinoids have been shown to inhibit chemically induced neoplasia of the breast, urinary bladder, skin, and lung in animals.

The committee concluded that the laboratory evidence shows that vitamin A itself and many of the retinoids are able to suppress chemically induced tumors. The epidemiological evidence is sufficient to suggest that foods rich in carotenes or vitamin A are associated with a reduced risk of cancer. The toxicity of vitamin A in doses exceeding those required for optimum nutrition, and the difficulty of epidemiological studies to distinguish the effects of carotenes from those of vitamin A, argue against increasing vitamin A intake by the use of supplements.

Vitamin C (Ascorbic Acid). The epidemiological data pertaining to the effect of vitamin C on the occurrence of cancer are not extensive. Furthermore, they provide mostly indirect evidence since they are based on the consumption of foods, especially fresh fruits and vegetables, known to contain high concentrations of the vitamin, rather than on actual measurements of vitamin C intake. The results of several case-control studies and a few correlation studies suggest that the consumption of vitamin-C-containing foods is associated with a lower risk of certain cancers, particularly gastric and esophageal cancer.

In the laboratory, ascorbic acid can inhibit the formation of carcinogenic N-nitroso compounds, both in vitro and in vivo. On the other hand, studies of its inhibitory effect on preformed carcinogens have not provided conclusive results. In recent studies, the addition of ascorbic acid to cells grown in culture prevented the chemically induced transformation of these cells and, in some cases, caused reversion of transformed cells.

Thus, the limited evidence suggests that vitamin C can inhibit the formation of some carcinogens and that the consumption of vitamin-C-containing foods is associated with a lower risk of cancers of the stomach and esophagus.

Vitamin E (α-Tocopherol). Because vitamin E is present in a variety of commonly consumed foods (particularly vegetable oils, whole grain cereal products, and eggs), it is difficult to identify population groups with substantially different levels of intake. Consequently, it is not surprising that there are no epidemiological reports concerning vitamin E intake and the risk of cancer.

Vitamin E, like ascorbic acid, inhibits the formation of nitrosamines in vivo and in vitro. However, there are no reports about the effect of this vitamin on nitrosamine-induced neoplasia. Limited evidence from studies in animals suggests that vitamin E may also inhibit the induction of tumorigenesis by other chemicals.

The data are not sufficient to permit any firm conclusion to be drawn about the effect of vitamin E on cancer in humans.

The B Vitamins. No specific information has been produced by epidemiological studies, and there have been only a few inadequate laboratory investigations to determine whether there is a relationship between various B vitamins and the occurrence of cancer. Therefore, no conclusion can be drawn.

Minerals

Of the many minerals present in the diet of humans, the committee reviewed the evidence for nine that have been suspected of playing a role in carcinogenesis. The assessment was severely limited by a paucity of relevant studies on all but two minerals--selenium and iron. Where data on dietary exposure and carcinogenesis were insufficient, the committee used information from studies of occupational exposure or laboratory experiments in which the animals were exposed through routes other than diet. Chapter 10 contains more detailed information on the evidence summarized below.

Selenium. Selenium has been studied to determine its role in both the causation and the prevention of cancer. The epidemiological evidence is derived from a few geographical correlation studies, which have shown that the risk of cancer is inversely related to estimates of per capita selenium intake, selenium levels in blood specimens, or selenium concentrations in water supplies. It is not clear whether this relationship applies to all types of cancer or only to cancer at specific sites such as the gastrointestinal tract. There have been no case-control or cohort studies.

Experiments in animals have also demonstrated an antitumorigenic effect of selenium. But the relevance of these results to cancer in humans is not apparent since the selenium levels used in most of the studies far exceeded dietary requirements and often bordered on levels that are toxic. Earlier reports suggesting that selenium was carcinogenic in laboratory animals have not been confirmed.

Therefore, both the epidemiological and laboratory studies suggest that selenium may offer some protection against the risk of cancer. However, firm conclusions cannot be drawn from the limited evidence. Increasing the selenium intake to more than 200 μg/day[1] by the use of supplements has not been shown to confer health benefits exceeding

---

[1]The upper limit of the Range of Safe and Adequate Daily Dietary Intakes published in the Recommended Dietary Allowances (see Chapter 10).

those derived from the consumption of a balanced diet. Such supplementation should be considered an experimental procedure requiring strict medical supervision and is not recommended for use by the public.

Iron. Iron deficiency has been related to an increase in the risk of Plummer-Vinson syndrome, which is associated with cancer of the upper alimentary tract. Some evidence suggests that iron deficiency may be related to gastric cancer, also through an indirect mechanism. Although epidemiological reports have suggested that inhalation exposures to high concentrations of iron increase the risk of cancer, there is no evidence pertaining to the effect of high levels of dietary iron on the risk of cancer in humans. The limited evidence from animal experiments suggests that a deficiency of dietary iron may increase susceptibility to some chemically induced tumors.

The data are not sufficient for a firm conclusion to be drawn about the role of iron in carcinogenesis.

Copper, Zinc, Molybdenum, and Iodine. Some epidemiological studies suggest that dietary zinc is associated with an increase in the incidence of cancer at certain sites; others suggest that blood and tissue levels of zinc in cancer patients are lower, and those of copper are higher, than in the controls. Results of experiments in animals are also inconclusive. Different levels of dietary zinc either enhance or retard tumor growth, depending on the specific test design. High levels of copper have been observed to protect against chemical induction of tumors.

There is some epidemiological evidence that a deficiency of molybdenum and other trace elements is associated with an increased risk of esophageal cancer. Limited experiments in animals suggest that dietary molybdenum supplementation may reduce the incidence of nitrosamine-induced tumors of the esophagus and forestomach.

Studies conducted in Colombia, Iceland, and Scotland indicated that iodine deficiency, and also excessive iodine intake, may increase the risk of thyroid carcinoma. These observations have not been confirmed in other countries or in other studies. In general, the results of studies in animals support the association between iodine deficiency and thyroid cancer.

The committee concluded that the data concerning dietary exposure to zinc, copper, molybdenum, and iodine are insufficient and provide no basis for conclusions about the association of these elements with cancer risk.

Arsenic, Cadmium, and Lead. Occupational exposure to these elements is associated with an increased risk of cancer at several sites. Exposure to high concentrations of arsenic in drinking water has been linked with skin cancer. However, the evidence for cancer risk resulting from exposure to the normally low levels of these elements in the diet is not conclusive. No carcinogenic effects of dietary cadmium and arsenic have been observed in laboratory experiments, whereas high intakes of certain lead compounds appear to increase the incidence of cancer in mice and rats.

On this basis, the committee believes that no firm conclusions can be drawn about the risk of cancer due to normal dietary exposure to arsenic, cadmium, and lead.

Inhibitors of Carcinogenesis

Foods and numerous nutritive and nonnutritive components of the diet have been examined for their potential to protect against carcinogenesis. In epidemiological studies, investigators have attempted to correlate the intake of specific foods (and by inference, certain vitamins and trace elements) and the incidence of cancer. In laboratory experiments, vitamins, trace elements, nonnutritive food additives, and other organic constituents of foods (e.g., indoles, phenols, flavones, and isothiocyanates) have been tested for their ability to inhibit neoplasia (see Chapter 15).

The committee believes that there is sufficient epidemiological evidence to suggest that consumption of certain vegetables, especially carotene-rich (i.e., dark green and deep yellow) vegetables and cruciferous vegetables (e.g., cabbage, broccoli, cauliflower, and brussels sprouts), is associated with a reduction in the incidence of cancer at several sites in humans. A number of nonnutritive and nutritive compounds that are present in these vegetables also inhibit carcinogenesis in laboratory animals. Investigators have not yet established which, if any, of these compounds may be responsible for the protective effect observed in epidemiological studies.

Alcohol

The effects of alcohol consumption on cancer incidence have been studied in human populations. In some countries, including the United States, excessive beer drinking has been associated with an increased risk of colorectal cancer, especially rectal cancer. This observation has not been confirmed in other studies. There is limited evidence that excessive alcohol consumption causes hepatic injury and cirrhosis, which in turn may lead to the formation of hepatomas (liver cancer). When consumed in large quantities, alcoholic beverages appear to act synergistically with inhaled cigarette smoke to increase the risk for cancers of the mouth, larynx, esophagus, and the respiratory tract. The studies of alcohol consumption and cancer are discussed in Chapter 11.

Naturally Occurring Carcinogens

In addition to nutrients, a variety of nonnutritive substances (e.g., hydrazines) are natural constituents of foods. Furthermore, metabolites of molds (e.g., mycotoxins such as the potent carcinogen aflatoxin) and of bacteria (e.g., carcinogenic nitrosamines) may contaminate foods. Many of these are occasional contaminants, whereas others are normal components of relatively common foods. In Chapter 12, the committee examines evidence linking consumption of some of these substances to carcinogenesis.

The committee concluded that certain naturally occurring contaminants in food are carcinogenic in animals and pose a potential risk of cancer to humans. Noteworthy among these are mycotoxins (especially aflatoxin) and N-nitroso compounds, for which there is some epidemiological evidence. Studies in animals indicate that a few nonnutritive constituents of some foods, such as hydrazines in mushrooms, are also carcinogenic.

The compounds thus far shown to be carcinogenic in animals have been reported to occur in the average U.S. diet in small amounts; however, there is no evidence that any of these substances individually makes a major contribution to the total risk of cancer in the United States. This lack of sufficient data should not be interpreted as an indication that these or other compounds subsequently found to be carcinogenic do not present a hazard.

Mutagens in Foods

Mutagens are substances that cause heritable changes in the genetic material of cells. If a chemical is mutagenic to bacteria or other organisms, it is generally regarded as a suspect carcinogen, although carcinogenicity must be confirmed in long-term tests in whole animals.

As is evident from the discussion in Chapter 13, considerable attention has recently been directed toward mutagenic activity in foods. Many vegetables contain mutagenic flavonoids such as quercetin, kaempferol, and their glycosides. Furthermore, some substances found in foods can enhance or inhibit the mutagenic activity of other compounds. Mutagens in charred meat and fish are produced during the pyrolysis of proteins that occurs when foods are cooked at very high temperatures. Mutagens can also be produced during normal cooking of meat at lower temperatures. Smoking of foods as well as charcoal broiling results in the deposition of mutagenic and carcinogenic polynuclear organic compounds such as benzo[a]pyrene on the surface of the food.

Most mutagens detected in foods have not been adequately tested for their carcinogenic activity. Thus, the committee believes that it is not yet possible to assess whether such mutagens are likely to contribute significantly to the incidence of cancer in the United States.

Food Additives

In the United States, nearly 3,000 substances are intentionally added to foods during processing. Another estimated 12,000 chemicals (e.g., vinyl chloride and acrylonitrile, which are used in food-packaging materials) are classified as indirect (or unintentional) additives, and are occasionally detected in some foods. Large amounts of some additives, such as sugar, are consumed by the general population, but the annual per capita exposure to most indirect additives represents only a minute portion of the diet. Although the Food Safety Provisions and, in many cases, the "Delaney Clause" of the Federal Food, Drug, and Cosmetic Act[2] prohibit the addition of known carcinogens to foods, only a small proportion of the substances added to foods have been tested for carcinogenicity according to protocols that are considered acceptable by current standards. Moreover, except for the studies on nonnutritive sweeteners, only a few epidemiological studies have been conducted to assess the effect of food additives on cancer incidence.

Chapter 14 contains detailed information on certain additives, i.e., selected nonnutritive sweeteners, antioxidants, and additives used in packaging or for promoting the growth of animals used for food. Particular attention is given to substances to which humans are widely exposed.

Of the few direct food additives that have been tested and found to be carcinogenic in animals, all except saccharin have been banned from use in the food supply. Only minute residues of a few indirect additives that are known either to produce cancer in animals (e.g., acrylonitrile) or to be carcinogenic in humans (e.g., vinyl chloride and diethylstilbestrol) are occasionally detected in foods.

The evidence reviewed by the committee does not suggest that the increasing use of food additives has contributed significantly to the overall risk of cancer for humans. However, this lack of detectable effect may be due to their lack of carcinogenicity, to the relatively recent use of many of these substances, or to the inability of epidemiological techniques to detect the effects of additives against the background of common cancers from other causes.

Environmental Contaminants

Very low levels of a large and chemically diverse group of environmental contaminants may be present in a variety of foods. The dietary levels of some of these substances are monitored by the Market Basket Surveys conducted by the Food and Drug Administration. Many of them have been extensively tested for carcinogenicity.

---

[2]Sec. 402(a)(2)(C) and Sec. 409(c)(1)(A), respectively.

In Chapter 14, the committee has summarized the evidence concerning exposure of humans to, and the carcinogenicity of, selected pesticides, some industrial chemicals, and other environmental contaminants. As with food additives, consideration was given primarily to compounds to which humans are widely exposed.

The results of standard chronic toxicity tests indicate that a number of environmental contaminants (e.g., some organochlorine pesticides, polychlorinated biphenyls, and polycyclic aromatic hydrocarbons) cause cancer in laboratory animals. The committee found no epidemiological evidence to suggest that these compounds individually make a major contribution to the risk of cancer in humans. However, the possibility that they may act synergistically and may thereby create a greater carcinogenic risk cannot be excluded.

Contribution of Diet to Overall Risk of Cancer

By some estimates, as much as 90% of all cancer in humans has been attributed to various environmental factors, including diet (see Chapter 18). Other investigators have estimated that diet is responsible for 30% to 40% of cancers in men and 60% of cancers in women. Recently, two epidemiologists suggested that a significant proportion of the deaths from cancer could be prevented by dietary means and that dietary modifications would have the greatest effect on the incidence of cancers of the stomach and large bowel and, to a lesser extent, on cancers of the breast, the endometrium, and the lung.

The evidence reviewed by the committee suggests that cancers of most major sites are influenced by dietary patterns. However, the committee concluded that the data are not sufficient to quantitate the contribution of diet to the overall cancer risk or to determine the percent reduction in risk that might be achieved by dietary modifications.

INTERIM DIETARY GUIDELINES

It is not now possible, and may never be possible, to specify a diet that would protect everyone against all forms of cancer. Nevertheless, the committee believes that it is possible on the basis of current evidence to formulate interim dietary guidelines that are both consistent with good nutritional practices and likely to reduce the risk of cancer. These guidelines are meant to be applied in their entirety to obtain maximal benefit.

1.   There is sufficient evidence that high fat consumption is linked to increased incidence of certain common cancers (notably breast and colon cancer) and that low fat intake is associated with a lower incidence of these cancers. The committee recommends that the consumption

of both saturated and unsaturated fats be reduced in the average U.S. diet. An appropriate and practical target is to reduce the intake of fat from its present level (approximately 40%) to 30% of total calories in the diet. The scientific data do not provide a strong basis for establishing fat intake at precisely 30% of total calories. Indeed, the data could be used to justify an even greater reduction. However, in the judgment of the committee, the suggested reduction (i.e., one-quarter of the fat intake) is a moderate and practical target, and is likely to be beneficial.

2. The committee emphasizes the importance of including fruits, vegetables, and whole grain cereal products in the daily diet. In epidemiological studies, frequent consumption of these foods has been inversely correlated with the incidence of various cancers. Results of laboratory experiments have supported these findings in tests of individual nutritive and nonnutritive constituents of fruits (especially citrus fruits) and vegetables (especially carotene-rich and cruciferous vegetables).

These recommendations apply only to foods as sources of nutrients--not to dietary supplements of individual nutrients. The vast literature examined in this report focuses on the relationship between the consumption of foods and the incidence of cancer in human populations. In contrast, there is very little information on the effects of various levels of individual nutrients on the risk of cancer in humans. Therefore, the committee is unable to predict the health effects of high and potentially toxic doses of isolated nutrients consumed in the form of supplements.

3. In some parts of the world, especially China, Japan, and Iceland, populations that frequently consume salt-cured (including salt-pickled) or smoked foods have a greater incidence of cancers at some sites, especially the esophagus and the stomach. In addition, some methods of smoking and pickling foods seem to produce higher levels of polycyclic aromatic hydrocarbons and N-nitroso compounds. These compounds cause mutations in bacteria and cancer in animals, and are suspected of being carcinogenic in humans. Therefore, the committee recommends that the consumption of food preserved by salt-curing (including salt-pickling) or smoking be minimized.

4. Certain nonnutritive constituents of foods, whether naturally occurring or introduced inadvertently (as contaminants) during production, processing, and storage, pose a potential risk of cancer to humans. The committee recommends that efforts continue to be made to minimize contamination of foods with carcinogens from any source. Where such contaminants are unavoidable, permissible levels should continue to be established and the food supply monitored to assure that such levels are not exceeded. Furthermore, intentional additives (direct and indirect) should continue to be evaluated for carcinogenic activity before they are approved for use in the food supply.

5.   The committee suggests that further efforts be made to identify mutagens in food and to expedite testing for their carcinogenicity. Where feasible and prudent, mutagens should be removed or their concentration minimized when this can be accomplished without jeopardizing the nutritive value of foods or introducing other potentially hazardous substances into the diet.

6.   Excessive consumption of alcoholic beverages, particularly combined with cigarette smoking, has been associated with an increased risk of cancer of the upper gastrointestinal and respiratory tracts. Consumption of alcohol is also associated with other adverse health effects. Thus, the committee recommends that if alcoholic beverages are consumed, it be done in moderation.

* * *

The committee suggests that agencies involved in education and public information should be encouraged to disseminate information on the relationship between dietary and nutritional factors and the incidence of cancer, and to publicize the conclusions and interim dietary guidelines in this report. It should be made clear that the weight of evidence suggests that what we eat during our lifetime strongly influences the probability of developing certain kinds of cancer but that it is not now possible, and may never be possible, to specify a diet that protects all people against all forms of cancer. The cooperation of the food industry should be sought to help implement the dietary guidelines described above.

Since the current data base is incomplete, future epidemiological and experimental research is likely to provide new insights into the relationship between diet and cancer. Therefore, the committee suggests that the National Cancer Institute establish mechanisms to review these dietary guidelines at least every 5 years.

2 Cancer: Its Nature and Relationship to Diet

Before discussing the effects of diet and nutrition on the incidence of cancer, it is useful to review what is known about the nature of cancer, the basis for suspecting a relationship between diet and cancer, and the stages of carcinogenesis at which diet may exert an effect.

The following review is meant for a general audience. To avoid being too long, it oversimplifies several issues. For a more complete coverage, the reader should turn to two books--Origins of Human Cancer (Hiatt et al., 1977) and Cancer: Science and Society (Cairns, 1978)--and a journal article entitled "The causes of cancer: Quantitative estimates of avoidable risks of cancer in the United States today" (Doll and Peto, 1981).

THE NATURE OF CANCER

Cancers are populations of cells in the body that have acquired the ability to multiply and spread without the normal restraints. To understand how such populations arise and the nature of their abnormality, it is necessary to understand how cells normally control their own behavior. This subject falls within a branch of basic biology that is still not well understood.

The Control of Cell Division During the Growth and Replacement of Normal Tissues

The adult human body contains about ten trillion (10^{13}) cells. Some of these cells (e.g., the neurons and striated muscle cells) are incapable of undergoing cell division; some (e.g., the cells of the marrow and the epithelial cells of the gut and skin) are actively dividing throughout our adult life; and others (e.g., the cells of the liver) retain the ability to divide, but multiply rapidly only when tissues are undergoing regeneration after having been damaged. During our entire adult life, the gross and microscopic anatomy of the body is preserved by precise systems that regulate cell division. Cancer develops from cells that escape such regulation.

Although developmental biologists have for many years studied the operation of these regulatory systems, few of the signals that control cell behavior in multicellular animals have been identified. Certain tissues (e.g., the endocrine glands, the liver, and the bone marrow) serve general (systemic) functions rather than local functions; their role is to add or substract substances or cells from blood. The extent of cell multiplication in such tissues must be under general control and therefore must be regulated by various hormones circulating in the blood. Many of these hormones have been identified, and the general features of their operation, if not the precise molecular mechanism, are now well understood. By contrast, local signals that influence each cell's reaction to its immediate environment have not been identified. Yet, these are the signals that are responsible for the microscopic architecture of each tissue. As the result of numerous experiments on tissue development and regeneration, we know that local signals pass between cells, but we still do not know much about their nature.

The entire network of signals serves to maintain the stability and integrity of each organ and tissue, and to protect the organism from any form of uncontrolled growth. For the organism as a whole, the forces of natural selection are inexorably at work: animals that multiply fastest win the race for survival. Within each multicellular organism, however, natural selection must be held at bay. Fortunately, the controls work very well. Although some 10^{16} cell divisions occur within each human being during his or her lifetime, only about one-third of the U.S. population will develop a clinically detectable cancer.

Various Abnormalities of Cell Behavior

Until the signalling systems that impose territoriality upon the cells of the body are better understood, it is going to be difficult to determine the way a cell must be altered to free it from these restraints and allow it to form a tumor. During the early days of cancer research, many people hoped that all cancer cells would prove to be defective in one particular, common feature (e.g., in their ability to respond to a specific restraining signal received by all tissues), but this now seems most unlikely. The different forms of uncontrolled growth that lead to the different varieties of benign and malignant (cancerous) tumors appear to have distinct causes.

The adult human body contains several hundred different classes of cell that can be distinguished by their morphology, their relationship to other cells, the chemistry of their products, and their response to various hormones and to changes in their environment. Cells in each of these classes are capable of uncontrolled growth and tumor formation, but cells in some classes seem more at risk than others. For example, cancers derived from nerve cells are confined almost entirely to young children, probably because neurons lose their ability to multiply when embryogenesis is complete. In humans of all ages, cancers are common in the epithelial cells of the gut and skin, perhaps because these cells are continually undergoing division and replacement throughout life. The epithelial cells in the breast seem to be particularly susceptible to certain ill-defined carcinogenic factors during the interval between onset of menstruation and the first pregnancy. In all, several hundred forms of uncontrolled growth are now recognized and, as the result of some 100 years of clinical study involving a vast number of patients, the usual behavior of each of these kinds of tumor is now well established.

The range of cell behavior is very great. At one extreme there are such trivial abnormalities as the localized growth of melanocytes, which creates the common freckle. (Indeed, in fair-skinned people who are frequently exposed to sunlight, freckles are regarded as a normal abnormality.) At the other extreme is malignant melanoma, a cancer arising from skin melanocytes. This form of cancer is often rapidly fatal because it has a marked tendency to undergo swift dissemination through the bloodstream to all organs of the body. Between these extremes, all levels of severity can be found. Many tumors vary little in their behavior from one patient to the next. For example, the commonest tumor of the uterus (the benign fibroma or leiomyoma) arises in the smooth muscle of the uterus and can grow to enormous size, but the cells of the tumor virtually never invade the surrounding tissue or spread to distant sites. Similarly, the commonest tumor of the facial skin (the basal cell carcinoma) is locally very invasive, but it also never spreads to distant sites. Other tumors, such as those in the breast, are much less predictable; some of them spread quickly and others do not.

The pathological classification of all these growth abnormalities (or neoplasias) depends on (1) the tissue of origin, (2) the type of cell involved, and (3) most importantly, whether the abnormal cells are confined to their original location (in which case the tumor is classified as benign) or have invaded the surrounding tissues or "metastasized" to distant sites (in which case the tumor counts as a cancer). Cancers that arise in the epithelial cells are called carcinomas, and they account for more than 90% of all human deaths from cancer. Cancers that arise in the progénitors of the circulating cells of the blood are called leukemias (if the abnormal cells are circulating) and lymphomas or myelomas (if the cancer affects lymphocytes that tend to be localized in the lymph nodes or the bone marrow, respectively). Cancers that arise in fibrous connective tissue or bone are called sarcomas. Together these nonepithelial cancers account for slightly less than 10% of deaths from cancer. The pathological classification goes further and subdivides the carcinomas according to the tissue of origin (e.g., hepatocarcinoma) or the behavior of the component cells (e.g., adenocarcinoma and squamous cell carcinoma).

Cancer and Cell Heredity

It seems likely that most cancers arise from the proliferation of a single altered cell. Every tissue of the body has been shown to be made up of a very large number of small hereditarily similar nests (families) of cells. Therefore, any large piece of tissue will contain cells that are members of several of these families (i.e., they come from different branches of the family tree of cells descended from the original fertilized egg). Cancers, however, prove almost without

exception to contain cells from only one family (i.e., they must have
arisen within a single family)--a finding that is most easily explained
by assuming that each cancer is descended from a single abnormal cell.
However, it is also clear that even though cancers are in this sense
clonal, a considerable amount of modification by variation and natural
selection can occur during the growth of each cancer. For example,
although a particular cancer may be marked, from the start, with a
particular chromosomal abnormality, further abnormalities may be added
during its subsequent growth. It is as if an early step had permitted
uncontrolled growth and the operation of natural selection, which in
turn allowed the progressive evolution of increasingly abnormal and more
rapidly multiplying types of cells. Because the average cancerous growth
will amount to many millions of cells before it becomes detectable, it
may already have undergone considerable selection for the fittest vari-
ants arising spontaneously within the population. So, even if two separate cancers were to start off with the same underlying abnormality,
they could have very different characteristics by the time the diagnosis
of cancer becomes possible. This makes it very difficult to be certain
whether the great diversity of phenotypic characteristics observed in
most forms of cancer means that there has to be great diversity in the
ways of producing cancer.

The Varying Incidence of Cancer

It is abundantly clear that the incidence of all the common cancers
in humans is being determined by various potentially controllable external factors, because people in different parts of the world suffer from
different kinds of cancer, depending on their habits, diet, and customs
rather than on their ethnic origins. Thus, when people migrate from one
country to another they tend to acquire the pattern of cancer that is
characteristic of their new home. This is surely the most comforting
fact to come out of all cancer research, for it means that cancer is, in
large part, a preventable disease.

Next, it is also clear that some carcinogens tend to be associated
with specific cancers. For example, cigarette smoke is the major cause
of the common bronchogenic carcinoma of the lung, but it does not cause
the less common mesothelioma of the lung. Asbestos causes both mesotheliomas and bronchogenic carcinomas. Certain aniline dyes (especially
2-naphthylamine) cause bladder cancer, but little of any other kind of
cancer. A similar specificity probably also applies to cancers whose
cause or causes have not yet been identified, because the incidences of
the different kinds of cancer tend to vary independently.

Although the causes of most cancers that are common in affluent industrialized nations have not yet been identified, epidemiological data
suggest certain general conclusions about the nature of these causes.
Apart from lung cancer (which has become much more prevalent during this
century as more and more people have taken up smoking), the only common

cancers to have changed much in incidence during the 20th century are stomach and uterine cancers, both of which have become much less common. So it seems probable that most cases of the cancers that are common today are not being caused by the products of modern industry. In fact, the same conclusion can be reached in quite a different way, because the incidence and age-specific death rate from many of the common nonrespiratory cancers has been found to be higher in certain nonindustrialized nations like New Zealand than in the United States. It seems likely, therefore, that the common cancers not attributable to smoking are related, for the most part, not to industrialization but to various other long-standing features of our lifestyle, especially diet.

Experimentally Induced Carcinogenesis

Before considering how ingredients of the diet (or any other factor that varies from one population to another) could determine the incidence of cancer, it would be helpful if we had more information about the kinds of event that can turn a normal cell into a cancer cell. In principle, this information can come from experimental studies of carcinogenesis.

Much of this report is concerned with certain experimental systems for producing (or preventing) cancer in animals. These experiments show that a variety of treatments and agents affect the incidence of cancer. If only one general class of agent or treatment had proved to be carcinogenic, it would then have been clear what kinds of substance we should, if possible, be trying to eradicate from our lifestyle or environment. In fact, a bewildering array of agents and treatments have been shown to influence the incidence of cancer in animals.

The most widely studied method for producing cancer is to expose an animal to repeated doses of any physical or chemical agent that damages DNA and causes mutations. In certain instances it has been possible to show that the cancers produced by these agents are indeed arising as the consequence of damage to DNA. This has led people to postulate that the substances that are the important determinants of cancer in humans will, for the most part, prove to be agents that produce mutations. The idea is attractive because the cancer cell plainly has a defect that can be inherited by all its descendents. Moreover, several quick and inexpensive methods have been developed for detecting mutagens in our environment. However, it is clear that many, perhaps most, examples of carcinogenesis in laboratory animals actually proceed by way of a sequence of steps, some of which are brought about by the mutagens, whereas other, later steps are driven by agents (promoters) that are not mutagenic.

One of the most fully studied examples of "multistep" carcinogenesis is the induction of skin cancer in mice. The first step, referred to as initiation, can be produced by any of a wide range of mutagens. The step appears to occur rapidly and to be essentially irreversible and is assumed to be a direct consequence of damage to the DNA of those cells in the skin that normally proliferate and differentiate to produce the scaly cells that protect the body surface. To complete the process, it is then necessary to expose the skin for a prolonged period to various promoting agents that modify or accelerate the normal process of cell turnover. Because initiation is essentially irreversible, the process of promotion will produce cancer, even if a long time is allowed to elapse between initiation and promotion.

The nature of the events taking place during these later stages of carcinogenesis is still very obscure. For example, it is not simply a matter of forcing the initiated cell to divide quickly, because certain agents that provoke cell proliferation do not act as promoters. Most promoting agents (e.g., the irritant phorbol esters in croton oil) have a wide range of effects on the physiological functions of cells, especially on reactions taking place in the cell membrane. But there is no reason to believe that they have any direct action on DNA. Unlike initiation, the steps driven by promoters must be to some extent reversible because the effects of prolonged exposure to a promoter such as croton oil are lost if too long an interval is allowed between each application. To complicate matters still further, there is good evidence that promotion can itself be divided into two classes of events, each of which can be driven and inhibited by specific agents. So far, however, the exact molecular biology of these later events in carcinogenesis remains obscure.

The predominant effects of the mutagens commonly used in experiments in animals are localized changes in DNA, usually affecting only one or two base pairs. There are, however, other ways to induce cancer in animals that do not involve local changes in base pair sequence. For example, approximately one-quarter of all viruses known to infect vertebrates are capable of causing cancer in some animal or other. Many of these viruses probably are carcinogenic because they lead to novel juxtapositions of genes from the virus and the host. Perhaps for this reason they tend to cause particular kinds of cancer (e.g., lymphomas, leukemias, or sarcomas) rather than act as general nonspecific carcinogens. Certainly, there is little evidence that they are acting as mutagens.

Certain cancers can be produced simply by transplanting cells to novel sites in the body where they can multiply without the usual restraint or by placing them next to inert solid surfaces such as plastic or metal. It seems unlikely that mutation plays any part in these processes, especially since certain of the cancers produced in this way will recover their normal restrained behavior when they are returned to their normal location.

One conspicuous (and neglected) group of cancers results from overfeeding--a treatment that is obviously not mutagenic. The incidence of these cancers can be reduced by reductions in food intake. These effects of nutrition on the incidence of several kinds of "spontaneous" cancer in animals are very much like some of the correlations between diet and cancer that have been observed by epidemiologists--correlations that involve most of the major forms of cancer.

Laboratory studies of carcinogenesis are therefore offering us a choice of possible mechanisms for the formation of the major cancers in humans. There appears to be no way of guessing which are likely to be the important mechanisms of carcinogenesis in humans until further epidemiological studies have been conducted to isolate and identify the variables that determine cancer rates in humans.

THE CAUSES OF CANCER

The commonest cancer in Western nations is lung cancer. Its incidence is related to each nation's consumption of cigarettes--not to its level of industrialization. Thus, it is safe to be a nonsmoker in the United States, but it is not safe to be a smoker anywhere, even in the clean air of a country like Finland. A somewhat similar observation has been made for the next two most common cancers: cancer of the large intestine and breast. Both of these cancers are associated in some way with long-standing affluence, but they are apparently not linked to industrialization. Thus, the incidence of both cancers in an industrialized country like Czechoslovakia is not nearly as high as it is in New Zealand, which has one of the highest rates for both cancers despite its lack of the oil and coal required for chemical and manufacturing industries and its dependence on dairy and agricultural products for income.

The incidence of the other major cancers also varies greatly from one nation to the next, but not in the way most of us must have been led to believe from reading the many news reports about newly discovered carcinogens in our environment. Apart from cigarettes, the causes of most of today's cancers do not bear any simple and direct relationship to the intended and unintended products of industry and to what might be called the more unnatural features of modern life. This is not to say that industrial exposure is harmless, but simply that relatively few of the middle-aged and older members of our current population have been exposed to great occupational hazards. For those who were exposed, the hazards are real and inexcusable. In addition, we have to remember that the time course of carcinogenesis commonly extends over 20 years or more. This means that we have to be very concerned about the possible long-term effects resulting from exposure to novel hazards.

Investigation of the causes of cancer has been an important branch of cancer research. Early in the course of such studies it became apparent that genetic factors were not responsible for international differences in cancer incidence. When groups of people migrate from one country to another, thereby changing their environment and way of life,

they tend to leave behind the cancers typical of their homeland and acquire those of their new country. It is almost as if they are offering
us the results of a calculated experiment; indeed, to make the experiment
more perfect, several migrant groups have tended to intermarry for several generations rather than to outbreed with the other inhabitants of
their new country. Although studies of migrants have some drawbacks,
they have made an invaluable contribution to research on cancer in humans.
For example, the fact that blacks and Japanese within the United States
develop the spectrum of cancers that is generally typical for the U.S.
population but different from that in Africa and Japan tells us that most
cancers must have external causes and, in principle, should therefore be
preventable.

Certain causes of cancer have been fairly obvious for a long time.
For example, it was not difficult to connect sunlight with skin cancer.
Similarly, it seemed likely that the ever-increasing number of lung
cancers would prove to be related to something that people were breath-
ing. For most cancers, however, likely candidates for the causes were
not immediately apparent.

The list of forces that play upon us, and are likely to change if
we move from one country to another, is not impossibly long. Such
forces obviously include the air we breathe, the water we drink, and
the food we eat, as well as the way we prepare the food and apportion
it into meals. The list should include the infectious diseases that
we contract and perhaps, in a more general sense, some measure of our
contact with other living creatures. In addition to the radiation in
sunlight, we are exposed to other forms of radiation that vary somewhat
in intensity from one region to another.

Lifestyles in various countries differ enormously. Cultures vary
in family size, in the age at which reproduction starts, in the stresses
and strains placed on their populations, and in many other ways. Some
of these variables can be precisely measured. For example, it is possible to estimate accurately the extent to which time spent indoors in cold
climates increases our exposure to the background radiation that emanates
from many building materials, and to speculate that this increased exposure might account for some of the extra incidence of cancer in the northeastern United States. Similarly, it is easy to measure exposures to infectious agents. Thus, it was a straightforward exercise to demonstrate
that Burkitt's lymphoma in Africa bears some relationship to a conjunction
of endemic malaria and infection with Epstein-Barr virus. At the opposite
end of the scale, certain other variables are virtually impossible to
quantitate. For example, some people have suggested that stress can cause
cancer, but this hypothesis cannot easily be tested, and there is, as yet,
no reason to think that it is true.

For most of the variables, however, measurements can be made, but
they are not straightforward. Thus, it will require some care to trace

all the threads of causality to their source. The cancers are fairly easy to record, in terms of either incidence or mortality, but the environmental variables are not. This is especially true for diet. During the past 200 years, there have been major changes in the nutritional content of our diet and in our exposure and response to infectious diseases. The effects can be seen most readily in migrants. For example, the children of migrants to the United States are, on average, taller and live longer than their parents, just as their parents were taller than their ancestors. Because nutrition has strong effects on growth, physiology, and longevity, it was natural to suspect that the effects could extend to cover susceptibility to cancer. This hypothesis has been examined in both epidemiological studies and laboratory experiments, but the investigation of the association between diet and cancer is far from complete.

Epidemiologists found it relatively easy to demonstrate a correlation between the diets consumed by modern affluent societies and the incidence of cancers in such organs as the breast, colon, and uterus. But it is much more difficult to determine exactly which, if any, of the dietary components are responsible. For example, certain interested parties formerly argued that the association between lung cancer and smoking was not causal; instead, they suggested that the kind of people who smoke are the kind of people who, for some quite independent reason, develop lung cancer. This argument had to be resolved by prospective studies of groups of people who had stopped smoking. Exactly the same questions now arise about components of our diet: are the associations causal or coincidental? Unfortunately, it is much harder to find out what someone is eating than whether or not they smoke. It is important therefore that we prepare ourselves for a period of uncertainty, between our present realization that diet affects cancer and our eventual ability to offer the public a precise formula for minimizing the incidence of cancer.

Although the formula is still not known, we do have some estimate of the benefits it would bestow. Judging from the observed differences in cancer rates among populations with different diets, it is highly likely that the United States will eventually have the option of adopting a diet that reduces its incidence of cancer by approximately one-third, and it is absolutely certain that another third could be prevented by abolishing smoking. Those reductions would be roughly equivalent to the reduction in mortality from the infectious diseases brought about by improved hygiene and better health care delivery during the 19th century.

This prediction can be made with confidence because some major cancers have already been controlled. For example, the mortality due to stomach cancer in the United States has dropped sharply during the past 50 years--from first to sixth place on the list of most common cancers--a change brought about presumably by some alterations in our diet that took place during that period.

What cannot be predicted is the exact way in which we will discover the precise changes that ought to be made in the nation's diet. As this report points out several times (especially in Chapter 3), it is not easy to determine precisely what people are eating now, and it is even more difficult to learn what they were eating many years ago when the seeds were presumably being sown for the cancers they now have.

As shown in later chapters, it has been possible to develop in laboratory animals reasonable facsimiles of the common cancers in humans. By studying these cancers, it may be possible for the experimentalist to uncover certain important variables that the epidemiologist would only discover with difficulty.

THE INFLUENCE OF DIET ON EXPERIMENTALLY INDUCED CANCERS

Most laboratory and domesticated animals have a significant incidence of cancer during old age. These cancers tend to be affected by changes in diet in the same way as cancer in their human counterparts. Thus, a reduction in total intake of food or specific food items tends to lower the incidence of both "spontaneous" and chemically induced cancer in most strains of rats and mice. The main exceptions to this rule occur when some dietary restriction leads to a deficiency disease involving some particular tissue, thereby raising the incidence of cancer in that tissue. For example, deficiency of methyl donors such as choline leads to liver damage and raises the incidence of "spontaneous" liver cancer in rats.

These examples of the influence of diet on experimentally induced cancers are not easily investigated because the underlying mechanisms and molecular biology of the cancers are not understood. Indeed, the effects of diet were often treated as if they were simply a nuisance, being yet another variable standing between the investigators and their assays for carcinogenicity.

The Early Stages of Carcinogenesis

As mentioned earlier, the most generally accepted concept of carcinogenesis is that it is a prolonged process that starts when an animal or human being is exposed to some mutagen (initiator) that can interact with the DNA. Because chemical initiators have to be reactive to interact in this way, they are usually unstable and cannot persist very long in the environment. Thus, a more usual carcinogenic sequence is exposure to a stable but toxic chemical (e.g., aflatoxin B_1) that has to be detoxified in an organ such as the liver and, in the process, is turned into a highly reactive derivative that interacts with the DNA of the liver cell. In short, most carcinogenic initiators are created within the body as the result of "metabolic activation." This opens the way for a number of very complicated effects during carcinogenesis.

For example, a chemical that is not itself a carcinogen can act as a cocarcinogen or an anticarcinogen by stimulating or inhibiting one of the enzymes involved in the metabolism of some carcinogen. An item in the diet could therefore determine the incidence of cancer not only because of the carcinogens that it contains but also because of its various cocarcinogens and anticarcinogens, which can modify the process of carcinogenesis.

Metabolic activation has one other important consequence. In some cases, a carcinogen can be partly metabolized in one tissue and then enter the blood and undergo its final activation in some other, distant tissue. Therefore, it is not uncommon to observe that a carcinogen fed to an animal can produce cancer in organs such as breast, brain, lung, or uterus, which are far from the gastrointestinal tract.

One other variable is also important in determining the course of initiation. Most cells possess effective methods for repairing DNA. They are therefore able to undo most of the damage caused by initiating carcinogens, if there is sufficient time before they have to duplicate their DNA. It follows that initiators are sometimes made more effective if administered at the same time as some agent that forces rapid cell multiplication. For example, the production of liver cancers in choline-deficient rats, mentioned earlier, proved on further investigation to result from the action of two separate stimuli--an unexpected (and unintended) initiating carcinogen in the diet and the intended deficiency of choline, which was acting as a cocarcinogen by destroying the liver and therefore forcing the remaining liver cells to continue regenerating. Thus, these cancers could have been prevented either by adding choline to the diet or by removing the carcinogen from the diet.

To summarize, the effect of diet on the initiation of cancer can be quite complex. The early stages of carcinogenesis can involve the simultaneous interaction of several independent variables operating in a variety of ways. But at least this means that the early steps in the formation of many kinds of cancer may be interceptable in any one of several ways.

The Late Stages of Carcinogenesis

The late stages of carcinogenesis tend to be even more obscure, because they involve reactions that are even less well understood than the biochemistry of metabolic activation, DNA damage, and DNA repair. For most chemically induced (as opposed to spontaneous) cancers in laboratory animals, the process of carcinogenesis seems to go through a succession of stages. The early initiatory steps require exposure to substances that usually are known to be mutagenic. The later stages are brought about by agents (promoters) that affect cell differentiation and provoke cell proliferation. These agents appear to act primarily on processes occurring in cell membranes, including the responses to certain signalling substances and free radicals. But the molecular biology of their action remains obscure despite extensive studies on the subject. This must surely be the outstanding lacuna in experimental cancer research. Many investigators believe that these later stages concern the gradual expression of all the mutations produced during the early stages, but several observations do not fit in well with this hypothesis.

Whenever dietary experiments discriminate between the early and late stages of carcinogenesis, they usually show that the late stages are most affected by changes in the diet. The mechanisms underlying such effects are not known, but it is clear that normal dietary components can either raise or lower the incidence of cancers that have been initiated by exposing animals to carcinogens in the diet or by other routes. The details of many such experiments are described in the body of this report.

One interesting feature of these experiments is that their results so closely mimic the human condition. Most laboratory animals fed ad libitum are grossly obese compared to their wild counterparts. If they are placed on diets to maintain their weight within the range that would be found in the wild, their cancer rate tends to drop to very low levels—unless, of course, they are simultaneously exposed to high levels of some carcinogen. Similarly, obesity has also been associated with higher rates of cancer at some sites in humans.

In principle, we should be at least as interested in the late stages of carcinogenesis as in the early stages. Although cancer could in principle be prevented by blocking events at any stage, only the young would receive much benefit if we removed the initiators from our environment, whereas everyone—old and young alike—could be benefited by blocking the late stages. Unfortunately, because the late events of carcinogenesis are so poorly understood, much more effort has been expended on the study of initiators. Furthermore, searches for environmental hazards and most cost-benefit analyses have centered on eradicating the initiators to which we are exposed, rather than seeking out the promoters.

REFERENCES

Cairns, J. 1978. Cancer: Science and Society. W. H. Freeman and
     Company, San Francisco, Calif. 199 pp.

Doll, R., and R. Peto. 1981. The causes of cancer: Quantitative esti-
     mates of avoidable risks of cancer in the United States today. J.
     Natl. Cancer Inst. 66:1191-1308.

Hiatt, H. H., J. D. Watson, and J. A. Winsten, eds. 1977. Origins of
     Human Cancer. Cold Spring Harbor Laboratory, Cold Spring Harbor,
     N.Y. 3 volumes, 1,889 pp.

3 Methodology

As might be judged from the preceding chapter's discussion of the nature of cancer, it will not be easy to determine what causes cancer. It is especially difficult to identify the connections between cancer and what people eat, not only because of the complex nature of the disease, but also because of the complex nature of the food supply, the variations in eating habits, and the limitations of scientific tools.

The classic diet-related disease is associated with a deficiency of one or more nutrients. The discoveries of the causes and cures of diseases such as scurvy (caused by a lack of ascorbic acid) and beriberi (caused by a lack of thiamine) led to the development of a specific model for nutrition research in which nutrient requirements were determined by producing deficiencies in laboratory animals or volunteers.

The relationships between diet and chronic disease did not emerge as a major interest to investigators until the causes of the principal deficiency diseases were identified. Just as it was once difficult for investigators to recognize that a symptom complex could be caused by the lack of a nutrient, so until recently has it been difficult for scientists to recognize that certain pathological conditions might result from an abundant and apparently normal diet. Adverse effects on health associated with nutrient excess in humans have long been recognized. Obesity is the most noticeable among them. Other adverse effects result, at least partly, from the availability (and overuse) of vitamin and mineral supplements. Certain vitamins and most of the minerals are known to be toxic above certain levels. But these known adverse (pathologic) effects of vitamin and mineral overdoses have, like the deficiency diseases, a conspicuously direct relationship with the nutrients in question. That is, the effects of denying or restoring a nutrient to an experimental subject, whether animal or human, are usually observable within a short time--at most, months. The links between diet and metabolic, degenerative, and malignant diseases are considerably less obvious. However, because such conditions as atherosclerosis or cancer are probably associated with dietary patterns that extend over a number of years, the causative agents are difficult to identify.

The possible relationships between diet and cancer have been investigated in studies of human populations and in laboratory experiments using various _in vitro_ systems (to check substances for their ability to mutate bacteria and mutate or transform other cells) or animal models (to test substances directly for carcinogenicity). This chapter provides a synopsis of the strengths and weaknesses that are inherent in the methods used

to study these relationships. It also explains the approach adopted by
the committee in evaluating the epidemiological and experimental evidence.

EPIDEMIOLOGICAL METHODS

General Approaches

In epidemiological research on cancer and diet, investigators seek to
associate exposure to dietary risk factors with the occurrence of cancer
in defined population groups. The studies are largely observational, and
may be of several different types:

Descriptive Studies. These studies describe the patterns of disease
occurrence in one or more populations, in components of the same population, or in a single population over time. The observed patterns may be
related to certain other environmental variables or characteristics of
the population, such as demographic factors, industrial pollution, or
diet. Data from descriptive studies are suggestive, rather than definitive, and serve primarily to identify population groups at risk and to
generate hypotheses for further investigation.

Correlation Studies. These studies, based on aggregate exposure
data and observed outcomes, provide the next step in establishing meaningful associations. The crudest of these studies are ecological studies
in which national per capita food intake is related to patterns of cancer incidence or mortality. This type of analysis is frequently able
to utilize existing data and is a valuable tool for generating new hypotheses. At a more refined level, interviews with carefully selected
individuals may be correlated either with group-specific cancer rates or
with regional differences in rates. In such analyses, the data on exposure and those on outcome may be representative of exposure of different groups in the population. Consequently, they often do not reflect
true individual associations and thus may be misleading. This is often
referred to as an ecological fallacy.

Case-Control Studies. Unlike descriptive and correlation studies,
case-control studies enable investigators to collect data for individuals
rather than for groups, and they are designed to control for confounding
variables. In these studies, exposure data (such as dietary intake) are
collected for cases with a specific type of cancer and are then compared
with similar exposure data for a suitably selected noncancer group,
usually referred to as "controls" or compeers. Differences in exposures
between the two groups that cannot be accounted for by chance occurrence
(random errors) or by known biases (systematic errors) represent true
associations between individual exposure and disease and may actually
reflect causal relationships (Ibrahim, 1979; MacMahon and Pugh, 1970).
The strength of the association can be measured by an odds ratio
calculated from a 2 by 2 contingency table.

Cohort Studies. Similar to case-control studies, cohort studies focus on individuals and control for confounding variables. Furthermore, they are less susceptible to bias than case-control studies because the exposure data are collected prior to the occurrence of the disease. In the simplest cohort studies, occurrence rates of disease (e.g., cancer) over time are compared between two groups of individuals with similar characteristics but with different histories of exposure (e.g., none vs. any; low vs. high) to the factors being studied. Higher or lower incidence of disease in one group relative to the other implicates the exposure variable as playing a role in the etiology of the disease. Cohort studies are reported relatively infrequently because the low incidence of the disease requires following large groups for long periods. This necessitates considerable expenditures of both time and money. Furthermore, even if a cohort study is prospective, it is limited in that the cohorts were self-selected and were not randomly assigned as in true clinical trials or intervention studies. However, dietary intake data from several cohort studies of coronary heart disease have enabled investigators to perform retrospective cohort analyses of diet and cancer (see Chapter 5).

Intervention Studies. In these studies, which are sometimes called experimental studies, the investigator randomly assigns the subjects to two (or more) groups, which are then exposed (or not exposed) to different levels of the substance being studied. Although such studies are ideal for establishing true causal relationships, opportunities for conducting this type of study are rare. In the past, intervention studies have most often been undertaken to test the effectiveness of vaccination programs or new treatments for disease. Their use in future research on diet and cancer will be discussed in a second report to be prepared by this committee.

Methods For Determining Dietary Intake

Several standard methods with markedly different levels of precision are used to determine what people eat. Some of these methods are based on government production statistics; others use information obtained from individuals about what they have purchased, prepared, or eaten.

Group Dietary Data. Comparisons of diets for different population groups are generally based on one or two types of data: national per capita food intakes (also called food disappearance data) or household food inventories.

Most cross-national studies of cancer incidence comparing national per capita "intake" of various foods or nutrients are based on figures derived from food balance sheets. The intakes are calculated by adding the total quantity of food produced in a country to the quantity of food imported, and then subtracting the sum of food exported, fed to livestock, put to nonfood uses, and lost in storage. These estimates are then divided by the total population to yield per capita intakes. Comparisons of cancer rates at various sites with national per capita intakes of, for example, fat, fiber, and animal protein are derived from data such as these. Although national per capita intakes have been very useful in providing leads for further research, they are inaccurate as measures of food that has actually been eaten. They really only measure food that has "disappeared" into the food supply--which is why they are sometimes called "food disappearance data." They do not account for food produced by individuals, for waste in stores, restaurants, or homes, or for differences in consumption within a country by different age and sex groups.

In this report, the term "per capita intake" is used synonymously with "food disappearance data."

Household food inventories are used in epidemiological studies to obtain data on the eating patterns of groups of persons who differ geographically, socioeconomically, ethnically, or in other ways. Food intake over a fixed period, usually 1 week, is estimated either by trained workers who visit individual homes or by the person in the household responsible for food preparation who is asked either to record purchases and menus or to recall household food use. Average per capita intakes of food and nutrients are calculated by dividing the total household intake by the number of persons in the family. A major limitation of this method is that it assumes uniform food distribution for members of the individual household.

Individual Dietary Data. Of necessity, individual food consumption data must be provided by individual assessments--usually reports from the subjects themselves, but occasionally reports from family members who share their living quarters. Such information is obtained from three basic sources: recent (e.g., 24-hour) recall, food records, or diet history.

The recent recall is used most frequently to measure individual consumption. In this method, subjects are asked what foods they consumed over a recent specified time--usually 1 to 7 days. The 1-day (or 24-hour) recall only requires that each person estimate the amounts of specific food items consumed during the preceding 24 hours. However, since the foods consumed may vary considerably from one day to the next, 24-hour recalls are more reliable as a source of group data than as a source of individual data, i.e., the average for an entire group is probably reasonably representative of the eating pattern for that group. A 24-hour recall may be recorded by the subject or, more often, by a trained interviewer. He or she may be asked to recall all items or only certain foods eaten during the specified period. One sampling problem is inherent in the 24-hour recall: diets during the weekend may differ greatly from those consumed during the week. To increase the representativeness of the 24-hour recall, this method is often combined with a consumption frequency questionnaire in which subjects are asked how often they eat selected groups of foods.

In studies based on <u>food records</u>, participants are asked to maintain an accurate diary of all foods consumed during a specified period (e.g., 1 week). The subjects must estimate the quantity or weigh or measure each food item eaten at home, allow for inedible portions and plate waste, and note and measure all ingredients in recipes. They must also record estimated amounts of foods consumed away from home. Although the weighed diet record was long viewed as the ideal standard in estimating dietary intake, it requires, at a minimum, a great deal of interest and cooperation on the part of the subjects and, hence, selects for certain types of people. Moreover, this method is likely to cause subjects to modify their eating patterns to some extent, if only for purposes of reducing their work load (e.g., by eating fewer mixed dishes). The accuracy of this method is also compromised in developed countries, where much of the food eaten is neither prepared nor consumed in the home. Finally, this method is unsuitable for very large-scale surveys or studies because of the time and effort involved in providing detailed instructions to the subjects, in making frequent follow-up contacts, and in coding the unstructured information from the records. Despite these limitations, the food record has been used to validate other methods used for collecting dietary intake data in the same study population.

Unlike the recent recall, the <u>diet history</u> method does not seek information on intake during a specified day or week but, rather, attempts to determine the average pattern of consumption during a particular period of the subject's life, e.g., just before the onset of an illness. The intake of selected items or the usual dietary pattern for total intake is obtained through interviews or, less often, by self-administered questionnaire. The information is recorded as frequencies of consumption or, preferably, as estimated total amounts for the period of study. The method requires very thorough training of interviewers (or subjects, if self-administered), careful standardization of the questionnaire, adequate allowances for differences in food preparation, and the provision of suitable <u>food models</u> to facilitate quantification.

Each of the methods for estimating individual intake has its strengths and weaknesses, but they share certain limitations. People vary in their abilities to estimate exactly how much of something they have eaten, and may sometimes fail to notice (or forget to report) their consumption of certain foods (e.g., side dishes at meals, peanuts taken from a readily available supply). Respondents may also know nothing about the ingredients of the dishes set before them. Furthermore, as mentioned above, they may alter their eating habits when asked to record their intake. In case-control studies, there is an additional problem: subjects who are ill (i.e., cases and sometimes controls) may have altered their diets as a result of their illness. Although patients are generally asked to recall what they ate before the onset of their illness, they may not be completely successful in this effort.

It is especially difficult to relate diet to a disease like cancer, which has a long time course, because we need to learn not only what people ate yesterday or during the previous week, but also what they consumed in the more distant past. (The length of time between exposure and onset of disease depends partly on whether the dietary component being studied is an initiator or promoter.) The notion that subjects can accurately report not only what they usually eat but also what they usually ate is, for the most part, untested, although limited data suggest that "recall" of a diet consumed 20 or more years ago may more closely reflect present food choices than past ones (Garland and Ibrahim, 1981).

There is considerable potential for variation in the technique used by interviewers and the introduction of bias during dietary interviews, especially when very detailed information is required as in studies of cancer. Depending on the hypothesis being tested, the interviewer may need to elicit careful descriptions of food preparation methods, of the fats and oils used for frying, of usual portion sizes, of seasonal variations in intake, etc. Eliciting such information requires considerable probing on the part of the interviewer. During this process, subjectivity may be introduced in the recording of responses. For these reasons, researchers active in this field spend considerable time training interviewers and developing effective instruments and aids (for example, see Morgan et al., 1978).

Asking subjects for the same information in two or more different ways by using several methods in conjunction with one another may also help to overcome some of these problems. Estimates of quantity can be improved by using realistic or abstract food models (Morgan et al., 1978), photographs of graded portion sizes (Hankin et al., 1975), and similar devices. The strengths and limitations of the major epidemiological methods to study effects of diet have been discussed extensively in a number of reports (Beaton et al., 1979; Graham and Mettlin, 1979; Graham et al., 1967; Hankin et al., 1975; Marr, 1973; Mettlin and Graham, 1978; Morgan et al., 1978; National Academy of Sciences, 1981; Nichols et al., 1976; Nomura et al., 1976; Reshef and Epstein, 1972).

Biological markers are also used to obtain indirect estimates of individual intakes. This method has the appeal of objectivity, since it entails the direct measurement of substances in serum, tissues, or body wastes as a reflection of actual dietary exposures. Apart from the difficulty in collecting such data from healthy controls, there are other reasons why this method has not been widely used in epidemiological studies of diet and cancer. Foremost is the difficulty of identifying an appropriate indicator of past intake. For example, serum levels of some dietary components, such as cholesterol, do not correlate with information on intake and may reflect homeostatic balances or long-term patterns of consumption (Pearson, 1967; Underwood et al., 1970). However, recent reports on vitamin A serum levels suggest that some such measurements may nevertheless be useful in predicting cancer risk in cohort studies (Cambien et al., 1980; Kark et al., 1980; Wald et al., 1980). A particularly troublesome aspect of case-control studies using biological markers (e.g., the relationship of fecal steroids to colon cancer) is that the markers may themselves reflect consequences rather than antecedents of the disease.

Analysis of Dietary Data. Regardless of the method used to collect food intake data, the reported foods must be grouped into categories before they can be analyzed. Before this can be done, some decision must be made concerning the kinds of variables that should be compared with data on the occurrence of cancer. The very first level of decision may be whether to classify the data in terms of foods or nutrients—e.g., whether the variable of interest is vitamin C or citrus fruits, carotene or grams of dark green and deep yellow vegetables. In principle, the important analytic variables should be identified at the outset of the study, since that decision will determine the nature and format of the data that are collected. For example, if the variable of interest is total calories from fat rather than the characteristics of specific fats, which may differ according to their sources and processing, then the interviewer need not help the respondent differentiate between animal fats and vegetable oils or between liquid and hydrogenated shortenings. If vitamin C is considered to be the relevant variable rather than fresh citrus fruit, then no effort need be made to sort out the various forms in which oranges might be consumed (e.g., as freshly squeezed or frozen juice, or as whole orange segments). Thus, the nature of the hypothesis determines the nature of the classification used for data collection. This explains much of the discrepant data from different investigations of the same cancer site, although the source of the discrepancy may not be immediately apparent from even the most careful perusal of the published reports.

Since much of the research on the relationship between diet and cancer has been based on hypotheses regarding the effects of nutrients, the raw data on foods consumed has most often been translated into nutrients, such as grams of protein, animal protein, total fat, saturated and unsaturated fat, cholesterol, and complex carbohydrates. The quantitative estimates are usually based on food composition tables, such as those developed by the U.S. Department of Agriculture. (For an example of these estimates, see Morgan et al., 1978.) Unfortunately, the mean values recorded in such sources as USDA Handbook No. 456 (U.S. Department of Agriculture, 1975) may not reflect the specific composition of the foods eaten by subjects in a particular study. For example, wide variations in the nutrient content of unprocessed and processed foods can result from modifications in processing procedures (e.g., the addition or removal of nutrients) over time. However, such inaccuracies will merely tend to weaken any detected association rather than introduce a spurious association.

Analyses based on individual foods or food groups are not encumbered by the need to estimate nutrient intake, but are often difficult to interpret because of the multiple comparisons involved. In such analyses, the specific substances responsible for an effect may be difficult to identify.

Overall Assessment of Epidemiological Approaches

The major strength of epidemiological studies is that their focus on human populations circumvents two important limitations of laboratory research. First, since humans are observed directly, the results do not have to be extrapolated from one species to another. Second, since the levels and patterns of exposure studied are those that actually occur among people, interpolation to low doses from the artificially high exposure levels frequently required in laboratory research can also be avoided. In addition, since the varieties of human experience produce a wide range of exposures to a given risk factor, epidemiological investigations are often able to examine directly the effects of different levels of exposure (i.e., dose-response).

On the other hand, epidemiological studies present some special difficulties. To begin with, such research is limited by its need to rely primarily on observational data, because it is difficult and often unethical to conduct experiments (i.e., intervention studies) on groups of humans. Furthermore, observational epidemiological studies are open to errors or bias. For example, persons who agree to participate in such studies or who are selected as participants by the investigator (e.g., hospitalized patients) may not comprise truly representative groups of subjects and may yield misleading findings.

Unlike studies of cancer among smokers and nonsmokers, dietary studies are confronted with the inherent difficulty of determining reasonably precise exposures. For example, the degree to which cases have been exposed to a particular dietary component may not be sufficiently different from that of controls to demonstrate any effect. Furthermore, it is often difficult to determine the specific dietary constituents to which study participants have been exposed.

Another difficulty inherent in epidemiological studies of diet and cancer is the long latency period between first exposure and overt manifestation of illness. In case-control studies, this delayed onset makes it necessary for investigators to learn what the subject ate during some period beginning long before the study began, or to assume that recent intakes reflect past exposures. In prospective cohort studies, the investigator must collect current dietary data and then either wait (for up to 20 to 30 years) for the disease to appear or identify sufficiently large groups of subjects for whom there are adequate retrospective dietary data.

Accuracy in the measurement of both the exposure and the outcome variables is especially difficult to attain in the studies of diet and cancer. For example, the frequent dependence on recall data from interviewed subjects virtually guarantees imprecise measurement of dietary exposure, which might mask small but real differences between cases and controls. Correlation studies may suffer from differences among countries such as completeness of cancer reporting, diagnostic practices, and terminology. Furthermore, because cancer incidence (occurrence) data are frequently not available for such studies, reliance must be placed on mortality data instead. Since mortality reflects survival as well as incidence, it is not an ideal measure for cancer etiology, particularly for sites where survival rates are high and have notable international variation. These and other considerations make it especially difficult to identify subtleties in the relationship between the degree of exposure and risk of disease.

Most of these deficiencies in epidemiological studies of diet and cancer are likely to result in nondifferential misclassification, thereby reducing the likelihood that a given study will be able to demonstrate true differences that exist between the groups compared. Therefore, the results of epidemiological studies may often be assumed to represent conservative estimates of the true risk for cancer associated with the dietary exposures of interest.

LABORATORY METHODS

As interest in the possible relationship between diet and cancer has grown in recent years, increasing attention has been paid to the chemical carcinogens in our diet. The foods that we eat contain a vast number of separate chemical entities: several thousand as additives and many times this number as natural constituents. Most of these chemicals are present in relatively low concentrations, but even small amounts of some potent carcinogens might be important if they are present in commonly consumed foods.

There are three major laboratory methods for detecting and identifying chemical carcinogens: analysis of molecular structure, short-term tests, and long-term bioassays in animals. The first two methods provide information about potential carcinogenicity, whereas the third provides direct evidence of carcinogenicity in laboratory animals.

Analysis of Molecular Structure

In a review of the large body of evidence pertaining to the role of structure-activity relationships in predicting carcinogenic activity, Miller (1970) suggested that most, if not all, chemical carcinogens are ultimately electron-deficient reactants (Miller, 1970). Carcinogens have been identified in more than a dozen chemical classes, which share no common structural features (Miller and Miller, 1971, 1979). Furthermore, even within classes, closely related chemicals may differ with respect to carcinogenicity--e.g., 2-acetylaminofluorene (2-AAF) is a well-known carcinogen in several species of animals, whereas its close relative 4-AAF is not carcinogenic (Office of Technology Assessment, 1981). The major utility of the analysis of molecular structure is to screen a variety of chemicals quickly and to treat the results as warnings rather than as definitive indicators of carcinogenic activity.

Short-Term Tests

Interest in establishing short-term, relatively quick and inexpensive procedures for the identification of chemical carcinogens has increased during the past several years as a result of the realization that the list of potential chemical carcinogens is growing faster than our capacity to test the materials (Bridges, 1976). Therefore, greater numbers of potentially hazardous compounds must be screened and placed into a priority system for further testing. This appears to be the primary role of short-term tests.

Since these tests can be conducted quickly (often in only a day or two) and inexpensively, they are useful for screening substances for potential carcinogenicity. For these tests to be useful, they must not only be faster, easier to interpret, more sensitive, and less expensive than the standard feeding studies, but they must also be reliable and relevant to the in vivo assay upon which they are modeled.

A number of validated short-term tests can be used to examine the capacity of a substance to cause mutations, other genetic alterations, or neoplastic transformation. These tests can be used with a variety of biological systems such as bacteria, yeast, mammalian cells, and intact animals.

To date, the most widely used method appears to be the Salmonella/ microsome assay (also called the Ames test), which utilizes several specifically constructed Salmonella typhimurium strains to detect various kinds of mutations and genetic damage (Ames et al., 1975). It is generally agreed, but not without considerable controversy, that there is a high degree of correlation between the mutagenicity of compounds in the Salmonella/microsome assay and their carcinogenicity in laboratory animals (McCann and Ames, 1976; Purchase et al., 1978; Sugimura et al., 1976). However, recent studies show that this correlation is dependent upon the class of chemical being investigated. For most aromatic amines, polycyclic aromatic hydrocarbons, and direct alkylating agents, there appears to be a high degree of correlation. On the other hand, chlorinated hydrocarbons are difficult to identify as mutagens in the Ames test, although they are known to be carcinogenic. In vitro mutagenicity tests have one major drawback: although they may provide a good indication of whether or not an agent is carcinogenic, they produce very little information on its relative carcinogenic potency.

Other short-term in vitro and in vivo tests in use include assays for the induction of DNA damage and repair or mutagenesis in bacteria, in yeast, in Drosophila melanogaster, or in mammalian cells in culture. Whole mammals can be used in the dominant lethal test, mouse spot test, tests for heritable translocations, and tests for chromosome aberrations. These mammalian mutagenesis bioassays offer promise as prescreening tools since they seem to provide both qualitative as well as quantitative data, but they are more expensive to perform and require more time than the other assays. The in vitro transformation systems are potentially useful for screening carcinogens, but they are also expensive and time-consuming. Moreover, the reliability of early markers of oncogenic transformation is unknown. If the in vitro transformation tests have to be carried out to the point of injecting presumably transformed cells into a syngeneic animal to determine if the cells develop into a tumor, then the expense and time involved are the same or possibly greater than required for some in vivo carcinogenicity test systems.

In general, short-term tests have a number of drawbacks:

● Carcinogens or modifiers of carcinogenesis may operate by mechanisms not involving DNA damage and repair. Thus, some agents, e.g., tumor promoters, which are particularly relevant when one considers diet, are not likely to be detected by these tests.

● The effects of absorption, transport, activation, detoxification, and excretion are not taken into account.

● Quantitative risk assessment cannot be made easily.

● Despite positive results for mutagenicity in a battery of such tests, many scientists do not accept such evidence alone as an indication of carcinogenicity. Long-term bioassays in whole animals are still necessary to make this determination (International Agency for Research on Cancer, 1980).

Long-Term Bioassays

These tests, which are conducted in animals, have been the most widely accepted methods for determining the carcinogenic effect of substances. In the absence of data on humans, all substances demonstrated to be carcinogenic in animals are regarded as potential carcinogens for humans, and the empirical evidence overwhelmingly supports this hypothesis.

The standard procedure in long-term bioassays is to feed substances at levels that are just below the maximum tolerated dose for a major portion of the lifespan of the animal (usually rodents, which have a lifespan of 2 to 3 years). The rationale for feeding very high doses of a substance in chronic bioassays is that the number of animals that develop cancer increases as the dose of the test substance is increased. To conduct a valid experiment at high doses, only a small number of animals (a few hundred) is required. An important variable that determines the outcome in these tests is the potency of the carcinogen: the greater its potency, the greater will be the number of animals that develop cancer at a particular dose or increase in the number of tumors per animal. Alternatively, a carcinogen can decrease the latency period or the lifespan without altering the tumor incidence. If a chemical produces cancer in test animals and if the route of administration is equivalent to the route by which humans are exposed, it is generally accepted that the compound is potentially carcinogenic in humans.

These bioassays also have some major drawbacks:

● An adequately performed feeding study takes several years to complete and analyze, and costs more than $500,000.

● The test lacks sensitivity to detect weak carcinogens. For example, if a carcinogen induces cancer in 1% of the test animals, then an experiment with 50 animals of each sex at each dose will not possess sufficient statistical power to detect the carcinogenicity of the test substance.

● False negatives can be obtained because some strains of test animals are more resistant than others. A negative result means that the test compound is not carcinogenic for that particular species and strain under the conditions of the test, but the chemical could be positive in another species or strain under the same or different conditions.

● Extrapolation from the high doses given to animals to predict risk to humans cannot be accomplished with any degree of confidence, even when the test compound has been shown to be carcinogenic in a full-scale study in animals.

Only recently has there been an attempt to standardize tests for carcinogenicity. Variables include animal species and strain, genetic characteristics of the test strains, the diet given to the animals, the chemical and physical characteristics of the test substances, the method of tissue examination, spontaneous rate of tumor formation in control animals, susceptibility to various carcinogens, dose response to a given carcinogen, and tissue specificity of a large number of carcinogens.

Difficulties in Studying the Carcinogenicity and Mutagenicity of Food Constituents

Because foods contain unidentified chemicals or mixtures of compounds, it is difficult to test them in long-term bioassays, which require precise physical and chemical characterization of the test substance. Furthermore, many foods that are not toxic to humans are toxic to laboratory animals, making it difficult to test these substances at high doses (Elias, in press).

Because of the mere volume involved, it would be difficult to test the major components of diets for carcinogenicity by exposing the animals to doses 100 or more times higher than the expected levels of human exposure. It is also difficult to use different doses because nutrient imbalance may result from feeding high levels of the dietary component being tested, and the supplementation of diet with micronutrients to avoid nutritional deficiencies has not always proved satisfactory.

It is especially difficult to select a valid control diet in these studies. Ideally, control animals must be fed a diet identical to the one fed to test animals except that the food or diet being tested should not contain the presumed carcinogen. If the carcinogen happens to be a naturally occurring constituent (e.g., aflatoxins), then the carcinogen will have to be removed from the control diet. However, this generally leads to many complications such as the introduction of new chemicals and/or the removal of others in addition to the carcinogen. If the carcinogen is generated as a result of food processing, then the control food must be subjected to an alternative type of processing, if possible, to achieve similar results without generating the carcinogen (Elias, in press).

Since many dietary carcinogens are probably present in very low amounts, it would be logical to expose a large number of laboratory animals to low levels of suspected carcinogens. This may be prohibitively expensive.

Alterations in the diet or nutritional status do not appear to cause cancer directly in laboratory animals, but are only believed to modify the spontaneous rate of tumor formation or the induction and growth of cancer by specific carcinogens. It is important to learn the background (spontaneous) rate of tumor formation in a given animal model so that changes induced by altered diets can be evaluated with confidence. It is also very important to know the dose-response characteristics of carcinogens in order to induce a 50% tumor incidence in tests to determine if a given dietary or nutritional change enhances or inhibits the induced response. For example, if a carcinogen induces a 90% tumor incidence, it would be difficult to determine if some change in diet had enhanced tumorigenesis. Alternatively, it would be difficult to determine if the dietary changes had a significant inhibitory effect on tumor response if the carcinogen induced only a low incidence of tumors. Assessment of risk as related to the time to tumor response is discussed in Chapter 18. Furthermore, it is important to select the test animal whose response to the carcinogen being tested most closely approximates the suspected response of humans. For example, if a high fat diet appears to be related to an increased risk for colon and breast cancer in humans, the animal models selected should be able to develop the same type of tumors.

Many laboratory studies of the effect of diet and nutrition on carcinogenesis have not been well controlled, especially with respect to the composition of the diets fed to the animals. This is an important consideration because diets are a potential source of naturally occurring carcinogens and may also contain contaminants with carcinogenic activity. Diets fed to test animals have ranged from various commercial laboratory chows to diets so purified that mixtures of individual amino acids are fed in place of protein. Specific nutrients may be administered at levels that range from the marginally deficient to the questionably excessive. As a consequence, it is difficult to compare results from these studies. Recent recommendations that standard diets [e.g., the AIN-76 diet (Anonymous, 1977)] be used should help considerably. Another drawback is the failure to insure isocaloric intakes by control and experimental groups. Caloric restriction and total food intake have been reported to be important determinants of tumor yield (Silverstone and Tannenbaum, 1949; Tannenbaum, 1944, 1945; Waxler, 1960). The difficulty in distinguishing between the effects from changes in total food intake and caloric intake is discussed in Chapter 4. For example, even an alteration in body size caused by a change in caloric or total food intake may affect tumor yield (Clayson, 1975). More insight can be gained by pair-feeding to control for total food intake, nutrient deficiencies, or weight gain.

The in vitro mutagenicity tests were originally developed to assess the mutagenicity of pure substances, which are much easier to test than the complex mixtures of compounds contained in foodstuffs. Testing is especially complicated if the nature and properties of the suspected substance presumed to be present in the food are not known. Until recently, this problem has been circumvented by using food extracts. However, this process is subject to numerous criticisms. For example, active mutagenic substances detected in food extracts may not be present in the animal during the normal digestive process. On the other hand, reactions during the digestive process can result in the formation of mutagens from previously innocuous substances. Furthermore, solvents used in the extraction procedures could conceivably react with food constituents, and solvent residues may persist in the extracts--resulting in erroneous conclusions (Elias, in press). In vivo mutagenicity testing of these foodstuffs is comparatively simpler, since the test substance can be fed to the animals in their diet for several days.

COMMITTEE'S APPROACH TO EVALUATION OF THE LITERATURE

The strengths and weaknesses inherent in the epidemiological and laboratory methods used to study the relationship between diet and cancer are described above. In the chapters that follow, the committee has refrained from presenting a detailed critique of the results and methodology of each report, because most of the criticisms that apply to individual studies are in fact limitations imposed by the design of various types of epidemiological studies, by the method selected to determine dietary intake, or by the laboratory tests used, all of which are described in this chapter. Furthermore, because no studies of this difficult subject are without limitations, the committee did not wish to place too much emphasis on the results, especially the precise quantitative data (e.g., relative risks in epidemiological studies or tumor incidence in animal experiments), from any single study. Rather, it reviewed all the data and

based its conclusions on the overall strength of all the evidence combined.

Although the committee considered the evidence from all types of
epidemiological studies, it had the most confidence in data derived from
case-control studies and from the few cohort studies that have been reported.   Instead of relying on aggregate correlation data, these studies
are based on the collection and analysis of data on individuals, and investigators can control for confounding variables.   Therefore, the committee concluded that the evidence on diet and cancer provided by these
two types of studies is more definitive and indicative of meaningful
associations than data derived from correlation and descriptive studies.
Particular emphasis was given to the results of case-control or cohort
studies that were designed to examine a specific hypothesis.

In evaluating laboratory evidence, the committee placed more confidence in data derived from studies on more than one animal species or
test system, on results that have been reproduced in different laboratories, and on the few data that indicate a gradient in response.

The preponderance of data and the degree of concordance between the
epidemiological and laboratory evidence determined the strength of the
conclusions in the report.

SUMMARY AND CONCLUSIONS

Both epidemiological studies and laboratory experiments have been
used to examine the relationship between dietary factors and carcinogenesis.   A number of different epidemiological methods have been used.
These include descriptive studies, correlation studies, case-control
studies, and cohort studies.   Accurate measurement of intake is funda-
mental to the success of most of these studies.   Both food disappearance
data and household food inventories are used to determine the intakes of
groups.   Methods used to measure individual nutrient intake are recent
recalls of intake, food records, and diet histories.

The major strength of epidemiological studies is their focus on human
populations.   They are the most direct way of investigating the possible
causes of human cancer, thereby avoiding the need to extrapolate data
from animals to humans.   Since the exposures studied are those that
actually occur among people, dose-response relationships can be deduced
because different people are exposed to different levels of the variable
under study.   Furthermore, interpolation from high doses to low doses,
which would be necessary in the laboratory, is also avoided.

The interpretation of epidemiological studies is complicated by the
heterogeneity of the human population, the wide variety of changing
lifestyles, and difficulties in the accurate measurement of both the
exposure and the outcome variables.   Moreover, ethical, social, and

political considerations preclude manipulating and arranging human affairs into simpler patterns for analysis. For example, differences among groups may be difficult to identify if there is little difference in the degree of exposure to a particular dietary variable. Their interpretation may be further jeopardized by the lack of specificity of the methods for measuring intake and the uncertainty about whether the data reflect nutrient intake or whether current intake correlates well with past dietary patterns (which may be more relevant to carcinogenesis).

Laboratory experimentation on animals is basically an effort to overcome the limitations of direct studies of cancer in humans. The laboratory provides a simplified and controlled environment, and laboratory animals can be regarded as uniform and controlled populations "standing in" for human beings. However, the animals are not human, and the etiology of the cancers they develop may not duplicate that for cancers in humans.

Laboratory tests to study neoplasia are conducted either with whole animals or with cell cultures in vitro, both of which have limitations. One general uncertainty lies in projections or extrapolations from laboratory data to humans. On the one hand, the biochemical similarity among many species means that what happens in one species is likely to occur in another; on the other hand, some responses may be peculiar to particular species. An attempted compromise is to assume that if two nonhuman species react similarly, then humans are likely to have the same reaction.

Compounds whose carcinogenicity was initially suspected in epidemiological studies can be more quickly and cheaply tested in short-term laboratory systems than in whole animals. These short-term systems may involve the use of bacterial cultures, human cells in culture, or even subcellular mixtures of cell components. Tests on bacteria measure genetic change (mutation) rather than carcinogenesis since the latter has no direct equivalent in bacteria. Their validity rests on the assumption, backed by considerable data, that carcinogenic substances are likely to be mutagenic and vice versa. This appears to be true for most compounds known to be carcinogenic in humans and for many mutagens tested for carcinogenicity in laboratory animals. However, there are many exceptions, particularly in establishing quantitative correlations between mutagenicity and carcinogenicity. Therefore, bacterial tests should be regarded as useful, especially for screening, but not as an exclusive method for determining carcinogenicity. Their basic function is the detection of initiator action—not the later stages of tumor promotion that may be more relevant for dietary factors, since nutrients have little or no mutagenic activity.

In summary, data obtained in laboratory tests are useful for evaluating the role of dietary and metabolic factors in the development of cancer in humans. The laboratory experiments tend to be better controlled and more precise than epidemiological investigations. However, they are costly in time and money, and they also depend upon simple assumptions that may not be valid for humans. The projection of such data to humans must be done cautiously and is most convincing when accompanied by confirmatory evidence from epidemiological studies. The two approaches are complimentary and should be used in conjunction with each other as often as possible.

The committee evaluated the evidence from all types of epidemiological studies and laboratory experiments, but had more confidence in data derived from case-control and cohort studies, in the results of experiments conducted in more than one animal species or test system, in results that had been reproduced in different laboratories, and in data that showed a dose response. The preponderence of data and the degree of concordance between the epidemiological and the laboratory evidence determined the strength of the conclusions in this report.

REFERENCES

Ames, B. N., J. McCann, and E. Yamasaki. 1975. Methods for detecting carcinogens and mutagens with the Salmonella/mammalian-microsome mutagenicity test. Mutat. Res. 31:347-364.

Anonymous. 1977. Report of the American Institute of Nutrition Ad Hoc Committee on Standards for Nutritional Studies. J. Nutr. 107:1340-1348.

Beaton, G. H., J. Milner, P. Corey, V. McGuire, M. Cousins, E. Stewart, M. de Ramos, D. Hewitt, P. V. Grambsch, N. Kassim, and J. A. Little. 1979. Sources of variance in 24-hour dietary recall data: Implications for nutrition study design and interpretation. Am. J. Clin. Nutr. 32:2546-2559.

Bridges, B. A. 1976. Short term screening tests for carcinogens. Nature 261:195-200.

Cambien, F., P. Ducimetiere, and J. Richard. 1980. Total serum cholesterol and cancer mortality in a middle-aged male population. Am. J. Epidemiol. 112:388-394.

Clayson, D. B. 1975. Nutrition and experimental carcinogenesis: A review. Cancer Res. 35:3292-3300.

Elias, P. S. In press. Methods for the detection of carcinogens and mutagens in food. An introductory review. In H. F. Stich, ed. Food Products, Carcinogens, and Mutagens in the Environment. Volume 1, Food Products. CRC Press, Boca Raton, Fla.

Garland, B., and M. A. Ibrahim. 1981. The reliability of retrospective dietary histories: Paper submitted to the Committee on Diet, Nutrition, and Cancer at the Workshop on Methodology for Dietary Studies in Cancer Epidemiology held at the National Academy of Sciences, Washington, D.C., May 20-21, 1981. National Academy of Sciences, Washington, D.C. (unpublished) 12 pp.

Graham, S., and C. Mettlin. 1979. Diet and colon cancer. Am. J. Epidemiol. 109:1-20.

Graham, S., A. M. Lilienfeld, and J. E. Tidings. 1967. Dietary and purgation factors in the epidemiology of gastric cancer. Cancer 20:2224-2234.

Hankin, J. H., G. G. Rhoads, and G. Glober. 1975. A dietary method for an epidemiologic study of gastrointestinal cancer. Am. J. Clin. Nutr. 28:1055-1060.

Ibrahim, M. A., ed. 1979. The case-control study: Consensus and controversy. J. Chronic Dis. 32:1-144.

International Agency for Research on Cancer. 1980. Long-Term and Short-Term Screening Assays for Carcinogens: A Critical Appraisal. IARC Monographs, Supplement 2. International Agency for Research on Cancer, Lyon, France. 426 pp.

Kark, J. D., A. H. Smith, and C. G. Hames. 1980. The relationship of serum cholesterol to the incidence of cancer in Evans County, Georgia. J. Chronic Dis. 33:311-322.

MacMahon, B., and T. F. Pugh. 1970. Case-control studies. Pp. 241-282 in Epidemiology. Principles and Methods. Little, Brown and Co., Boston, Mass.

Marr, J. W. 1973. Dietary survey methods: Individual and group aspects. Proc. R. Soc. Med. 66:639-641.

McCann, J., and B. N. Ames. 1976. Detection of carcinogens as mutagens in the Salmonella/microsome test: Assay of 300 chemicals: Discussion. Proc. Natl. Acad. Sci. U.S.A. 73:950-954.

Mettlin, C. J., and S. Graham. 1978. Methodological issues in etiologic studies of diet and colon cancer. Nutr. Cancer 1(4):46-55.

Miller, J. A. 1970. Carcinogenesis by chemicals: An overview-- G. H. A. Clowes Memorial Lecture. Cancer Res. 30:559-576.

Miller, J. A., and E. C. Miller. 1971. Guest editorial: Chemical carcinogenesis: Mechanisms and approaches to its control. J. Natl. Cancer Inst. 47(3):v-xiv.

Miller, J. A., and E. C. Miller. 1979. Perspectives on the metabolism of chemical carcinogens. Pp. 25-50 in P. Emmelot and E. Kriek, eds. Environmental Carcinogenesis. Occurrence, Risk Evaluation and Mechanisms. Elsevier/North-Holland Biomedical Press, Amsterdam, New York, and Oxford.

Morgan, R. W., M. Jain, A. B. Miller, N. W. Choi, V. Matthews, L. Munan, J. D. Burch, J. Feather, G. R. Howe, and A. Kelly. 1978. A comparison of dietary methods in epidemiologic studies. Am. J. Epidemiol. 107:488-498.

National Academy of Sciences. 1981. Assessing Changing Food Consumption Patterns. Committee on Food Consumption Patterns, Food and Nutrition Board. National Academy Press, Washington, D.C. 284 pp.

Nichols, A. B., C. Ravenscroft, D. E. Lamphiear, and L. D. Ostrander, Jr. 1976. Daily nutritional intake and serum lipid levels. The Tecumseh study. Am. J. Clin. Nutr. 29:1384-1392.

Nomura, A., J. H. Hankin, and G. G. Rhoads. 1976. The reproducibility of dietary intake data in a prospective study of gastrointestinal cancer. Am. J. Clin. Nutr. 29:1432-1436.

Office of Technology Assessment. 1981. Assessment of Technologies for Determining Cancer Risks from the Environment. Office of Technology Assessment, U.S. Congress, Washington, D.C. 242 pp.

Pearson, W. N. 1967. Blood and urinary vitamin levels as potential indices of body stores. Am. J. Clin. Nutr. 20:514-525.

Purchase, I. F. H., E. Longstaff, J. Ashby, J. A. Styles, D. Anderson, P. A. Lefevre, and F. R. Westwood. 1978. An evaluation of 6 short-term tests for detecting organic chemical carcinogens. Br. J. Cancer 37:873-959.

Reshef, A., and L. M. Epstein. 1972. Reliability of a dietary questionnaire. Am. J. Clin. Nutr. 25:91-95.

Silverstone, H., and A. Tannenbaum. 1949. Influence of thyroid hormone on the formation of induced skin tumors in mice. Cancer Res. 9:684-688.

Sugimura, T., S. Sato, M. Nagao, T. Yahagi, T. Matsushima, Y. Seino, M. Takeuchi, and T. Kawachi. 1976. Overlapping of carcinogens and mutagens. Pp. 191-213 in P. N. Magee, S. Takayama, T. Sugimura, and T. Matsushima, eds. Fundamentals in Cancer Prevention. University Park Press, Baltimore, London, and Tokyo.

Tannenbaum, A. 1944. The dependence of the genesis of induced skin tumors on the caloric intake during different stages of carcinogenesis. Cancer Res. 4:673-677.

Tannenbaum, A. 1945. The dependence of tumor formation on the composition of the calorie-restricted diet as well as on the degree of restriction. Cancer Res. 5:616-625.

Underwood, B. A., H. Siegel, R. C. Weisell, and M. Dolinski. 1970. Liver stores of vitamin A in a normal population dying suddenly or rapidly from unnatural causes in New York City. Am. J. Clin. Nutr. 23:1037-1042.

U.S. Department of Agriculture. 1975. Nutritive Value of American Foods in Common Units. Agriculture Handbook No. 456. Agricultural

Research Service, U.S. Department of Agriculture, Washington, D.C. 291 pp.

Wald, N., M. Idle, J. Boreham, and A. Bailey. 1980. Low serum-vitamin A and subsequent risk of cancer--preliminary results of a prospective study. Lancet 2:813-815.

Waxler, S. H. 1960. Obesity and cancer susceptibility in mice. Am. J. Clin. Nutr. 8:760-765.

Section A The Relationship Between Nutrients and Cancer

The foods comprising the diets of humans are complex mixtures of chemicals modified by many events that occur between the field and the table. Only a small proportion of these chemicals have specific nutritional functions. However, much research and, therefore, much of this report--especially the eight chapters that follow--are focused on the relationships between rates of cancer at different sites and consumption of specific nutrients.

This focus is not surprising since diet-related diseases have characteristically been associated with deficiencies of one or more nutrients (e.g., scurvy results from a deficiency of vitamin C). The conquest of such diseases encouraged investigators to look at the metabolic and degenerative diseases (often called diseases of affluence) in relation to the same constituents of food consumed in excess.

Yet, as the data reviewed in Chapters 13 and 15 indicate, at least some of the compounds in food (e.g., flavones, isothiocyanates) that have been implicated in the causation or prevention of cancer are food constituents other than nutrients (or additives, or contaminants). This fact suggests (1) that some food classifications other than the presently obvious nutrient-based ones may need to be regularly considered in epidemiological studies and (2) that changes in the chemical composition of the food supply may need to be monitored and controlled, even if they do not appear to affect the per capita supply of compounds classed as nutrients.

CHANGES IN THE FOOD SUPPLY

Table A-1 lists the daily per capita intake of nutrients during certain years between 1909 and 1976. These estimates, based on food disappearance data reported by Page and Friend (1978), show that if nutrients alone are measured, the food supply appears to have undergone little overall change during this period. There has been a slight decline in total calories available for consumption, essentially no change in total protein, and a moderate increase in total fat, balancing a similar decline in total carbohydrate. The available supply of most of the vitamins and minerals measured has remained essentially unchanged. The exceptions are iron and vitamins B_1, B_2, and niacin, which have increased, and magnesium, which has decreased. The increases probably reflect the enrichment of a variety of flour-based products. Since magnesium is lost during the refining of flour, as are a number of trace minerals, the decline in magnesium intake might reflect a general decline in trace minerals, especially those derived from whole grains. If one were relating U.S. trends

TABLE A-1

Daily Per Capita Intake of Nutrients in the United States[a]

Year	Calories	Energy Sources			Minerals				Vitamins						
		Protein (g)	Fat (g)	CHO[b] (g)	Ca (mg)	P (mg)	Fe (mg)	Mg (mg)	B1 (mg)	B2 (mg)	Niacin (mg)	B6 (mg)	B12 (μg)	A (μg)	C (mg)
1909	3,480	102	125	492	820	1,560	15.2	408	1.64	1.86	19.2	2.26	8.4	2,280	104
1927	3,460	95	134	476	860	1,510	14.1	388	1.55	1.87	18.0	2.05	8.1	2,400	106
1948	3,230	95	140	403	1,000	1,550	18.6	369	1.91	2.30	21.4	1.99	9.0	2,640	114
1965	3,150	96	144	372	960	1,520	16.7	339	1.81	2.30	21.9	2.02	9.1	2,310	97
1976	3,300	101	157	376	930	1,550	18.6	344	2.04	2.46	25.2	2.26	9.6	2,430	118

[a]Adapted from Page and Friend, 1978.
[b]Carbohydrate.

in per capita intake to trends in cancer incidence, these data suggest that the relatively stable nutrient composition of the diet is being reflected in the relatively stable cancer rates at most sites.

However, these figures on the availability of a limited group of nutrients tend to obscure the extensive changes that have taken place in the food supply during the past 50 years. Some of these can be seen by examining the changes that have occurred in the contribution of various food groups to total calories (Figure A-1). For example, the percentage of calories derived from grain products has been halved. As shown in Table A-2, most of this change can be attributed to a decline in per capita intake of flour: from approximately 131 kg per capita in 1909 to 63 kg in 1976. The intake of fat has also changed in a manner that is not evident in Table A-1. Although total per capita fat intake increased only 27% during this period, fat as a percentage of calories increased by 35%. There was also a 56% increase in the intake of separated fats, most of them from vegetable sources. In other words, as attention shifts from nutrients to food groups and from there to specific food substances, it becomes increasingly evident that there have been extensive changes in the composition of what is actually available to eat.

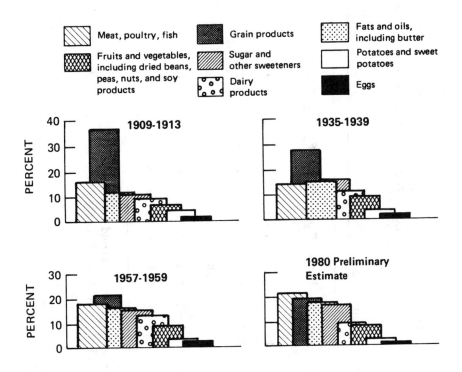

FIGURE A-1. Contribution of various food groups to per capita supply of food energy (calories). Adapted from Page and Friend, 1978.

A-3

TABLE A-2

Annual Per Capita Intake of Food in the United States[a]

	Annual Consumption kg/Person											liters/Person[b]
Year	Meat	Poultry	Fish	Eggs	Fats	Fruits	Vegetables	Potatoes	Beans	Flour	Sugar	Dairy Products
1909	63.5	8.1	5.9	16.7	18.5	79.2	91.4	92.3	7.2	131.0	40.1	168.2
1927	58.1	7.7	6.3	18.0	21.6	84.6	97.7	72.9	7.7	106.7	53.6	181.5
1948	63.5	9.9	5.9	21.2	20.7	81.9	104.4	55.4	7.7	77.0	49.5	224.2
1965	66.6	18.5	6.3	18.0	23.0	74.7	92.7	38.7	7.2	64.8	50.4	223.3
1976	74.3	23.9	6.8	15.8	26.6	84.6	95.9	36.0	8.1	63.0	53.6	210.9

[a]Adapted from Page and Friend, 1978.
[b]Based on milk equivalent. Excludes butter, which is included among fats.

There are some data indicating the magnitude of the changes in per capita intake of certain food items and constituents; however, many of the changes are not adequately documented. For example, there are no data on the consumption of whole wheat flour, commercial baby food, or home-produced vegetables. Moreover, there is no indication whether fresh vegetables eaten in the Northeast were grown in that region or whether they were shipped by train from California or by air from Mexico (Brewster and Jacobson, 1978). A variety of differences in their chemical composition (e.g., in their vitamin and mineral content) can result from differences in the way in which these vegetables were grown, transported, and stored.

Between 1940 and 1977, per capita intake of food color additives increased tenfold. Soft drink consumption increased 1.5 times in just 16 years--between 1960 and 1976 (Brewster and Jacobson, 1978). Although total intake of fruits and vegetables increased slightly between 1909 and 1976 (Table A-2), the intake of fresh fruits and vegetables[1] actually declined (Table A-3), a major portion of that decline having occurred after 1948. Changes in the per capita intake of certain individual commodities are especially striking. For example, the intake of fresh potatoes is more than two-thirds lower than it was at the turn of the century and more than one-half lower than it was 30 years ago, whereas the intake of processed potatoes has increased by a factor of 44 during the same 30 years. The per capita intake of processed citrus fruit juice--which accounts for much of the increase in overall fruit intake--increased dramatically from an average of less than one 4-oz (120-ml) serving per person annually in 1948 to 117 4-oz servings per person in 1976 (Brewster and Jacobson, 1978). Similarly, the intake of canned or bottled tomato products (e.g., paste, sauce, catsup, and chili sauce) increased from 2.25 kg per capita in 1920 to 10.1 kg per capita in 1976 (Brewster and Jacobson, 1978). All of these changes reflect the proliferation of food products on the market--from less than 1,000 at the end of World War II to well over 10,000 at present (Molitor, 1980).

---

[1]The term "fresh" applied to fruits and vegetables commonly refers to produce that has been, at most, washed, trimmed, and chilled. The term "processed" has many meanings; for example, preservation by canning and freezing, which result in some chemical but little structural change; extraction and dehydration such as the preparation of orange juice concentrate, which produce significant structural and possibly major chemical changes including nutrient loss; and processes that involve extensive separation of foods into components, or the fabrication of new foods such as "chips" made from molded rehydrated potato flakes, which result in marked structural changes that may have equally marked effects on the chemical composition of foods.

TABLE A-3

Annual Per Capita Intake of Fresh and Processed Fruits,
Potatoes, and Other Vegetables in the United States[a]

| | Annual Consumption, kg/Person | | | | | |
| | Fruits | | Vegetables (Excluding Potatoes) | | Potatoes | |
Year	Fresh	Processed	Fresh	Processed	Fresh	Processed
1909	75.6	3.61	83.7	7.7	81.9	0.2
1927	76.5	8.1	85.5	11.7	63.9	0.2
1948	73.8	19.8	82.8	21.15	50.0	0.2
1965	47.3	27.5	63.5	29.7	30.6	5.4
1976	52.7	36.5	65.3	31.1	24.3	9.9

[a]Adapted from Page and Friend, 1978.

These striking changes in the food supply need to be taken into
account when one examines the relationship between diet and cancer.
On the one hand, any change in cancer incidence resulting from major
changes in food processing that occurred before 1900 (e.g., roller
milling of grain) or up to 40 years ago (e.g., flour enrichment) would
probably have been observed long before now. Conversely, because of
the long latent period between exposure and manifestation of cancer,
effects from changes introduced less than 10 years ago might not yet be
evident. If, as is often the case, changes in food-processing methods
are poorly monitored, the extent of exposure to substances resulting
from those processes will not be known. In such cases, it will be
difficult to make any associations between those substances and cancer
incidence.

A more difficult problem is encountered in case-control studies:
here one must determine what foods were consumed by subjects one or
more decades in the past. It is necessary to make one of two assumptions when collecting such information: that people can accurately
remember their typical dietary patterns of 10 or more years ago, or
that present diets adequately reflect diets consumed in the past. Both
of these assumptions are most subject to inaccuracies when there have
been continual shifts in the numbers, types, and varieties of available
foodstuffs. Even when the kinds and amounts of foods consumed in the
past can be accurately determined, their chemical composition remains
unknown and may have changed significantly over the decades. For
example, a frozen pizza made with imitation cheese, tomato extender,
and soy-protein "pepperoni" is composed of a very different collection
of chemicals than the apparently similar product made 10 years earlier
with mozzarella cheese, tomato paste, and meat sausage.

The proportion of manufactured products in the average diet has been increasing, especially in developed countries, but the detailed composition of many of these products is not known. Manufacturers often consider it proprietary information. Figures on the production of ascorbic acid illustrate both the scale of the potential effects of processing and the difficulty of monitoring such effects (Table A-4). During the past 20 years, there has been a sixfold increase in the tonnage of ascorbic acid produced. But in standard food composition tables prepared by the U.S. Department of Agriculture, only the amount of ascorbic acid used for food fortification is recorded. The disposition of the remainder is unknown. Most of the imbalance is probably consumed in the form of vitamin supplements. Nonetheless, the fact remains that large amounts of ascorbic acid, as well as other nutrients, are added to foods for "technical" reasons, e.g., for their antioxidant properties, as opposed to "nutritional" reasons. These amounts do not show up on tables of nutritional value, although vitamins are monitored more carefully than most other components of the food supply. Most non-nutritive substances are not monitored at all, and as a consequence almost nothing is known about their presence or fluctuations over time. Saccharin, for example, is a nonnutritive substance intentionally added to food--by manufacturers or by the consumers themselves--and, to a very large extent, it is knowingly consumed. Yet, in epidemiological studies it has proved very difficult to obtain reliable data on individual saccharin intake. Obviously, it is even more difficult to obtain consumption data for substances that are neither monitored, as are the nutrients, nor consumed intentionally, as is saccharin.

TABLE A-4

Production of Ascorbic Acid in the United States[a]

Year	Amount Produced (Metric Tons)
1960	2,392
1965	3,914
1970	5,470
1974	10,054
1982	14,800 (estimated)

[a]Data from U.S. International Trade Commission, 1980.

Because of this paucity of information, it is possible to make only the crudest assessments of factors that may affect the composition of foods. For example, one can determine whether fruits are available fresh, frozen, or canned, whether potatoes are available fresh or dried, but not whether macaroni contains soy flour or whether tomato paste contains modified starch, β-carotene (for color), and added vitamin C--among other things.

It is not clear whether all the changes in the food supply have increased, decreased, or had no effect on the incidence of cancer. Overall U.S. cancer rates at most sites other than lung and stomach have remained relatively stable for several decades. This might suggest that the food supply has contained an unchanging cluster of cancer-causing or protective substances throughout much of this period, despite the extensive changes in the composition and quantity of many of the foods consumed. It is also possible that any changes capable of affecting cancer rates (positively or negatively) have occurred too recently to be reflected in cancer statistics. But even if cancer rates rise or fall in the future, it may prove very difficult to identify which, if any, specific compositional modifications are involved, since so many different changes are going on simultaneously. This is illustrated in Figures A-2 and A-3, which show the changing sources of fat in the U.S. diet. These figures reveal that the relatively stable consumption of "total table spreads" and "total cooking fats" masks a dramatic shift in the sources and, hence, the composition of the fats involved. The use of butter and lard has decreased sharply, whereas margarine and shortening (usually based on vegetable oil) have come into much wider use (Brewster and Jacobson, 1978).

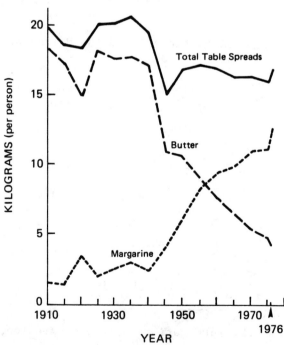

FIGURE A-2.   Intake of butter and margarine.   From Brewster and Jacobson, 1978.

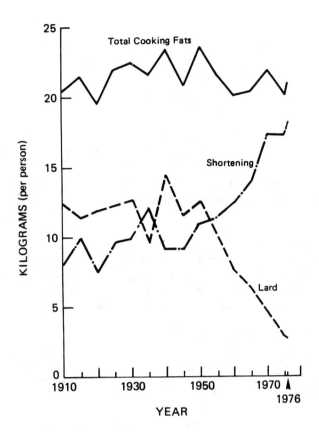

FIGURE A-3. Intake of cooking fat. From Brewster and Jacobson, 1978.

At any particular time, cancer rates probably reflect the sum of many changes, some producing positive and others negative effects. For example, the introduction and subsequent wide use of refrigeration and the increased use of mold-inhibitors and antioxidants have probably had positive effects. Together, these changes have markedly decreased the population's exposure to rancid and/or moldy foods and to foods preserved by salting, smoking, or drying.

The effect of other changes is less clear. Although there has been relatively little change in the overall percentage of calories derived from fat, protein, and carbohydrate, there have been marked shifts in consumption patterns from vegetable to animal protein, from complex to simple carbohydrates, and, as already noted, from animal to vegetable fats. The increase in per capita intake of fat from meat has compensated for a decline in the intake of dairy fats. In addition, there has been a marked increase in the intake of separated vegetable oils that have been structurally altered by hydrogenation and other treatments.

There have also been changes in the nature of the fat-soluble contaminants present in the diet. In federal inspections for pesticide residues, contaminants have been found most frequently in meats and fats (U.S. Food and Drug Administration, 1980). The Comptroller General (1979) reported that "of 143 drugs and pesticides likely to leave residues in raw meat and poultry, 42 were known to cause or suspected of causing cancer." Twenty years ago, fats were much less likely to carry such residues since the use of both drugs in animals and pesticides has increased markedly in the interim (Smith, 1980).

A fivefold increase in the per capita intake of french-fried potatoes is part of a trend toward a much greater consumption of products crisped by exposure to heated fat or to extreme dry heat. Such products include potato chips, fried snacks, crackers, and ready-to-eat breakfast cereals. Many products of such browning reactions have proved to be mutagenic in laboratory tests as have the by-products resulting from the frying and broiling of meat and fish (see Chapter 13). Hence, products in this category must be regarded as potential contributors to carcinogenesis.

Several other changes may also be important, but their effects on carcinogenesis are not known. For example, there has been a documented decline in the consumption of certain types of vegetables, especially in their fresh state. The effect, if any, of the marked increase in the consumption of cooked (and often burned) tomatoes is also unclear as is the effect of the documented decline in the consumption of fresh cabbage, since the total long-term consumption of other cruciferous vegetables (e.g., broccoli, cabbage, and kale) is impossible to calculate given the lack of accurate data on home production. However, the documented decrease in the annual per capita intake of sweet potatoes, from 11.1 kg per person during 1976 to 2.4 kg during 1980, combined with the declining consumption of fresh dark green and deep yellow vegetables, has very likely decreased the intake of dietary fiber and naturally occurring β-carotene, which recently have been studied for their possibly protective roles in carcinogenesis (Chapters 8 and 9).

Despite (or perhaps because of) the paucity of information pertaining to the composition of our contemporary food supply, foods have been most often used in epidemiological studies as indicators of the presence of particular nutrients or they have been grouped for analysis according to certain nutrients they have in common. Given the multitude of other chemicals present in the diet, it is notable that epidemiological studies have found significant relationships between the occurrence of cancer and estimated intakes of such nutrients as fat, vitamins A and C, or protein (see Chapters 5, 6, and 9). This would seem to indicate either that these nutrients must play a role in the development of cancer or that they serve as indicators of other substances that do.

Epidemiological associations between cancer and nutrients are often based on the presence in the diet of certain foods. For example, citrus fruits have sometimes been used as indicators of the presence of vitamin C, although they obviously have much more in common than ascorbic acid. They contain, among other substances, flavonoids (Chapters 13 and 15). The dietary presence of vitamin A has often been based on green and yellow vegetable consumption (Chapter 9), although the active agent in those foods may not actually be vitamin A. Peto et al. (1981) suggested that carcinogenesis may be inhibited by β-carotene (the plant constituent that can be converted to vitamin A in the body), rather than by the vitamin itself. Their report suggests that, when examining naturally occurring compounds in foods, we should not limit our attention to those already identified as having a nutritional role.

Until fairly recently, fiber was also overlooked as a possible protective factor in carcinogenesis. For many years, fiber was regarded as a collection of inert substances in foods, even though it was known to be present in relatively large amounts, compared to vitamins and minerals. These substances were even regarded as a nuisance factor that might interfere with the absorption of minerals in unrefined diets. Since most traditional diets contain large amounts of such indigestible residues, fiber came to scientific attention as a result of observations that peoples consuming "primitive" diets high in complex carbohyates (including fiber) appear to be spared a number of maladies, including bowel cancer, that are common to populations consuming more refined diets.

These simple observations have led to ongoing investigations concerning which components of carbohydrate should "count" as fiber, which of them might play a role in carcinogenesis, and how (or whether) fiber affects the incidence of certain diseases or whether it acts merely by displacing other dietary substances that are either carcinogens or promoters of carcinogenesis.

The recent findings concerning fiber remind us again that substances in food other than those presently classified as nutrients may be instrumental in the development of cancer. Milk is one major food that is difficult to classify in cancer studies. As a source of vitamin A (Mettlin and Graham, 1979), whole milk may be a beneficial component of the diet; but as a source of fat (Blair and Fraumeni, 1978; Howell, 1974), it may have deleterious consequences. The category "dairy products" or "milk products" may combine milk products such as butter, cheese, cream, yogurt, low-fat milk, and cottage cheese, some of which are very different from each other in composition. In a case-control study conducted by Phillips (1975), dairy products other than milk were associated with breast cancer. Hirayama (1977) reported that the ingestion of two glasses of milk daily was associated with a lower risk of gastric cancer in a large cohort.

There have been surprisingly few studies linking specific foods with either increases or decreases in cancer rates. Where there have been such studies, e.g., those on cruciferous vegetables, the data underscore the fact that it will be difficult for epidemiologists to sort out the specific chemicals of concern. For example, the constituents of cruciferae responsible for their apparent effect on the occurrence of cancer may be, as Chapter 15 suggests, indoles, isothiocyanates, or other nonnutritive substances demonstrated to affect carcinogenesis in the laboratory. But it is not yet possible to attribute the epidemiological associations to any such substances simply because of the simultaneous presence in these vegetables of such other constituents as fiber, β-carotene, ascorbic acid, or calcium.

Moreover, the identification of these associations is complicated not only by the composite nature of single foods but also by the interrelated variations in the intakes of a number of foods in any given diet. By eating more broccoli, one ordinarily eats less of something else. More broadly, those who increase their consumption of vegetable products must, of necessity, simultaneously reduce their consumption of animal products since these are the only two classes of substances (other than table salt and water) ordinarily consumed by humans. A reduced intake of animal products will normally result in a decreased consumption of nutrients such as animal fat, animal protein, heme iron, preformed vitamin A, and zinc; of mutagens formed during the cooking of meat; and of such fat-soluble contaminants as pesticides and drugs used for animals. This tendency for certain nutrients and other substances to occur together in certain types of foods accounts for the strong direct correlations among such dietary variables as beef, all meats, animal fat, and animal protein in epidemiological studies. Moreover, a reduced intake of animal products is necessarily accompanied by an increased intake of substances such as starches, fibers, and certain vitamins and minerals that are present in the substituted vegetable foods. Since all these dietary constituents increase and decrease simultaneously, it is difficult to determine which ones, if any, are involved when, for example, consumption of animal products and cancer rates decrease simultaneously or when control subjects consume more animal products than do cancer cases.

Individual diets are not composed of isolated substances or even isolated foods but, rather, they contain thousands of unique combinations of nutrients and other compounds that comprise the individual food items. From the standpoint of public education and public health, therefore, it is considerably less important to identify isolated compounds that cause or protect against certain cancers than it is to identify dietary patterns that enhance or minimize overall risk. The conclusions and recommendations contained in Chapter 1 reflect this committee's assessment of the evidence regarding some components of these patterns.

SUMMARY AND CONCLUSIONS

Since the turn of the century, there have been extensive changes in foodstuffs consumed by the U.S. population. Only a few of these changes have been measured, and then only crudely. Levels of nutrient intake that have been monitored have remained relatively constant between 1909 and the present, but data indicate that this constancy obscures major unmeasured changes in intake of other substances resulting from the declining consumption of certain commodities; changes in the forms in which foods are consumed; or the introduction of entirely new products and substances.

The relationship between these changes in the food supply and the incidence of cancer is not yet clear. The fact that the food supply has undergone major changes while the rates of cancer at most sites have been relatively constant may suggest that none of the changes has an effect on cancer incidence, that the changes have occurred too recently to produce an effect, or, more likely, that some changes have had a positive and some a negative impact. Data reviewed in this report indicate that a number of substances in food other than nutrients may play a role in the causation or the prevention of cancer. Thus, it may be important in epidemiolgical studies to consider a variety of food classifications and to monitor changes in the food supply in addition to those that affect nutrients.

REFERENCES

Blair, A., and J. F. Fraumeni, Jr. 1978. Geographic patterns of prostate cancer in the United States. J. Natl. Cancer Inst. 61:1379-1384.

Brewster, L. M., and M. Jacobson. 1978. The Changing American Diet. Center for Science in the Public Interest, Washington, D.C. 80 pp.

Comptroller General. 1979. Problems in Preventing the Marketing of Raw Meat and Poultry Containing Potentially Harmful Residues. Comptroller General's Report to the Congress of the United States, No. HRD-79-10, April 17, 1979. General Accounting Office, Washington, D.C. 87 pp.

Hirayama, T. 1977. Changing patterns of cancer in Japan with special reference to the decrease in stomach cancer mortality. Pp. 55-75 in H. H. Hiatt, J. D. Watson, and J. A. Winsten, eds. Origins of Human Cancer, Book A: Incidence of Cancer in Humans. Cold Spring Harbor Laboratory, Cold Spring Harbor, N.Y.

Howell, M. A. 1974. Factor analysis of international cancer mortality data and per capita food consumption. Br. J. Cancer 29:328-336.

Mettlin, C., and S. Graham. 1979. Dietary risk factors in human bladder cancer. Am. J. Epidemiol. 110:255-263.

Molitor, G. T. T. 1980. The food system in the 1980s. J. Nutr. Educ. 12 (Suppl. 1):103-111.

Page, L., and B. Friend. 1978. The changing United States diet. BioScience 28:192-197.

Peto, R., R. Doll, J. D. Buckley, and M. B. Sporn. 1981. Can dietary carotene materially reduce human cancer rates? Nature 290:201-208.

Phillips, R. L. 1975. Role of life-style and dietary habits in risk of cancer among Seventh-Day Adventists. Cancer Res. 35:3513-3522.

Smith D. T. 1980. Antibiotic additives: The prospect of doing without. Farmline 1(9):14-15.

U.S. Food and Drug Administration. 1980. Compliance Program Report of Findings. FY 77 Total Diet Studies--Adult (7320.73). Bureau of

Foods, Food and Drug Administration, U.S. Department of Health, Education, and Welfare, Washington, D.C. [33] pp.

U.S. International Trade Commission. 1980. Synthetic Organic Chemicals. United States Production and Sales, 1980. USITC Publication 1183. Office of Industries, U.S. International Trade Commission, Washington, D.C. 327 pp.

4 Total Caloric Intake

This chapter reviews the many experiments in which the variable studied is the total amount of food humans or animals eat, rather than the precise composition of their diet. It is entitled "Total Caloric Intake," although it is difficult to determine whether the effects brought about by changing the quantity of a diet are due to the resulting changes in caloric intake or to the changed distribution of specific nutrients.

A number of factors complicate the interpretation of the effect of caloric intake on cancer incidence. Caloric density can be modified either by modifying the ratio of fat (9.5 kcal/g) to carbohydrate (4.0 kcal/g) or by varying the concentration of nonnutritive bulk (fiber). Since dietary fat and fiber may also affect carcinogenesis, it becomes difficult to measure any independent effect of calories.

It is also not possible to identify the effect of caloric intake on cancer incidence in studies of humans. Although total caloric intake by two populations can be compared, the interpretation of the data is limited by the same considerations that apply to experiments in animals. It is also difficult to interpret studies in which the prevalence of obesity is compared with cancer incidence. Obesity is related to the balance between caloric intake and caloric expenditure. However, the proportional contributions of caloric intake and caloric expenditure to cancer risk are not known. Furthermore, there is evidence that obesity is related to the consumption of diets with increased caloric density. Thus, the contributions of fat, fiber, and carbohydrate cannot be readily measured independently.

EPIDEMIOLOGICAL EVIDENCE

There are few epidemiological data relating total caloric intake to cancer risk, partly because most dietary studies have been based on preselected food lists, which do not permit the quantification of total dietary intake.

Berg (1975) pointed out that the international distribution of hormone-dependent cancers has generated suspicion that these cancers may be related to affluence. He suggested that diets typical of affluent populations, when ingested since childhood, could overstimulate the endocrine system, lead to aberrations in metabolic processes, and result in cancer.

Gregor et al. (1969) analyzed data on caloric intake and the incidence of gastric and intestinal cancers. They concluded that as the per capita food intake (or gross national product) increases, the mortality rates for gastric cancers fall and those for intestinal cancer rise. Hill et al. (1979), who studied mortality from colorectal cancer in three socioeconomic groups in Hong Kong, found that the most affluent group had more than twice the mortality of the poorest group, i.e., 26.7/100,000 vs. 11.7/100,000. The relative proportions of nutrients in their diets were similar, but estimated daily caloric intake was 2,700 in the lowest socioeconomic group and 3,900 in the highest.

In a correlation study conducted by Armstrong and Doll (1975), per capita total caloric intake was examined in relation to cancer incidence in 23 countries and to cancer mortality in 32 countries. Significant correlation coefficients ($r \geqslant 0.70$) were found for total calories and rectal cancer incidence in males, leukemia in males, and mortality from breast cancer in females. Notably, the per capita intake of calories was highly correlated with intakes of total fat, total protein, and animal protein. The finding for breast cancer was reproduced by Gaskill et al. (1979), who analyzed data on mortality from breast cancer in relation to per capita intake for foods by state within the United States. However, there was no correlation when they controlled for age at first marriage (to reflect age at first pregnancy) in the analysis.

In two case-control studies, a number of dietary variables, including total caloric and fat intake, were estimated for subjects with cancer of the breast (Miller et al., 1978), for subjects with cancer of the colon and rectum (Jain et al., 1980), and for matched controls. For breast cancer cases, Miller and colleagues found no association with caloric intake and a weak association with total dietary fat. Jain and coworkers reported direct associations with caloric intake for both colon and rectal cancer, but the associations were not as strong as they were for intake of saturated fat. The authors concluded that the relevant variable in each study was more likely to be dietary fat than caloric intake.

Independent associations of breast cancer with body weight and height were found by de Waard and Baanders-van Halewijn (1974) in a cohort study of postmenopausal women in the Netherlands. Also, differentials in weight between cases of breast cancer and controls were found in Taiwan (Lin et al., 1971) and in São Paulo, Brazil (Mirra et al., 1971). Thus, de Waard (1975) suggested that susceptibility to breast cancer could be related to body mass (which, in turn, could be related to nutrition), but this hypothesis has not been accepted universally (MacMahon, 1975). Subsequently, de Waard et al. (1977) examined the influence of height and weight on age-specific incidence of breast cancer in the Netherlands and Japan and computed age-specific incidence curves for different height and weight groups. The heavier and taller postmenopausal women had the highest incidence of breast cancer. However, there appeared to be little independent effect of weight if there was an adjustment for its correlation with height. In his earlier study, de Waard (1975) suggested that lean body mass may be the important variable. However, if height is critical (and it is critical to the calculation of lean body mass), nutritional factors, if relevant, must begin to operate during adolescence or earlier, as was pointed out by MacMahon (1975). De Waard et al. (1977) suggested that approximately one-half of the differences in incidence of breast cancer between Holland and Japan can be attributed to differences in body weight and height.

In an analysis based on a long-term prospective study conducted by the American Cancer Society from 1959 to 1972, Lew and Garfinkel (1979) examined the relationship between mortality from cancer and other diseases and variation in weight among 750,000 men and women selected from the general population. Cancer mortality was significantly elevated in both sexes only among those 40% or more overweight. For men, most of the excess mortality resulted from cancer of the colon and rectum; for women, cancer of the gallbladder and biliary passages, breast, cervix, endometrium, and ovary were the major sites. It was not possible to evaluate the relative importance of overweight in comparison to total caloric intake or intake of other nutrients. Therefore, it cannot be assumed that obesity as such is the major risk factor. Nonetheless, most studies confirm a relationship between obesity and caloric intake, and in the absence of definitive information from studies that have separated the effects of caloric intake and fat intake, e.g., Miller et al. (1978) and Jain et al. (1980) (discussed above), it is reasonable to assume that high total caloric intake is a risk factor for some sites identified in other studies.

EXPERIMENTS IN ANIMALS

Tannenbaum (1942a,b, 1944, 1945a,b) examined the effects of caloric restriction upon the development of spontaneous and chemically induced tumors in several strains of mice. Growth of benzo[a]pyrene-induced tumors was inhibited by caloric restriction to different extents in ABC, Swiss, or DBA mice (Tannenbaum, 1942a). The level of dietary fat affected growth of skin tumors or spontaneous and chemically induced breast tumors, but not of sarcomas or lung tumors (Tannenbaum, 1942b). Caloric intake was restricted by controlling the amount of starch added to a diet containing commercial ration and skim milk powder. Mice whose daily dietary intake was 11.7 calories exhibited 25% more spontaneous mammary tumors than mice whose intake was 9.6 calories (Tannenbaum, 1945a). The incidence of benzpyrene-induced tumors was similar in mice ingesting 11.7 and 9.6 calories per day, but when caloric intake dropped to 8.1 calories daily, tumor incidence fell by 38% (Tannenbaum, 1945a). Among mice ingesting 11.7 calories daily, those receiving 18% of the calories from fat developed 70% more spontaneous mammary tumors than those whose diets contained only 2% (approximately 4% of calories) fat. Tannenbaum concluded that dietary fat exerted a specific influence over and above its caloric contribution (Tannenbaum, 1945b).

The influence of caloric restriction was also tested in a study of 3-methylcholanthrene-induced skin tumors in mice fed ad libitum and in a control group on a restricted diet. The carcinogen was painted on the skin for 10 weeks, and the mice were then observed for 1 year. On the basis of this experiment and earlier studies, Tannenbaum (1944, 1945b) concluded that the carcinogen-induced changes occur regardless of diet, but that the ad libitum ingestion of diet promotes tumor development.

Lavik and Baumann (1943) studied the promoting action of different levels of dietary fat on 3-methylcholanthrene-induced skin tumors in mice. A low fat, low calorie diet resulted in the fewest tumors. Lard with high (saturated) and low (unsaturated) melting points produced similar results, and the addition of riboflavin to the diet had a slight promoting effect; but the principal effect on carcinogenesis was produced by high caloric intake.

The studies of Tannenbaum and those by Lavik and Baumann could be profitably extended since we have identified a variety of possible carcinogens and promoters and have gained a greater understanding of food composition in recent decades.

SUMMARY AND CONCLUSIONS

Epidemiological Evidence

The epidemiological evidence supporting total caloric intake as a risk factor for cancer is slight and largely indirect. Much of it is based on associations between body weight or obesity and cancer. Studies that have evaluated both caloric and fat intake suggest that fat intake is the more relevant variable.

Experimental Evidence

Studies in animals to examine the effect of caloric intake on carcinogenesis have been few and are difficult to interpret. In these experiments, animals on restricted diets developed fewer tumors and their lifespan far exceeded that of animals fed ad libitum, thereby indicating a decrease in the age-specific incidence of tumors. However, because the intake of all nutrients was simultaneously depressed in these studies, the observed reduction in tumor incidence or delayed onset of tumors might have been due to the reduction of other nutrients such as fat. It is also difficult to interpret experiments in which caloric intake has been modified by varying dietary fat or fiber, both of which may by themselves exert effects on tumorigenesis.

Thus, neither the epidemiological nor the experimental studies permit a clear interpretation of the specific effect of caloric intake on the risk of cancer. Nonetheless, the studies conducted in animals show that a reduction in total food intake decreases the age-specific incidence of cancer. The evidence for humans is less clear.

REFERENCES

Armstrong, B., and R. Doll. 1975. Environmental factors and cancer incidence and mortality in different countries, with special reference to dietary practices. Int. J. Cancer 15:617-631.

Berg, J. W. 1975. Can nutrition explain the pattern of international epidemiology of hormone-dependent cancers? Cancer Res. 35:3345-3350.

de Waard, F. 1975. Breast cancer incidence and nutritional status with particular reference to body weight and height. Cancer Res. 35:3351-3356.

de Waard, F., and E. A. Baanders-van Halewijn. 1974. A prospective study in general practice on breast-cancer risk in postmenopausal women. Int. J. Cancer 14:153-160.

de Waard, F., J. P. Cornelis, K. Aoki, and M. Yoshida. 1977. Breast cancer incidence according to weight and height in two cities of the Netherlands and in Aichi prefecture, Japan. Cancer 40:1269-1275.

Gaskill, S. P., W. L. McGuire, C. K. Osborne, and M. P. Stern. 1979. Breast cancer mortality and diet in the United States. Cancer Res. 39:3628-3637.

Gregor, O., R. Toman, and F. Prušová. 1969. Gastrointestinal cancer and nutrition. Gut 10:1031-1034.

Hill, M., R. MacLennan, and K. Newcombe. 1979. Letter to the Editor: Diet and large-bowel cancer in three socioeconomic groups in Hong Kong. Lancet 1:436.

Jain, M., G. M. Cook, F. G. Davis, M. G. Grace, G. R. Howe, and A. B. Miller. 1980. A case-control study of diet and colo-rectal cancer. Int. J. Cancer 26:757-768.

Lavik, P. S., and C. A. Baumann. 1943. Further studies on the tumor-promoting action of fat. Cancer Res. 3:749-756.

Lew, E. A., and L. Garfinkel. 1979. Variations in mortality by weight among 750,000 men and women. J. Chronic Dis. 32:563-576.

Lin, T. M., K. P. Chen, and B. MacMahon. 1971. Epidemiologic characteristics of cancer of the breast in Taiwan. Cancer 27:1497-1504.

MacMahon, B. 1975. Formal discussion of "Breast cancer incidence and nutritional status with particular reference to body weight and height." Cancer Res. 35:3357-3358.

Miller, A. B., A. Kelly, N. W. Choi, V. Matthews, R. W. Morgan, L. Munan, J. D. Burch, J. Feather, G. R. Howe, and M. Jain. 1978. A study of diet and breast cancer. Am. J. Epidemiol. 107:499-509.

Mirra, A. P., P. Cole, and B. MacMahon. 1971. Breast cancer in an area of high parity: São Paolo, Brazil. Cancer Res. 31:77-83.

Tannenbaum, A. 1942a. The genesis and growth of tumors. II. Effects of caloric restriction per se. Cancer Res. 2:460-467.

Tannenbaum, A. 1942b. The genesis and growth of tumors. III. Effects of a high-fat diet. Cancer Res. 2:468-475.

Tannenbaum, A. 1944. The dependence of the genesis of induced skin tumors on the caloric intake during different stages of carcinogenesis. Cancer Res. 4:673-677.

Tannenbaum, A. 1945a. The dependence of tumor formation on the degree of caloric restriction. Cancer Res. 5:609-615.

Tannenbaum, A. 1945b. The dependence of tumor formation on the composition of the calorie-restricted diet as well as on the degree of restriction. Cancer Res. 5:616-625.

5 Lipids (Fats and Cholesterol)

EPIDEMIOLOGICAL EVIDENCE

Fats

Of all the dietary factors that have been associated epidemiologically with cancers of various sites, fat has probably been studied most thoroughly and produced the greatest frequency of direct associations. However, since dietary fat is highly correlated with the consumption of other nutrients that are present in the same foods, especially protein in Western diets, it is not always possible to attribute these associations to fat intake per se with absolute certainty.

Breast Cancer. Several international correlation studies have shown direct associations between per capita fat intake and breast cancer incidence or mortality (Armstrong and Doll, 1975; Carroll, 1975; Drasar and Irving, 1973; Gray et al., 1979; Hems, 1978; Knox, 1977). In general, the correlations were higher for total fat than for the other dietary factors considered (e.g., animal protein, meat, specific fat components, and oils). Some of the similarities in the findings undoubtedly reflect the overlapping data sets used in these studies rather than reproduced results.

In other correlation studies, intracountry data sets have been used to compare dietary fat intake and breast cancer. Gaskill et al. (1979) compared per capita intake of various foods by state within the United States with corresponding breast cancer mortality rates and found a significant direct correlation with fat intake when results from all states studied were combined. The correlation disappeared, however, when the southern states were excluded from the analysis or when they controlled for age at first marriage (as a reflection of age at first pregnancy) or median income. Their results suggested that dairy products as a class increased the risk of breast cancer. Hems (1980) noted that time trends for breast cancer mortality in England and Wales from 1911 to 1975 correlated best with corresponding per capita intake patterns for fat, sugar, and animal protein one decade earlier. In studies based on personal interview data, Kolonel et al. (1981) correlated individual consumption of fat with ethnic patterns of breast cancer incidence in Hawaii. These investigators found significant associations with total fat, with animal fat, and with both saturated and unsaturated fats.

The findings of three case-control studies support a role for dietary fat in the risk for breast cancer. Phillips (1975) reported a direct association between frequency of consumption of high-fat foods and breast cancer in a study of 77 breast cancer cases and matched controls among

73

Seventh-Day Adventists in California. Miller et al. (1978) also found a weak direct association, but no evidence of a dose response, between total fat consumption (based on quantitative dietary histories) and breast cancer in a study of 400 cases and 400 matched neighborhood controls in Canada.

In the third case-control study, Lubin et al. (1981) found significant increasing trends in relative risk with more frequent consumption of beef and other red meat, pork, and sweet desserts. Analysis of computed mean daily nutrient intake supported a link between breast cancer and consumption of animal fat and protein.

Nomura et al. (1978) compared the diets consumed by husbands of women with and without breast cancer. (The men were participants in a prospective cohort study of Japanese men in Hawaii.) These investigators reported a direct association between consumption of high fat diets by the husbands and breast cancer in their wives, who were assumed to have adhered to similar eating patterns.

Prostate Cancer. Prostate cancer has also been associated epidemiologically with fat intake. International data on mortality, but not incidence, indicate that there is a strong direct correlation of per capita total fat intake and cancer at this site (Armstrong and Doll, 1975). Howell (1974) reported similar results from a study based on a rank correlation with mortality in 41 countries. In Hawaii, the incidence of prostate cancer in four ethnic groups was highly correlated with consumption of both animal and saturated fat (Kolonel et al., 1981). In the mainland United States, Blair and Fraumeni (1978) correlated prostate cancer mortality by county with dietary variables. They observed that counties with a high risk for prostate cancer among whites had correspondingly high per capita fat intakes among the same population. Hirayama (1977) observed that one of the most notable dietary changes in Japan since 1950 is increased per capita fat intake and that this change parallels a striking increase in mortality from prostate cancer.

Prostate cancer has been associated with dietary fat in two case-control studies. In an ongoing study based on 111 cases with prostate cancer and 111 matched hospital controls, Rotkin (1977) has found that the cases had consumed high fat foods with greater frequency than had the controls. Schuman et al. (1982) also reported a more frequent consumption of foods with high animal fat content by cases than by controls.

Cancer of Other Reproductive Organs. Other reproductive organs for which there have been associations between dietary fat and cancer include the testes, corpus uteri, and ovary. Armstrong and Doll (1975) found direct correlations between per capita intake of total fat and incidence of cancer of the testes and corpus uteri and mortality from ovarian cancer. Lingeman (1974) also correlated mortality from ovarian cancer with international data on fat intake. Kolonel et al. (1981) found a direct association between ethnic patterns of total, animal, saturated, and unsaturated fat consumption in Hawaii and incidence of cancer of the corpus uteri.

Gastrointestinal Tract Cancer. Dietary fat has also been associated with cancer at several sites in the gastrointestinal tract. In only one case-control study, however, has an association of stomach cancer with dietary fat been suggested. In that study, Higginson (1966) reported more frequent consumption of fried foods and greater use of animal fats in cooking by gastric cancer cases than by controls. Graham et al. (1972) failed to confirm this finding in a subsequent study of 168 gastric cancer cases matched to hospital controls.

Although time-trend data in Japan (Hirayama, 1977) and one international correlation study (Lea, 1967) have shown associations of fat intake with pancreatic cancer, most epidemiological data pertain to cancers of the large bowel. Armstrong and Doll (1975) reported direct correlations between colon and rectal cancer incidence and mortality and per capita intake of total fat, based on international data. Knox (1977) also reported a strong correlation between mortality from cancer of the large intestine (excluding rectum) and per capita total fat intake, and only a slightly weaker correlation between mortality from rectal cancer and intake of total fat and animal fat.

After reviewing their data from an earlier study, Enig et al. (1979) retracted their original suggestion that colon cancer was directly correlated with intake of total, saturated, and vegetable fat, but not with animal fat. Bingham et al. (1979) calculated average intakes of nutrients by populations in different regions of Great Britain. They found no significant association of fat intake with mortality from colon and rectal cancers. Lyon and Sorenson (1978) also reported little difference in fat intake between the population of Utah (with a low risk for colon cancer) and that of the United States as a whole.

The contrast between the strong international correlations and the lack of associations within countries is striking. One possible explanation is that the regional food intake data within a country are based on means of individual consumption data and, thus, may be too uniform to demonstrate any strong association with risk of colon or rectal cancer. In contrast, the variation in fat intake among countries is much greater, thereby facilitating the demonstration of associations.

MacLennan et al. (1978) compared the diets of adult men in two Scandinavian populations with different risks for colon cancer (high risk for Danes in Copenhagen and low risk for Finns in Kuopio). These studies, which were based on food diaries, indicated that the consumption of fat was similar for both groups, but that there were differences in fiber intake (see Chapter 8). Reddy et al. (1978) also studied this low risk Finnish population and compared their diets to those of a high risk population in New York. They too found no difference between groups in total fat intake, but noted that a higher proportion of total fat was consumed as dairy products by the Finns and as meat by the New Yorkers. This observation raises the possibility that the source as well as the quantity of dietary fat may be relevant.

In a case-control study conducted in parallel with the study on breast cancer (described above), Phillips (1975) found a direct association between colon cancer and the frequent consumption of high-fat foods by Seventh-Day Adventists. In a study of cases and hospital controls among blacks in California, Dales et al. (1978) observed a direct association between risk of colon cancer and frequent consumption of foods high in saturated fat. The association was strongest for those who consumed diets high in saturated fat and low in fiber content. Total fat consumption, estimated from frequency data, was also reported to be higher among large bowel cancer cases than among controls in a study conducted in Puerto Rico (Martínez et al., 1979).

Dietary histories were used to estimate nutrient intake in a case-control study conducted by Jain et al. (1980) in Canada. They reported a direct association (including a dose response) between risk of both colon and rectal cancer and consumption of fat, especially saturated fat. The elevated risks persisted after adjustment for other nutrients in the diet.

Several reports on meat consumption are relevant to this discussion since meat can be an important source of dietary fat, especially saturated fat. Berg and Howell (1974) and Howell (1975) reported a high correlation between colon cancer mortality and meat intake (particularly beef), based on international per capita intake data. In Hawaii, investigators reported a direct association between frequency of meat, especially beef, consumption and large bowel cancer among Japanese cases and hospital controls (Haenszel et al., 1973). This finding was not reproduced in studies conducted in Buffalo, New York (Graham et al., 1978) and in Japan (Haenszel et al., 1980), nor in parallel cohorts followed prospectively in Minnesota and Norway (Bjelke, 1978). Furthermore, Enstrom (1975) has noted that trends in beef intake in the United States do not correlate with trends in the incidence of and mortality from colorectal cancer.

Meat consumption has also been associated with pancreatic cancer. In a case-control study conducted in Japan, Ishii et al. (1968) found a direct association between meat consumption by men and mortality from pancreatic cancer. Their findings were based on responses to mailed questionnaires, most of which were completed by relatives of deceased cases. Hirayama (1977) reported a relative risk of 2.5 for daily meat intake and incidence of pancreatic cancer in a prospective cohort study of 265,118 Japanese.

Summary. The results from a substantial number of epidemiological studies have indicated an association between dietary fat and cancers of the gastrointestinal tract (especially the large bowel) and of endocrine target organs (especially the breast and prostate). Some studies of large bowel cancer were conducted on groups of relatively homogeneous populations, and some were not specifically designed to test the hypothesis that fat consumption is associated with colon cancer. The studies designed specifically to test this hypothesis (e.g., Dales et al., 1978; Jain et al., 1980) tended to show the most striking direct associations, especially when the possible confounding effects of dietary fiber were considered. The evidence for cancer of the breast and prostate is more consistent than that for large bowel cancer. The results of the most thorough case-control study of breast cancer yet reported (Miller et al., 1978) were only weakly positive, however, partly reflecting the fact that recent food consumption was measured rather than dietary intake patterns earlier in life, which may have been the more relevant exposure period. (Studies of changing breast cancer incidence among Japanese migrants to the United States and their descendents, for example, suggest that early-life exposures are important determinants of breast cancer risk.)

Cholesterol

High-fat diets have been associated with atherosclerosis--a condition that has also been associated with elevated serum cholesterol levels. Therefore, there has been interest in studying the relationship of serum cholesterol levels as well as cholesterol intake to the incidence of cancer. Most of the studies described below were designed to examine the association between cholesterol and cardiovascular disease, and were not specifically intended to measure cancer incidence or mortality. However, the opportunity provided by these long-term studies of cardiovascular disease in which serum cholesterol levels of the subjects were determined at the beginning of the study has resulted in a number of different reports on observed associations.

Using per capita food intake data from 20 industrialized nations and simple correlation analysis, Liu et al. (1979) showed that there was a strong direct correlation between per capita intake of total fat and cholesterol and the mortality rate for colon cancer, but that there was an inverse correlation for fiber intake. Cross-classification showed a highly significant association for cholesterol, but not for fat or fiber. These investigators suggested that the data support a causal relationship between dietary cholesterol and colon cancer.

Pearce and Dayton (1971) conducted an 8-year clinical trial in which groups of 422 and 424 men were fed a conventional diet or one containing high levels of polyunsaturated fat (to lower cholesterol levels), respectively. Incidence of cancer deaths in the groups on the experimental diet was higher. In a similar experiment conducted in Finland, Miettinen et al. (1972) also found more carcinomas in the test group. A study group, convened to examine cancer incidence in men from five controlled trials of cholesterol-lowering diets, found little difference in relative risks (Ederer et al., 1971).

In other studies, clofibrate, a hypolipidemic agent, or a placebo was administered to more than 10,000 volunteers between 30 to 54 years of age whose serum cholesterol levels were in the top tertile (Committee on Principle Investigators, 1978). The total mortality from causes other than ischemic heart disease was substantially higher in the clofibrate group: there was a disproportionately large number of neoplasms of the gastrointestinal tract and a few more neoplasms in the respiratory tract. However, there were too few cancer deaths to demonstrate a statisticially significant difference among the test groups.

In another study of the relationship between colon cancer and serum cholesterol, Rose et al. (1974) observed that the initial levels of serum cholesterol in colon cancer patients were lower than expected. They also reported that serum cholesterol levels were higher in patients with cancer of the stomach, pancreas, liver, bile ducts, and rectum than in the controls. Bjelke (1974) reported a similar correlation between colon cancer and low levels of serum cholesterol. Nydegger and Butler (1972) examined total serum cholesterol levels in 186 controls and 122 subjects with malignant tumors. Their data also generally showed lower cholesterol levels in the cancer patients.

Beaglehole et al. (1980) studied the relationship between serum cholesterol concentration and mortality in New Zealand Maoris over a period of 11 years. They found significant inverse relationships between serum cholesterol concentrations and cancer mortality.

In a 7.5-year follow-up study of London civil servants, Rose and Shipley (1980) observed that mortality from cancer at all sites was associated with a progressive decline in plasma cholesterol levels. These investigators grouped cancer deaths into those that occurred less than 2 years after the subjects entered the study and those that occurred from 2 to 7.5 years afterward. For the group in which deaths occurred within 2 years, the age-adjusted mortality rate for those with the lowest plasma cholesterol levels was more than double the rate for those with the highest levels. However, cancer deaths among those followed for longer than 2 years occurred at the same rate, regardless of plasma cholesterol level at entry into the study. The investigators concluded that the decline in cholesterol levels was probably a metabolic consequence of cancer, which, while unsuspected, was present when the subjects entered the study.

In more than 5,000 subjects studied for 24 years in the Framingham Heart Study (Williams et al., 1981), an inverse relationship between serum cholesterol levels and cancer of the colon and other sites was observed in men but not in women.

Kark et al. (1980) related serum cholesterol levels to cancer incidence in more than 3,000 individuals followed for as long as 14 years in Evans County, Georgia. Patients diagnosed as having cancer at any site at least 1 year following entry into the study had had entry serum cholesterol levels significantly lower than those in the noncancer patients.

This association was the same for black and white females and for black and white males, but was stronger in males of both races. The possibility that the presence of cancer may have been responsible for the lower serum cholesterol levels was investigated. Patients were categorized into three groups, depending on when evidence of cancer was first observed after entry into the study: within 1 year, from 1 to 6 years, and from 7 to 13 years. Initial serum cholesterol levels were <u>higher</u> in the first group than in the other two groups, but no differences were noted between the latter groups. Kark and colleagues also observed little difference in cholesterol levels in cases and controls when various cancer sites were grouped together. However, they did report low serum cholesterol levels in lung cancer patients, whereas Stamler <u>et al.</u> (1968) observed that serum cholesterol levels were higher in lung cancer cases than in controls. A study conducted in Norway indicated that there was no over-all relationship between serum cholesterol levels and total cancer incidence (Westlund and Nicolaysen, 1972).

In the Honolulu Heart Study, 598 deaths were observed in 7,961 men whose cholesterol levels had been determined and who were followed for 9 years (Kagan <u>et al.</u>, 1981). The baseline serum cholesterol levels were directly associated with mortality from coronary heart disease but inversely associated with total cancer mortality, mortality from cancers of the esophagus, colon, liver, and lung, and malignancies of the lymphatic and hematopoietic systems.

In Yugoslavia, Kozarevic <u>et al.</u> (1981) related baseline serum cholesterol levels to mortality in 11,121 males over a 7-year period. The inverse association between cancer deaths and serum cholesterol levels was not statistically significant.

In the Puerto Rico Heart Health Programme, 9,824 men were followed for 8 years (Garcia-Palmieri <u>et al.</u>, 1981). Serum cholesterol levels measured at the first examination were found to vary inversely with subsequent mortality from cancer.

Peterson <u>et al.</u> (1981) followed 10,000 men in Sweden for a mean of 2.5 years. They found that deaths from neoplastic disease and other noncoronary heart disease peaked at low levels of serum cholesterol.

In contrast, serum cholesterol was not associated with overall risk of death from cancer in three epidemiological studies of Chicago men (Dyer <u>et al.</u>, 1981). When cancer deaths were evaluated by site, there was a significant inverse association between serum cholesterol and deaths from sarcoma, leukemia, and Hodgkin's disease in the nearly 2,000 men studied for 17 years, but not for deaths from lung cancer, colorectal cancer, cancer of the oral cavity, pancreatic cancer, or all other cancers combined. There was, however, a suggestion of a direct association for breast cancer in women.

These studies have been assessed by Lilienfeld (1981) and by others, who concluded that the observed inverse correlations do not substantiate any direct cause-and-effect relationship between low blood cholesterol levels and cancer.

Only one case-control study has specifically evaluated serum cholesterol levels in cases of colon cancer and matched controls (Miller et al., 1981). In 133 pairs matched by age and sex, serum cholesterol levels were lower for cases than for controls. However, following stratification by tumor stage, significant differences in cholesterol levels persisted only between cases with advanced tumors and controls. Furthermore, only women, not men, had significantly lower serum cholesterol levels with advancing disease. The lack of an association in early disease supports the concept that low serum cholesterol levels observed in colon cancer patients may be the result of a metabolic change accompanying tumor growth and may not necessarily precede tumor formation.

Miller et al. (1978) studied the association of dietary levels of cholesterol and breast cancer. They found no significant differences in estimated cholesterol consumption between cases and controls. In another case-control study, the same group found that cholesterol intake for males with rectal cancer and females with colon and rectal cancer was higher than for controls (Jain et al., 1980). Although the relative risk for dietary cholesterol was significant at higher intakes for all male and female cases, compared to all controls, it was substantially less than the estimates of risk for other nutrients associated with intake of fat, especially saturated fat.

There is an apparent conflict in the evidence, i.e., that an increased risk of cancer of the colon and other sites has been associated not only with dietary cholesterol (and simultaneous intake of other, possibly more relevant lipid components) but also with very low serum cholesterol levels. A possible explanation might be that a high intake of dietary fat (and/or cholesterol) by persons whose metabolism maintains low serum cholesterol results in reduced biosynthesis of cholesterol and a high rate of excretion for cholesterol breakdown products in the intestine (Lin and Connor, 1980). These breakdown products could serve as substrates for the intraluminal production of carcinogens by intestinal bacteria (Hill et al., 1971). However, in metabolic studies conducted in hospital wards, low serum cholesterol is usually accompanied by excretion of low levels of bile acid. This observation is not compatible with the mechanisms normally proposed for the carcinogenic effect of dietary lipids.

In summary, data pertaining to the association between serum cholesterol levels and total cancer incidence and mortality are inconsistent. An inverse correlation between serum cholesterol levels and colon cancer in men has been noted in some studies, but not in all. It is not clear whether lower than normal serum cholesterol levels are the cause, or whether they reflect the metabolic consequences, of cancer. Thus, the data are inconclusive and do not point to a causal relationship between low cholesterol levels and risk of colon cancer. However, since they do suggest that low serum cholesterol levels may be a clue to some unknown factor, possibly something that is transported in the low density lipoprotein fraction of serum, these data and future findings should be examined carefully.

RELATIONSHIP OF FECAL STEROID EXCRETION TO BOWEL CARCINOGENESIS

The possibility that metabolites in the colon could provide a clue to the presence of malignancy has stimulated a number of investigators to study the level and spectrum of steroids in the feces of populations at low or high risk for colon cancer, as well as of animals fed colon carcinogens together with various dietary regimens. The amounts of neutral and acidic fecal steroids correspond to the level of fat intake. However, studies of the ratios of primary to secondary bile acids or the ratio of cholesterol to its metabolic products (i.e., coprostanol and coprostanone) have revealed no significant differences among the populations studied (Moskovitz et al., 1979; Mower et al., 1979; Reddy, 1979).

Recent comparisons of high risk and low risk populations, e.g., three socioeconomic groups in Hong Kong (Hill et al., 1979) and Finns and New Yorkers (Reddy, 1979), suggest that the concentration of bile acids is elevated in feces of the groups that are at higher risk.

Pioneering efforts by Hill and his colleagues (1971) pointed to an association between rates of mortality from colon cancer and fecal excretion of bile acids as well as the fecal degradation of cholesterol and its metabolites. They revived an earlier concept, based on structural and steric similarities, that bile acids might be transformed to the carcinogen 3-methylcholanthrene by anaerobic gut bacteria. In the studies leading to these earlier theories, deoxycholic acid was converted chemically to 3-methylcholanthrene by Wieland and Dane (1933) and by Cook and Haslewood (1933). Later, Fieser and Newman (1935) derived the same carcinogen from cholic acid. The chemical steps used in these studies were all reactions known to occur naturally, i.e., oxidation, hydrogenation, cyclization, and dehydrogenation, although laboratory conditions for the synthesis did not reproduce normally encountered biological conditions.

Through the efforts of Hill, Reddy, Mastromarino, Narisawa, Nigro, their coworkers, and others, the concept has evolved that fecal bile acids and metabolites of cholesterol may function as cocarcinogens, carcinogens, or promoters in tumorigenesis of the large bowel (Hill et al., 1971; Mastromarino et al., 1976; Narisawa et al., 1974; Nigro et al., 1973; Reddy and Wynder, 1973; Reddy et al., 1977a). To date, however, no active carcinogen derived from bile acids has been isolated from human or animal feces.

Reddy et al. (1977a) demonstrated that a fourfold increase in dietary fat (from 5% to 20%) given to rats increased the 24-hour fecal excretion of neutral and acid sterols by 30% to 40% (based on body weight). Bacterial conversion of primary to secondary bile acids occurred more extensively in rats fed the high fat diet than in those fed the low fat diet.

The possibility that bile acids may have tumor-promoting effects is supported to some extent by the finding that bile acids affect cell kinetics in the intestinal epithelium. Diversion of biliary and pancreatic secretions from the intestine decreases DNA synthesis and cell proliferation (Fry and Staffeldt, 1964; Ranken et al., 1971; Roy et al., 1975), whereas the administration of secondary bile acids increases cell proliferation in liver bile ducts and the biliary tract epithelium (Bagheri et al., 1978). Inhibition of DNA synthesis and cell proliferation has also been observed in the rat colon following biliary diversion (Deschner and Raicht, 1979).

Possible promotional effects of bile acids on bowel tumorigenesis were suggested in studies initiated by Narisawa et al. (1974) and completed, with a large sampling of bile acids, by Reddy and colleagues (see review by Reddy et al., 1980). In these studies, N-methyl-N'-nitro-N-nitrosoguanidine (MNNG), which is a direct-acting carcinogen, was administered intrarectally to conventional or germfree rats for 2 weeks. During the subsequent 16 weeks, 20 mg doses of sodium cholate, sodium chenodeoxycholate, or sodium lithocholate in 0.5 ml of peanut oil were administered intrarectally to rats 3 times a week. No tumors were detected in the control groups. The total number of large bowel tumors in each of the conventional and germfree rats given intrarectal instillations of bile salts was greater than in rats given MNNG without bile salts. These data also suggest that gut microflora was not required for the effect of bile acids to be manifested. In this study, the quantity of bile salts administered intrarectally was approximately 20 to 60 times higher than that normally excreted in the feces during a 24-hour period. Perhaps more importantly, the instillations at levels of approximately 100 mM were at least 10 times higher than the normal concentrations of these salts within the lumen of the bowel.

Palmer (1979) observed that bile salts interact readily with membranes from artificial liposomes, bacteria, and mammalian cells. The well-studied cytotoxic effects of bile salts are invariably preceded by alterations in membrane permeability in red blood cells, in a variety of tissues, and in mucosal cells of both the large and the small intestine (Dawson and Isselbacher, 1960; Dietschy, 1967; Hoffman, 1967). In one study, the effects of these salts upon permeability (and presumably cytotoxicity) in the gut were minimized when conjugated bile salts were added to the unconjugated bile salts in sufficiently high concentrations (Low-Beer et al., 1970). Thus, it cannot be determined whether the effects of intrarectally instilled unconjugated bile salts demonstrated classic tumor promotional activity or resulted from nonspecific damage and repair activity associated with increased cellular proliferation of the colonic mucosa induced by the high intraluminal concentration of the salts.

Cohen and associates studied the effect of bile acid on colon tumors induced by nitrosomethylurea (NMU) by feeding rats lab chow pellets with and without added bile acid. They observed that 0.2% cholic acid (Cohen et al., 1978), but not chenodeoxycholic acid (Raicht et al., 1975), increased the number of NMU-induced colon tumors, as compared to the number of tumors in rats fed nonsupplemented pellets. In the dimethylhydrazine (DMH) model, no effect on colon tumorigenesis was observed in rats fed 0.3% cholic acid in a semisynthetic diet (Broitman, 1981).

Evidence that increased quantities of bile acids in the colonic lumen were associated with an increase in azoxymethane (AOM)-induced colon tumorigenesis in rats was provided by Chomchai et al. (1974). Williamson et al. (1979) showed that bile initiated prompt ileal hyperplasia in rats following intestinal resection with diversion of the pancreatic and biliary ducts to the terminal ileum, i.e., pancreatobiliary diversion.

Feeding cholestyramine to rats given AOM for tumor induction increased the average number of tumors in the large bowel but not in the small bowel (Nigro et al., 1973, 1977). Vahouny et al. (1981) demonstrated that intraluminal infusion of 165 μM of cholic, deoxycholic, and chenodeoxycholic acids 1:1:1 twice daily for 5 days resulted in severe topological changes in the colonic mucosa.

Thus, the enhancement of tumorigenesis observed at high concentrations of bile acids may be related to nonspecific effects of tissue injury. Tumor-enhancing effects of nonspecific injury have been attributed to increased cellular proliferation, which accompanies inflammation and repair (Ryser, 1971).

EXPERIMENTAL EVIDENCE

The first demonstration that dietary fat could influence tumorigenesis was reported by Watson and Mellanby (1930). Most of these studies were conducted by increasing the level of dietary fat, which also led to an increase in the total intake of calories. Addition of 12.5% to 25.0% butter to a basal (3% fat) diet given to coal-tar-treated mice increased the incidence of skin tumors from 34% to 57%. Similarly, Lavik and Baumann (1941, 1943), who administered 3-methylcholanthrene topically to mice found that a basal diet, when supplemented with 15% fat (shortening), increased the yield of skin tumors from 12% to 83%. Fat was especially effective when fed 6 to 12 weeks after treatment with a carcinogen. Comparing diets containing 10% corn oil, 10% coconut oil, or 10% lard for their ability to enhance tumors, these investigators observed a minor effect of unsaturation: the incidence of tumors at 5 months was 33% (for control diets), 61% (for added lard diets), 66% (for added coconut oil diets), and 76% (for added corn oil diets).

Mammary Tumors

Tannenbaum (1942) demonstrated that dietary fat enhanced the development of either chemically or spontaneously induced mammary tumors in mice.

The incidence of spontaneous tumors was greater when the high fat diets were instituted at 24 weeks of age than when they were fed beginning at 38 weeks. Tannenbaum and Silverstone (1957) noted that tumor incidence was greater in obese mice than in normal mice and that caloric restriction inhibited mammary tumorigenesis in normal mice. This was also observed by Waxler and colleagues, who induced obesity in mice with gold thioglucose and observed that spontaneous mammary carcinomas developed more quickly in obese mice than in controls (Waxler, 1954; Waxler et al., 1953). After reducing the weight of the obese mice below that of controls (which were also treated with gold thioglucose) by limiting their dietary intake, they observed a decrease in mammary tumors compared to controls. The effects of caloric restriction on reducing the incidence of chemically induced tumors can be negated by increasing the dose of the carcinogen (King et al., 1949; Tannenbaum and Silverstone, 1957; White, 1961; White et al., 1944). By feeding mice isocaloric high and low fat diets, Tannenbaum (1942) provided evidence that fat, rather than calories per se, was responsible for enhancing tumorigenesis. This observation differed from the findings of Lavik and Baumann (1943), who reported that the caloric content of the diet had a greater effect than the level of fat on the induction of skin tumors in mice by 3-methylcholanthrene. These earlier studies have been comprehensively reviewed by Tannenbaum (1959), Tannenbaum and Silverstone (1957), and Carroll and Khor (1975).

In 1970, Carroll and Khor again pointed out that the level of dietary fat was as important as the amount of 7,12-dimethylbenz[a]anthracene (DMBA) administered to induce breast cancer. They studied the effect of both high and low doses of the carcinogen fed to rats in corn oil. At the low dose (1 mg), rats fed a 20% corn oil diet exhibited more tumors and a shorter latent period, but no difference in the number of tumors per tumor-bearing rat, as compared to rats fed a 0.5% corn oil diet. When the dose of DMBA was increased to 2.5 mg, the high fat diet increased tumor incidence and the number of tumors, but did not alter the latent period.

The quality or type of lipid was also shown to be an important factor in the induction of breast cancer by DMBA (Carroll and Khor, 1971). The incidence of tumors at this site was uniformly high with all dietary fats tested at a level of 20% in the diet, but the number of tumors per group and per tumor-bearing rat was proportionally greater in the rats fed unsaturated fats. Furthermore, it was apparent that the yield of tumors per group was also influenced by the level of essential fatty acid-- linoleic acid--present in the fat. Groups of rats fed tallow or coconut oil (which are inadequate sources of linoleate) had significantly fewer tumors than groups fed polyunsaturated fats (which are adequate sources of linoleate). Because the enhancement of breast tumorigenesis by high fat diets was observed when the diets were fed after tumor initiation by DMBA, the investigators concluded that dietary fat exerted its effect during the promotional phase (Carroll, 1980). As the dose of carcinogen was increased, the promotional effect of high fat diets became stronger. There is a limit to the promotional effects of dietary fats, however, since diets containing fat at levels greater than 20% were no more effective than those containing 20%.

The enhancement of DMBA-induced mammary tumorigenesis in rodents by high fat diets (especially those containing polyunsaturated fats) has been observed by a number of investigators (Carroll and Khor, 1971; Hopkins and West, 1976; Ip, 1980; King et al., 1979). More recently, Carroll and coworkers found that saturated fat was as effective as polyunsaturated fat in enhancing tumorigenesis when a small quantity of polyunsaturated fat (3% sunflower seed oil) was added to the saturated fat (17% coconut oil) (Carroll, 1975; Carroll and Hopkins, 1979; Hopkins and Carroll, 1979). They also learned that the polyunsaturated fat used must provide sufficient amounts of essential fatty acids and that the diet must contain high levels of total fat to increase the yield of breast tumors. Whether these two requirements are interrelated is not certain. But studies in rats have shown that essential fatty acid metabolism and accumulation of polyunsaturated fat in tissues is influenced by dietary fat (Mohrhauer and Holman, 1967; Peifer and Holman, 1959).

Providing support for an association between dietary fat and DMBA-induced breast cancer are findings from studies in rats with the known breast carcinogen NMU. Chan et al. (1977) observed a significant reduction in the latent period for the development of NMU-induced breast tumors in female Fischer 344 rats fed high fat diets compared to rats fed low fat diets. However, unlike the studies using the DMBA model of breast carcinogenesis, high fat diets increased only the incidence and not the multiplicity of NMU-induced breast tumors.

In a study of the relationship of dietary fat levels to x-ray-induced and NMU-induced mammary carcinogenesis, Silverman et al. (1980) reported similar effects. The incidence and multiplicity of breast tumors induced by 350 rads of total body irradiation were increased in Sprague-Dawley rats fed a calorie-controlled, 20% lard diet, compared to rats fed a 5% lard diet. The high fat diet increased the multiplicity of NMU-induced tumors, but not the incidence.

Both the level and the quality of dietary fat appear to influence the growth rate of DMBA-induced breast tumors, according to studies by McCay et al. (1980). Rats fed a diet containing a high level of polyunsaturated fat (20% corn oil) exhibited an average tumor growth rate that was considerably greater than that for rats fed a diet containing high levels of saturated fat (18% coconut oil and 2% linoleic acid). In animals fed a low fat diet (2% linoleic acid), the average tumor growth rate was markedly lower than the rates for the other two groups. Thus, the tumor growth rate appears to be determined in part by the total dietary fat and in part by the polyunsaturated fat content. Therefore, a given dose of DMBA could produce a similar number of initiated cells in the mammary gland, independent of the dietary regimen used, and the number of tumors that are palpable within a fixed time would depend on the growth rate of the initiated clones. Consequently, if a higher level of total dietary

5-13

fat or of polyunsaturated fat accelerated clonal growth, the number of tumors reaching palpable size within a fixed time would be greater.

Growth of transplantable tumors is also influenced by dietary fat. A transplantable mammary adenocarcinoma developed much more readily in host mice fed a high level of polyunsaturated fat than in mice fed an equivalent level of saturated fat (Hopkins and West, 1977). In a study by Abraham and Rao (1976), as little as 1.0% corn oil added to the diet stimulated the growth of a transplantable mammary tumor in mice. By using inhibitors of prostaglandin biosynthesis, these investigators concluded that this effect was related to the level of essential fatty acids, rather than to synthesis of prostaglandin. Pure linoleic acid in the diet at 0.1% was as effective as 15% corn oil in enhancing the growth of a transplantable mammary adenocarcinoma (Hillyard and Abraham, 1979). In studies of cell cultures with and without added polyunsaturated fat, Kidwell et al. (1978) and Wicha et al. (1979) demonstrated that polyunsaturated fat enhanced the growth of both normal and neoplastic mammary epithelial cells from rats. Corwin et al. (1979) measured the tumorigenicity of Kirsten sarcoma virus-transformed murine cell line, AK3T3, which was grown in delipidized tissue culture media. Its tumorigenicity (incidence of tumors following implantation of a constant number of cells) in BALB/c mice was compared to that in a conventional line of FK3T3 cells maintained in a complete tissue culture medium. Although sarcomas in general are not responsive to diet, an increase in tumorigenicity was observed with AK3T3 cells as the level of dietary polyunsaturated fats was increased from 4% to 8%, whereas an opposite effect on tumorigenicity was noted with the FK3T3 cells. Thus, lipid supply in vitro affected the expression of the transformed phenotype of a transplantable tumor. This, in turn, altered the response of the tumor to dietary lipids in the host.

Rogers (1975) and Newberne and Zeiger (1978) observed that the effects of a high fat diet on breast carcinogenesis could be modified when the diet was marginal in lipotrope (choline and methionine) content. In Sprague-Dawley rats given 2-acetylaminofluorene (AAF) or DMBA to induce breast tumors, the tumor incidence was lower and death from the tumors occurred later in marginally lipotrope-deficient rats than in controls.

Hepatic and Pancreatic Cancer

When administered to Fischer rats, which are resistant to breast cancer, AAF induced hepatic carcinomas (Newberne and Zeiger, 1978). Under these conditions, a high fat diet that was marginally deficient in lipotropes significantly increased the incidence of hepatic carcinomas, as compared to the incidence in rats fed a high fat diet with adequate lipotropes. Thus, the effect of marginal lipotrope deficiency on the relationship between dietary fat and carcinogen-induced tumorigenesis appeared to differ from one target organ to another.

An increase in dietary fat increased the incidence of AAF-induced hepatomas in male rats (Sugai et al., 1962). Farber (1973) suggested that chronic feeding of AAF resulted in the cloning of hepatic cells with resistance to AAF toxicity. Hyperplastic nodules that result from the regenerative activity of such clones ultimately progress to form hepatomas. McCay et al. (1980) studied the influence of dietary fat in the early stages of hyperplastic nodule formation and during the later stages of hepatoma development. Hyperplastic nodules formed from AAF more frequently and the latent period was shorter in rats fed a low fat diet (2% linoleic acid) than in rats fed diets with high saturated fat (18% coconut oil and 2% linoleic acid) or with a high polyunsaturated fat content (20% corn oil). In contrast, there was a 100% incidence of hepatomas in the rats fed the high polyunsaturated fat diet, a 20% incidence in those fed the low fat diet, and high mortality among those fed the high saturated fat diet because of the excessive toxicity of AAF under these conditions. These studies illustrate the differing effects of dietary fat upon the various stages of hepatoma development.

Dietary lipids also modify aflatoxin-B_1-induced liver tumors in rats (Newberne et al., 1979). When beef fat was fed to rats, the number of tumors induced was the same, regardless of whether the beef fat was fed only after induction (51%) or both before and after induction (53%). Feeding of polyunsaturated fat (corn oil) before and after induction resulted in a 100% tumor yield, but when the oil was fed only after tumor induction, the yield was 66%. The authors concluded that unsaturated fats increase the tumor yield more effectively than do saturated fats, but that this effect may occur during the initiation or early promotional phase of hepatic carcinogenesis.

Dietary fat may modify the incidence of pancreatic adenocarcinomas induced in rats by azaserine (Longnecker et al., 1981; Roebuck et al., 1981). In Lewis rats fed diets containing either 20% corn oil or 20% safflower oil, the number of pancreatic neoplasms was higher than in animals fed the same percentage of saturated fat. The animals fed the control diet (5% corn oil) and treated with azaserine exhibited the same incidence and numbers of pancreatic neoplasms as did animals fed an 18% saturated fat diet. Compared to controls, there was a marked increase in hepatocellular carcinomas in rats given azaserine but maintained on a lipotrope-deficient diet.

Intestinal Cancer

A variety of compounds that are carcinogenic in the bowel have been used in a number of animal models to study the effect of dietary fat on tumorigenesis at that site. Nigro et al. (1975) demonstrated that Sprague-Dawley rats treated with AOM developed more intestinal tumors and more metastatic lesions when fed a diet containing 35% beef fat than when fed regular chow. Since the caloric density of the beef fat diet was significantly greater than that of the laboratory chow, it is difficult to sort out the effect of calories from that of fat on tumorigenesis. Nevertheless, the report provided a model for studying diet-responsive intestinal tumorigenesis.

Reddy et al. (1974) used DMH to induce tumors of the colon (and, to a lesser extent, small intestine) in rats fed 5% or 20% lard or corn oil diets. Rats fed the 5% corn oil diets had a greater tumor incidence and higher average number of tumors per animal than those fed the 5% lard diet. Tumor incidence and multiplicity increased with the higher levels of dietary fat. However, rats fed the 20% fat diets exhibited essentially the same incidence and multiplicity of tumors whether the fat was polyunsaturated or saturated. In a repeat study with animals maintained on these diets for two generations before tumor induction with DMH, findings were essentially the same (Reddy et al., 1977a). Measurements indicated that there were no differences in the quantities of diet consumed daily among all the dietary groups. Since the caloric density of low and high fat diets differed, rats eating the high fat diets consumed, in addition to more fat, approximately 20% more calories.

In a study by Broitman et al. (1977), atherogenic diets containing 5% or 20% coconut oil were fed to rats given DMH to induce tumors of the bowel. These investigators also observed that rats fed the 20% saturated fat diet had a greater incidence and multiplicity of tumors than those fed the 5% saturated fat diet. However, they pointed out that rats fed the low fat diet consumed fewer calories, gained much less weight, and thus received less of the carcinogen than did rats fed the high fat diets.

Studies with a number of strains of rats and various carcinogens have illustrated that intestinal tumorigenesis is enhanced as the quantity of dietary fat is increased. Bansal et al. (1978), using Wistar Furth rats and DMH for tumor induction, noted that rats fed 30% lard developed more large bowel tumors than did those fed a low fat standard diet. To induce colon tumorigenesis in Fischer 344 rats, Reddy and associates (1977b, 1980) administered DMH or methylazoxymethanol (MAM) acetate systemically on a weight basis or gave the animals constant intrarectal doses of 2',3-dimethyl-4-aminobiphenyl (DMAB) or NMU. These investigators demonstrated that the tumor incidence in rats fed 20% beef fat was greater than that in those fed 5% beef fat, irrespective of the carcinogen used to induce the intestinal tumors. Since the routes of metabolic activation for some of these carcinogens differ, it is more likely that the effects of increased levels of dietary fat were manifested following activation of the carcinogen, rather than during the various steps leading to activation.

Promoting effects of dietary fat were suggested by studies in which high fat diets increased the frequency of small and large bowel tumors when fed to rats after administration of AOM but not before or during administration of the carcinogen (Bull et al., 1979). The high fat diet (30% beef fat) used in these studies had a caloric density that was approximately 34% greater than the low fat diet (5% beef fat), and was considered by the authors to be responsible for the differences in weight gains between groups fed the high and low fat diets.

Cruse et al. (1978) suggested that dietary cholesterol may be cocarcinogenic. Rats given DMH and fed a diet of liquid Vivonex (an amino acid hydrolysate) with added cholesterol had shorter lifespans, decreased time to tumor appearance, and more colonic tumors per rat than did the animals fed Vivonex alone. Because these dietary regimens are so different from those consumed by humans, the applicability of these findings to human health is not clear.

Broitman et al. (1977) studied effects of serum cholesterol levels on DMH-induced tumorigenesis in the bowel. Sprague-Dawley rats were fed isocaloric cholesterol-containing diets supplemented with either 20% coconut oil to promote hypercholesterolemia and vascular lipidosis or 20% safflower oil to maintain lower serum cholesterol levels and, presumably, to shunt cholesterol through the gut. Rats fed the 20% polyunsaturated fat diet experienced less vascular lipidosis but developed more bowel tumors than did rats fed the saturated fat diet. It could not be ascertained from these studies whether the enhanced bowel tumorigenesis was due to the polyunsaturated fat per se or whether the effects were related to its hypocholesterolemic action. Reddy and Watanabe (1979) observed that the intrarectal administration of cholesterol, cholesterol-5,6-epoxide, or cholestane-3,5,6-triol did not exert or lead to any tumor-promoting activity in rats given MNNG to induce bowel tumors.

The number of DMH-induced intestinal tumors was greater in rats fed diets marginally deficient in the lipotropes choline and methionine than in rats fed high fat diets with adequate amounts of lipotropes (Rogers and Newberne, 1973).

To date, an active carcinogen derived from bile acids has not been isolated from human or animal feces. The proposed mechanisms for the action of bile acids on bowel tumorigenesis are discussed earlier in this chapter.

SUMMARY

Epidemiological Evidence

Fats. There is some epidemiological evidence for an association between dietary fat and cancer at a number of sites, but most of the evidence pertains to three sites: the breast, the prostate, and the large bowel. In various populations, both the high incidence of and mortality from breast cancer have been shown to correlate strongly with higher per capita fat intake; the few case-control studies conducted have also shown this association with dietary fat. Like breast cancer, increased risk of large bowel cancer has been associated with higher fat intake in both correlation and case-control studies. The data on prostate cancer are more limited, but they too suggest that an increased risk is related to high levels of dietary fat. In general, it is not possible to identify specific components of fat as being clearly responsible for the observed effects, although total fat and saturated fat have been associated most frequently.

The epidemiological data are not entirely consistent. For example, the magnitude of the association of fat with breast cancer appears greater in the correlation data than in the case-control data. This may reflect the fact that recent dietary intake was assessed in the case-control studies, whereas dietary patterns much earlier in life may have had a greater influence on breast cancer risk. Furthermore, some studies of large bowel cancer did not show an association with dietary fat, possibly because they either focused on relatively homogeneous populations or were not specifically designed to test the hypothesis that fat intake is associated with cancer. Indeed, the studies designed specifically to test this hypothesis tended to show the most striking direct correlations, especially when the possible confounding effects of dietary fiber were taken into consideration.

Cholesterol. The relationship between dietary cholesterol and cancer in humans is not yet clear. Many studies of serum cholesterol levels and cancer mortality have indicated that there is an inverse association with colon cancer in males, but the evidence is inconsistent and is not sufficient to establish a causal relationship. Furthermore, other explanations for the observations are possible. For example, low serum levels could be the result rather than the cause of the cancer.

Relationship of Fecal Steroid Excretion to Bowel Carcinogenesis

In most reports on the association of dietary fat and bowel carcinogenesis, it is generally assumed that dietary fat acts as a promoter. To date, this effect has been examined in only one report, which suggested that high lipid diets may promote bowel tumorigenesis. High fat diets increased tumor yields more effectively than low fat diets when fed after the administration of a bowel carcinogen but not before. It is not clear if the effects observed were related to consumption of lipids or calories.

Increasing the quantity of dietary fat fed to rats increases the total quantity of bile acids and neutral sterols excreted in the feces. There is no evidence that bile acids or neutral sterols per se can be converted in vivo to carcinogens or cocarcinogens by the fecal flora under any dietary conditions.

Regardless of the carcinogen used to initiate bowel tumors, exposures of the colonic lumen to a direct flow of bile, resin-bound salts, or direct intrarectal instillation of bile salts have been consistently associated with a higher number of tumors than in control animals.

Colonic tissue damage may result from exposure to the abnormally high quantities and/or concentrations of bile salts used in these studies. Thus, it is not possible to determine whether the enhancing effect of bile salts on colon tumorigenesis is promotion or the result of nonspecific tissue injury.

Although most of the data suggest that dietary fat has promoting activity, there is little or no knowledge concerning the specific mechanisms involved in tumor promotion. Furthermore, there is not enough evidence to warrant the complete exclusion of an effect on initiation.

Experimental Evidence

Mammary Tumors. In studies of breast cancer, the influence of lipid nutriture on tumorigenesis follows a consistent pattern, regardless of whether the tumors are chemically induced, occur spontaneously, or result from tumor cell implantation.

Increasing the level of dietary fat from 5% to 20% increases the yield and/or incidence of chemically induced breast tumors, depending on the carcinogen used. Breast tumorigenesis is enhanced when high fat diets are fed after, but not before, tumor initiation. This is consistent with the concept that dietary fat exerts a promoting effect on tumorigenesis rather than an effect at the initiation stage. At low doses of the carcinogen, high fat diets decrease the latent period and increase tumor incidence. At high doses of carcinogen, high fat diets increase the incidence and numbers of tumors, but have no effect on latency.

In a few studies using isocaloric diets, various levels of dietary fat have been administered. It is possible that enhanced tumorigenesis, associated with increasing levels of dietary fat, may be related to a nonspecific increase in caloric intake. Mammary tumorigenesis is enhanced by obesity and is inhibited by restriction of total food intake.

Diets containing 20% polyunsaturated fat enhance tumorigenesis more effectively than saturated fat, provided that it serves as an adequate source of essential fatty acids. Supplementation of a high saturated fat diet with 3% polyunsaturated fat provides the same tumor-enhancing effects as a 20% polyunsaturated fat diet. Thus, the possible promoting effects of high-lipid diets on breast carcinogenesis depend upon the total quantity of fat in the diet (with the maximum effect achieved at 20%) and sufficient polyunsaturated fat to serve as an adequate source of essential fatty acids. Lipid requirements for enhanced growth of transplantable breast adenocarcinomas are essentially the same as those described above. Limited data on normal and neoplastic rat mammary epithelial cells in cell culture also indicate that essential fatty acids are required for maximal cell growth.

Hepatic and Pancreatic Cancer. Increasing dietary lipids increases the incidence of carcinogen-induced hepatomas. Differing effects of the quality and quantity of dietary fat depend upon the stage of hepatoma development at the time of exposure. Hepatic tumorigenesis, unlike breast carcinogenesis, is enhanced by lipotrope deficiency. Limited data indicate that the tumor yield of hepatomas and pancreatic neoplasms is increased more effectively by polyunsaturated fat than by saturated fat.

Intestinal Cancer. Increasing the quantity of dietary fat (generally from 5% to 20%) increases the incidence and yield of bowel tumors induced by a variety of carcinogens, including DMH, AOM, MAM acetate, DMAB, MNNG, and NMU. Data on the association of dietary lipids and tumorigenesis are more consistent for the large bowel than for the small intestine. Studies comparing the effects of high and low dietary fat on tumorigenesis in the bowel rarely used isocaloric diets or pair-feeding studies. Consequently, it is equally possible that the tumor-enhancing effect of high fat diets at this site may be related to increased consumption of calories. At dietary fat levels of 5%, polyunsaturated fat appears to have a greater tumor-enhancing effect than does the equivalent level of saturated fat. At 20% dietary fat levels, there is no clear difference between the effects of polyunsaturated fat and saturated fat on bowel tumorigenesis.

General Summation of Experimental Evidence. In summary, numerous experiments on animals have shown that dietary lipid influences tumorigenesis in the breast and the colon. Its effects on the liver and the pancreas have been studied in a few experiments. An increase in total dietary fat from 5% to 20% of the weight of the diet (i.e., approximately 10% to 40% of total calories) is associated with a higher tumor incidence in each of these tissues; conversely, animals consuming low fat diets have a lower tumor incidence. When total fat intake is low, polyun-unsaturated fats appear to be more effective than saturated fat in enhancing tumorigenesis; however, the effect of polyunsaturated fats becomes less prominent as total dietary fat is increased to 20% of the diet. Dietary fat appears to affect tumor promotion rather than tumor initiation, although an effect on initiation cannot be excluded. The specific mechanism involved in tumor promotion is not known, although some evidence suggests that colon cancer is associated with enhanced secretion of certain bile steroids and bile acids.

Experimental data on cholesterol and cancer risk are too limited to permit any inferences to be drawn.

CONCLUSIONS[1]

The committee concluded that of all the dietary components it studied, the combined epidemiological and experimental evidence is most

---

[1]The Committee on Diet, Nutrition, and Cancer judged the evidence associating high fat intake with increased cancer risk to be sufficient to recommend that consumption of fat be reduced (see Chapter 1). Two years ago, the Food and Nutrition Board stated in its report Toward Healthful Diets (National Academy of Sciences, 1980) that "there is no basis for making recommendations to modify the proportions of these macronutrients [e.g., fat] in the American diet at this time."

suggestive for a causal relationship between fat intake and the occurrence of cancer. Both epidemiological studies and experiments in animals provide convincing evidence that increasing the intake of total fat increases the incidence of cancer at certain sites, particularly the breast and colon, and, conversely, that the risk is lower with lower intakes of fat. Data from studies in animals suggest that when total fat intake is low, polyunsaturated fats are more effective than saturated fats in enhancing tumorigenesis, whereas the data on humans do not permit a clear distinction to be made between the effects of different components of fat. In general, however, the evidence from epidemiological and laboratory studies is consistent.

REFERENCES

Abraham, S., and G. A. Rao. 1976. Lipids and lipogenesis in a murine mammary neoplastic system. Pp. 363-378 in W. E. Criss, T. Ono, and J. R. Sabine, eds. Progress in Cancer Research and Therapy. Volume 1, Control Mechanisms in Cancer. Raven Press, New York.

Armstrong, B., and R. Doll. 1975. Environmental factors and cancer incidence and mortality in different countries, with special reference to dietary practices. Int. J. Cancer 15:617-631.

Bagheri, S. A., M. G. Bolt, J. L. Boyer, and R. H. Palmer. 1978. Stimulation of thymidine incorporation in mouse liver and biliary tract epithelium by lithocholate and deoxycholate. Gastroenterology 74:188-192.

Bansal, B. R., J. E. Rhoads, Jr., and S. C. Bansal. 1978. Effects of diet on colon carcinogenesis and the immune system in rats treated with 1,2-dimethylhydrazine. Cancer Res. 38:3293-3303.

Beaglehole, R., M. A. Foulkes, I. A. M. Prior, and E. F. Eyles. 1980. Cholesterol and mortality in New Zealand Maoris. Br. Med. J. 280:285-287.

Berg, J. W., and M. A. Howell. 1974. The geographic pathology of bowel cancer. Cancer 34:807-814.

Bingham, S., D. R. R. Williams, T. J. Cole, and W. P. T. James. 1979. Dietary fibre and regional large-bowel cancer mortality in Britain. Br. J. Cancer 40:456-463.

Bjelke, E. 1974. Letter to the Editor: Colon cancer and blood-cholesterol. Lancet 1:1116-1117.

Bjelke, E. 1978. Dietary factors and the epidemiology of cancer of the stomach and large bowel. Aktuel. Ernaehrungsmed. Klin. Prax. (Suppl. 2):10-17.

Blair, A., and J. F. Fraumeni, Jr. 1978. Geographic patterns of prostate cancer in the United States. J. Natl. Cancer Inst. 61:1379-1384.

Broitman, S. A. 1981. Cholesterol excretion and colon cancer. Cancer Res. 41:3738-3740.

Broitman, S. A., J. J. Vitale, E. Vavrousek-Jakuba, and L. S. Gottlieb. 1977. Polyunsaturated fat, cholesterol and large bowel tumorigenesis. Cancer 40:2455-2463.

Bull, A. W., B. K. Soullier, P. S. Wilson, M. T. Hayden, and N. D. Nigro. 1979. Promotion of azoxymethane-induced intestinal cancer by high-fat diet in rats. Cancer Res. 39:4956-4959.

Carroll, K. K. 1975. Experimental evidence of dietary factors and hormone-dependent cancers. Cancer Res. 35:3374-3383.

Carroll, K. K. 1980. Lipids and carcinogenesis. J. Environ. Pathol. Toxicol. 3(4):253-271.

Carroll, K. K., and G. J. Hopkins. 1979. Dietary polyunsaturated fat versus saturated fat in relation to mammary carcinogenesis. Lipids 14:155-158.

Carroll, K. K., and H. T. Khor. 1970. Effects of dietary fat and dose level of 7,12-dimethylbenz(α)anthracene on mammary tumor incidence in rats. Cancer Res. 30:2260-2264.

Carroll, K. K., and H. T. Khor. 1971. Effects of level and type of dietary fat on incidence of mammary tumors induced in female Sprague-Dawley rats by 7,12-dimethylbenz(α)anthracene. Lipids 6:415-420.

Carroll, K. K., and H. T. Khor. 1975. Dietary fat in relation to tumorigenesis. Prog. Biochem. Pharmacol. 10:308-353.

Chan, P.-C., J. F. Head, L. A. Cohen, and E. L. Wynder. 1977. Influence of dietary fat on the induction of mammary tumors by N-nitrosomethylurea: Associated hormone changes and differences between Sprague-Dawley and F344 rats. J. Natl. Cancer Inst. 59:1279-1283.

Chomchai, C., N. Bhadrachari, and N. D. Nigro. 1974. The effect of bile on the induction of experimental intestinal tumors in rats. Dis. Colon Rectum 17:310-312.

Cohen, B. I., R. F. Raicht, E. E. Deschner, E. Fazzini, M. Takahashi, and A. Sarwal. 1978. Effects of bile acids on induced colon cancer in rats. Proc. Am. Assoc. Cancer Res. Am. Soc. Clin. Oncol. 19:48. Abstract 190.

Committee on Principle Investigators. 1978. A co-operative trial in the primary prevention of ischaemic heart disease using clofibrate. Br. Heart J. 1069-1118.

Cook, J. W., and G. A. D. Haslewood. 1933. The conversion of a bile acid into a hydrocarbon derived from 1:2-benzanthracene. J. Soc. Chem. Ind. London Rev. Sect. 52:758-759.

Corwin, L. M., F. Varshavsky-Rose, and S. A. Broitman. 1979. Effect of dietary fats on tumorigenicity of two sarcoma cell lines. Cancer Res. 39:4350-4355.

Cruse, J. P., M. R. Lewin, G. P. Ferulano, and C. G. Clark. 1978. Cocarcinogenic effects of dietary cholesterol in experimental colon cancer. Nature 276:822-825.

Dales, L. G., G. D. Friedman, H. K. Ury, S. Grossman, and S. R. Williams. 1978. A case-control study of relationships of diet and other traits to colorectal cancer in American blacks. Am. J. Epidemiol. 109:132-144.

Dawson, A. M., and K. J. Isselbacher. 1960. Studies on lipid metabolism in the small intestine with observations on the role of bile salts. J. Clin. Invest. 39:730-740.

Deschner, E. E., and R. F. Raicht. 1979. The influence of bile on the kinetic behavior of colonic epithelial cells of the rat. Gastroenterology 76:1120. Abstract.

Dietschy, J. M. 1967. Effects of bile salts on intermediate metabolism of the intestinal mucosa. Fed. Proc. Fed. Am. Soc. Exp. Biol. 26:1589-1598.

Drasar, B. S., and D. Irving. 1973. Environmental factors and cancer of the colon and breast. Br. J. Cancer 27:167-172.

Dyer, A. R., J. Stamler, O. Paul, R. B. Shekelle, J. A. Schoenberger, D. M. Berkson, M. Lepper, P. Collette, S. Shekelle, and H. A. Lindberg. 1981. Serum cholesterol and risk of death from cancer and other causes in three Chicago epidemiological studies. J. Chronic Dis. 34:249-260.

Ederer, F., P. Leren, O. Turpeinen, and I. D. Frantz, Jr. 1971. Cancer among men on cholesterol-lowering diets: Experience from five clinical trials. Lancet 2:203-206.

Enig, M. G., R. J. Munn, and M. Keeney. 1979. Response to letters. Fed. Proc. Fed. Am. Soc. Exp. Biol. 38:2437-2439.

Enstrom, J. E. 1975. Colorectal cancer and consumption of beef and fat. Br. J. Cancer 32:432-439.

Farber, E. 1973. Carcinogenesis--cellular evolution as a unifying thread: Presidential address. Cancer Res. 33:2537-2550.

Fieser, L. F., and M. S. Newman. 1935. Methylcholanthrene from cholic acid. J. Am. Chem. Soc. 57:961.

Fry, R. J. M., and E. Staffeldt. 1964. Effect of a diet containing sodium deoxycholate on the intestinal mucosa of the mouse. Nature 203:1396-1398.

Garcia-Palmieri, M. R., P. D. Sorlie, R. Costas, Jr., and R. J. Havlik. 1981. An apparent inverse relationship between serum cholesterol and cancer mortality in Puerto Rico. Am. J. Epidemiol. 114:29-40.

Gaskill, S. P., W. L. McGuire, C. K. Osborne, and M. P. Stern. 1979. Breast cancer mortality and diet in the United States. Cancer Res. 39:3628-3637.

Graham, S., W. Schotz, and P. Martino. 1972. Alimentary factors in the epidemiology of gastric cancer. Cancer 30:927-938.

Graham, S., H. Dayal, M. Swanson, A. Mittleman, and G. Wilkinson. 1978. Diet in the epidemiology of cancer of the colon and rectum. J. Natl. Cancer Inst. 61:709-714.

Gray, G. E., M. C. Pike, and B. E. Henderson. 1979. Breast-cancer incidence and mortality rates in different countries in relation to known risk factors and dietary practices. Br. J. Cancer 39:1-7.

Haenszel, W., J. W. Berg, M. Segi, M. Kurihara, and F. B. Locke. 1973. Large-bowel cancer in Hawaiian Japanese. J. Natl. Cancer Inst. 51:1765-1779.

Haenszel, W., F. B. Locke, and M. Segi. 1980. A case-control study of large bowel cancer in Japan. J. Natl. Cancer Inst. 64:17-22.

Hems, G. 1978. The contributions of diet and childbearing to breast-cancer rates. Br. J. Cancer 37:974-982.

Hems, G. 1980. Associations between breast-cancer mortality rates, child-bearing and diet in the United Kingdom. Br. J. Cancer 41:429-437.

Higginson, J. 1966. Etiological factors in gastrointestinal cancer in man. J. Natl. Cancer Inst. 37:527-545.

Hill, M. J., B. S. Drasar, V. Aries, J. S. Crowther, G. Hawksworth, and R. E. O. Williams. 1971. Bacteria and aetiology of cancer of large bowel. Lancet 1:95-100.

Hill, M., R. MacLennan, and K. Newcombe. 1979. Letter to the Editor: Diet and large bowel cancer in three socioeconomic groups in Hong Kong. Lancet 1:436.

Hillyard, L. A., and S. Abraham. 1979. Effect of dietary polyunsaturated fatty acids on growth of mammary adenocarcinomas in mice and rats. Cancer Res. 39:4430-4437.

Hirayama, T. 1977. Changing patterns of cancer in Japan with special reference to the decrease in stomach cancer mortality. Pp. 55-75 in H. H. Hiatt, J. D. Watson, and J. A. Winsten, eds. Origins of Human Cancer, Book A: Incidence of Cancer in Humans. Cold Spring Harbor Laboratory, Cold Spring Harbor, N.Y.

Hoffman, A. F. 1967. The syndrome of ileal disease and the broken enterohepatic circulation: Cholerheic enteropathy. Gastroenterology 52:752-757.

Hopkins, G. J., and K. K. Carroll. 1979. Relationship between amount and type of dietary fat in promotion of mammary carcinogenesis induced by 7,12-dimethylbenz(a)anthracene. J. Natl. Cancer Inst. 62:1009-1012.

Hopkins, G. J., and C. E. West. 1976. Possible roles of dietary fats in carcinogenesis. Life Sci. 19:1103-1116.

Hopkins, G. J., and C. E. West. 1977. Effect of dietary polyunsaturated fat on the growth of a transplantable adenocarcinoma in C3HA^{vy}fB mice. J. Natl. Cancer Inst. 58:753-756.

Howell, M. A. 1974. Factor analysis of international cancer mortality data and per capita food consumption. Br. J. Cancer 29:328-336.

Howell, M. A. 1975. Diet as an etiological factor in the development of cancers of the colon and rectum. J. Chronic Dis. 28:67-80.

Ip, C. 1980. Ability of dietary fat to overcome the resistance of mature female rats to 7,12-dimethylbenz(a)anthracene-induced mammary tumorigenesis. Cancer Res. 40:2785-2789.

Ishii, K., K. Nakamura, H. Ozaki, N. Yamada, and T. Takeuchi. 1968. [In Japanese.] [Epidemiological problems of pancreas cancer.] Jpn. J. Clin. Med. 26:1839-1842.

Jain, M., G. M. Cook, F. G. Davis, M. G. Grace, G. R. Howe, and A. B. Miller. 1980. A case-control study of diet and colo-rectal cancer. Int. J. Cancer 26:757-768.

Kagan, A., D. L. McGee, K. Yano, G. G. Rhoads, and A. Nomura. 1981. Serum cholesterol and mortality in a Japanese-American population. Am. J. Epidemiol. 114:11-20.

Kark, J. D., A. H. Smith, and C. G. Hames. 1980. The relationship of serum cholesterol to the incidence of cancer in Evans County, Georgia. J. Chronic Dis. 33:311-322.

Kidwell, W. R., M. E. Monaco, M. S. Wicha, and G. S. Smith. 1978. Unsaturated fatty acid requirements for growth and survival of a rat mammary tumor cell line. Cancer Res. 38:4091-4100.

King, J. T., C. B. Casas, and M. B. Visscher. 1949. The influence of estrogen on cancer incidence and adrenal changes in ovariectomized mice on calorie restriction. Cancer Res. 9:436-437.

King, M. M., D. M. Bailey, D. D. Gibson, J. V. Pitha, and P. B. McCay. 1979. Incidence and growth of mammary tumors induced by 7,12-dimethylbenz[a]anthracene as related to the dietary content of fat and antioxidant. J. Natl. Cancer Inst. 63:657-663.

Knox, E. G. 1977. Foods and diseases. Br. J. Prev. Soc. Med. 31:71-80.

Kolonel, L. N., J. H. Hankin, J. Lee, S. Y. Chu, A. M. Y. Nomura, and M. W. Hinds. 1981. Nutrient intakes in relation to cancer incidence in Hawaii. Br. J. Cancer. 44:332-339.

Kozarevic, D., D. McGee, N. Vojvodic, T. Gordon, Z. Racic, W. Zukel, and T. Dawber. 1981. Serum cholesterol and mortality. The Yugoslavia cardiovascular disease study. Am. J. Epidemiol. 114:21-28.

Lavik, P. S., and C. A. Baumann. 1941. Dietary fat and tumor formation. Cancer Res. 1:181-187.

Lavik, P. S., and C. A. Baumann. 1943. Further studies on tumor-promoting action of fat. Cancer Res. 3:749-756.

Lea, A. J. 1967. Neoplasms and environmental factors. Ann. R. Coll. Surg. Engl. 41:432-438.

Lilienfeld, A. M. 1981. The Humean fog: Cancer and cholesterol. Am. J. Epidemiol. 114:1-4.

Lin, D. S., and W. E. Connor. 1980. The long term effects of dietary cholesterol upon the plasma lipids, lipoproteins, cholesterol absorption, and the sterol balance in man: The demonstration of feedback inhibition of cholesterol biosynthesis and increased bile acid excretion. J. Lipid Res. 21:1042-1052.

Lingeman, C. H. 1974. Etiology of cancer of the human ovary: A review. J. Natl. Cancer Inst. 53:1603-1618.

Liu, K., J. Stamler, D. Moss, D. Garside, V. Persky, and I. Soltero. 1979. Dietary cholesterol, fat, and fibre, and colon-cancer mortality. Lancet 2:782-785.

Longnecker, D. S., D. B. Roebuck, J. D. Yager, Jr., H. S. Lilja, and B. Siegmund. 1981. Pancreatic carcinoma in azaserine-treated rats: Induction, classification and dietary modulation of incidence. Cancer 47:1562-1572.

Low-Beer, T. S., R. E. Schneider, and W. O. Dobbins. 1970. Morpho-logical changes of the small-intestinal mucosa of guinea pig and hamster following incubation in vitro and perfusion in vivo with unconjugated bile salts. Gut 11:486-492.

Lubin, J. H., P. E. Burns, W. J. Blot, R. G. Ziegler, A. W. Lees, and J. F. Fraumeni, Jr. 1981. Dietary factors and breast cancer risk. Int. J. Cancer 28:685-689.

Lyon, J. L., and A. W. Sorenson. 1978. Colon cancer in a low-risk population. Am. J. Clin. Nutr. 31:5227-5230.

MacLennan, R., O. M. Jensen, J. Mosbech, and H. Vuori. 1978. Diet, transit time, stool weight, and colon cancer in two Scandinavian populations. Am. J. Clin. Nutr. 31:S239-S242.

Martínez, I., R. Torres, Z. Frías, J. R. Colón, and N. Fernández. 1979. Factors associated with adenocarcinomas of the large bowel in Puerto Rico. Pp. 45-52 in J. M. Birch, ed. Advances in Medical Oncology, Research and Education. Volume 3, Epidemiology. Pergamon Press, Oxford, New York, Toronto, Sydney, Paris, and Frankfurt.

Mastromarino, A., B. S. Reddy, and E. L. Wynder. 1976. Metabolic epidemiology of colon cancer: Enzymic activity of fecal flora. Am. J. Clin. Nutr. 29:1455-1460.

McCay, P. B., M. King, L. E. Rikans, and J. V. Pitha. 1980. Inter-actions between dietary fats and antioxidants on DMBA-induced mammary carcinomas and on AAF-induced hyperplastic nodules and hepatomas. J. Environ. Pathol. Toxicol. 3(4):451-465.

Miettinen, M., O. Turpeinen, M. J. Karvonen, R. Elosuo, and
    E. Paavilainen. 1972. Effect of cholesterol-lowering diet on
    mortality from coronary heart-causes and other causes: A
    twelve-year clinical trial in men and women. Lancet 2:835-838.

Miller, A. B., A. Kelly, N. W. Choi, V. Matthews, R. W. Morgan,
    L. Munan, J. D. Burch, J. Feather, G. R. Howe, and M. Jain. 1978.
    A study of diet and breast cancer. Am. J. Epidemiol. 107:499-509.

Miller, S. R., P. I. Tartter, A. E. Papatestas, G. Slater, and A. H.
    Aufses, Jr. 1981. Serum cholesterol and human colon cancer. J.
    Natl. Cancer Inst. 67:297-300.

Mohrhauer, H., and R. T. Holman. 1967. Metabolism of linoleic acid
    in relation to dietary saturated fatty acids in the rat. J. Nutr.
    91:528-534.

Moskovitz, M., C. White, R. N. Barnett, S. Stevens, E. Russell,
    D. Vargo, and M. H. Floch. 1979. Diet, fecal bile acids, and
    neutral sterols in carcinoma of the colon. Dig. Dis. Sci.
    24:746-751.

Mower, H. F., R. M. Ray, R. Shoff, G. N. Stemmermann, A. Nomura,
    G. A. Glober, S. Kamiyama, A. Shimada, and H. Yamakawa. 1979.
    Fecal bile acids in two Japanese populations with different colon
    cancer risks. Cancer Res. 39:328-331.

Narisawa, T., N. E. Magadia, J. H. Weisburger, and E. L. Wynder.
    1974. Promoting effect of bile acids on colon carcinogenesis after
    intrarectal instillation of N-methyl-N'-nitro-N-nitrosoguanidine in
    rats. J. Natl. Cancer Inst. 53:1093-1097.

National Academy of Sciences. 1980. Pp. 13-15 in Toward Healthful
    Diets. Report prepared by the Food and Nutrition Board, National
    Academy of Sciences, Washington, D.C.

Newberne, P. M., and E. Zeiger. 1978. Nutrition, carcinogenesis, and
    mutagenesis. Pp. 53-84 in W. G. Flamm and M. A. Mehlman, eds.
    Advances in Modern Toxicology. Volume 5, Mutagenesis. John Wiley
    and Sons, New York, London, Sydney, and Toronto.

Newberne, P. M., J. Weigert, and N. Kula. 1979. Effects of dietary fat
    on hepatic mixed-function oxidases and hepatocellular carcinoma
    induced by aflatoxin B_1 in rats. Cancer Res. 39:3986-3991.

Nigro, N. D., N. Bhadrachari, and C. Chomchai. 1973. A rat model for
    studying colonic cancer: Effect of cholestyramine on induced
    tumors. Dis. Colon Rectum 16:438-443.

Nigro, N. D., D. V. Singh, R. L. Campbell, and M. S. Pak. 1975. Effect of dietary beef fat on intestinal tumor formation by azoxymethane in rats. J. Natl. Cancer Inst. 54:439-442.

Nigro, N. D., R. L. Campbell, J. S. Gantt, Y. N. Lin, and D. V. Singh. 1977. A comparison of the effects of the hypocholesteremic agents, cholestyramine and candicidin, on the induction of intestinal tumors in rats by azoxymethane. Cancer Res. 37:3198-3203.

Nomura, A., B. E. Henderson, and J. Lee. 1978. Breast cancer and diet among the Japanese in Hawaii. Am. J. Clin. Nutr. 31:2020-2025.

Nydegger, U. E., and R. E. Butler. 1972. Serum lipoprotein levels in patients with cancer. Cancer Res. 32:1756-1760.

Palmer, R. H. 1979. Editorial: Bile acid heterogeneity and the gastrointestinal epithelium: From diarrhea to colon cancer. J. Lab. Clin. Med. 94:655-660.

Pearce, M. L., and S. Dayton. 1971. Incidence of cancer in men on a diet high in polyunsaturated fat. Lancet 1:464-467.

Peifer, J. J., and R. T. Holman. 1959. Effect of saturated fat upon essential fatty acid metabolism of the rat. J. Nutr. 68:155-168.

Peterson, B., E. Trell, and N. H. Sternby. 1981. Low cholesterol level as risk factor for noncoronary death in middle-aged men. J. Am. Med. Assoc. 245:2056-2057.

Phillips, R. L. 1975. Role of life-style and dietary habits in risk of cancer among Seventh-Day Adventists. Cancer Res. 35:3513-3522.

Raicht, R. F., E. Deschner, and G. Salen. 1975. Bile acids regulate intestinal cell turnover. Gastroenterology 68:979. Abstract.

Ranken, R., R. Wilson, and P. M. Bealmear. 1971. Increased turnover of intestinal mucosal cells of germfree mice induced by cholic acid. Proc. Soc. Exp. Biol. Med. 138:270-272.

Reddy, B. S. 1979. Nutrition and colon cancer. Adv. Nutr. Res. 2:199-218.

Reddy, B. S., and K. Watanabe. 1979. Effect of cholesterol metabolites and promoting effect of lithocholic acid in colon carcinogenesis in germ-free and conventional F344 rats. Cancer Res. 39:1521-1524.

Reddy, B. S., and E. L. Wynder. 1973. Large bowel carcinogenesis: Fecal constituents of populations with diverse incidence rates of colon cancer. J. Natl. Cancer Inst. 50:1437-1442.

Reddy, B. S., J. H. Weisburger, and E. L. Wynder. 1974. Effects of dietary fat level and dimethylhydrazine on fecal acid and neutral sterol excretion and colon carcinogenesis in rats. J. Natl. Cancer Inst. 52:507-511.

Reddy, B. S., S. Mangat, A. Sheinfil, J. H. Weisburger, and E. L. Wynder. 1977a. Effect of type and amount of dietary fat and 1,2-dimethylhydrazine on biliary bile acids, fecal bile acids, and neutral sterols in rats. Cancer Res. 37:2132-2137.

Reddy, B. S., K. Watanabe, and J. H. Weisburger. 1977b. Effect of high-fat diet on colon carcinogenesis in F344 rats treated with 1,2-dimethylhydrazine, methylazoxymethanol acetate, or methylnitrosourea. Cancer Res. 37:4156-4159.

Reddy, B. S., A. R. Hedges, K. Laakso, and E. L. Wynder. 1978. Metabolic epidemiology of large bowel cancer: Fecal bulk and constituents of high-risk North American and low-risk Finnish population. Cancer 42:2832-2838.

Reddy, B. S., L. A. Cohen, G. D. McCoy, P. Hill, J. H. Weisburger, and E. L. Wynder. 1980. Nutrition and its relationship to cancer. Adv. Cancer Res. 32:237-345.

Roebuck, B. D., J. D. Yager, Jr., and D. S. Longnecker. 1981. Dietary modulation of azaserine-induced pancreatic carcinogenesis in the rat. Cancer Res. 41:888-893.

Rogers, A. E. 1975. Variable effects of a lipotrope-deficient, high-fat diet on chemical carcinogenesis in rats. Cancer Res. 35:2469-2474.

Rogers, A. E., and P. M. Newberne. 1973. Dietary enhancement of intestinal carcinogenesis by dimethylhydrazine in rats. Nature 246:491-492.

Rose, G., and M. J. Shipley. 1980. Plasma lipids and mortality: A source of error. Lancet 1:523-526.

Rose, G., H. Blackburn, A. Keys, H. L. Taylor, W. B. Kannel, O. Paul, D. D. Reid, and J. Stamler. 1974. Colon cancer and blood-cholesterol. Lancet 1:181-183.

Rotkin, I. D. 1977. Studies in the epidemiology of prostatic cancer: Expanded sampling. Cancer Treat. Rep. 61:173-180.

Roy, C. C., G. Laurendeau, G. Doyon, L. Chartrand, and M. R. Rivest. 1975. The effect of bile and of sodium taurocholate on the epithelial cell dynamics of the rat small intestine. Proc. Soc. Exp. Biol. Med. 149:1000-1004.

Ryser, H. J.-P. 1971. Chemical carcinogenesis. N. Engl. J. Med.
285:721-734.

Schuman, L. M., J. S. Mandell, A. Radke, U. Seal, and F. Halberg. 1982.
Some selected features of the epidemiology of prostatic cancer:
Minneapolis-St. Paul, Minnesota case-control study, 1976-1979.
Pp. 345-354 in K. Magnus, ed. Trends in Cancer Incidence: Causes
and Practical Implications. Hemisphere Publishing Corp., Washington,
New York, and London.

Silverman, J., C. J. Shellabarger, S. Holtzman, J. P. Stone, and
J. H. Weisburger. 1980. Effect of dietary fat on X-ray-induced
mammary cancer in Sprague-Dawley rats. J. Natl. Cancer Inst.
64:631-634.

Stamler, J., D. M. Berkson, H. A. Linber, W. A. Miller, C. R. Soyugene,
T. Tokish, and T. Whipple. 1968. Does hypercholesterolemia
increase risk of lung cancer in cigarette smokers? Circulation
Suppl. 6:188. Abstract.

Sugai, M., L. A. Witting, H. Tsuchiyama, and F. A. Kummerow. 1962.
The effect of heated fat on the carcinogenic activity of
2-acetylaminofluorene. Cancer Res. 22:510-519.

Tannenbaum, A. 1942. The genesis and growth of tumors. III. Effects
of a high-fat diet. Cancer Res. 2:468-475.

Tannenbaum, A. 1959. Nutrition and cancer. Pp. 517-562 in F. F.
Homburger, ed. The Physiopathology of Cancer, Second edition.
Paul B. Hoeber, Inc., New York.

Tannenbaum, A., and H. Silverstone. 1957. Nutrition and the genesis
of tumours. Pp. 306-334 in R. W. Raven, ed. Cancer, Volume 1.
Butterworth and Co., Ltd., London.

Vahouny, G. V., M. M. Cassidy, F. Lightfoot, L. Grau, and D.
Kritchevsky. 1981. Ultrastructural modifications of intestinal
and colonic mucosa induced by free or bound bile acids. Cancer Res.
41:3764-3765.

Watson, A. F., and E. Mellanby. 1930. Tar cancer in mice; Condition of
skin when modified by external treatment or diet, as factors in
influencing cancerous reaction. Br. J. Exp. Pathol. 11:311-322.

Waxler, S. H. 1954. The effect of weight reduction on the occurrence
of spontaneous mammary tumors in mice. J. Natl. Cancer Inst.
14:1253-1256.

Waxler, S. H., P. Tabar, and L. R. Melcher. 1953. Obesity and the time of appearance of spontaneous mammary carcinoma in C3H mice. Cancer Res. 13:276-278.

Westlund, K., and R. Nicolaysen. 1972. Ten-year mortality and morbidity related to serum cholesterol. Scand. J. Clin. Lab. Invest. Suppl. 127:1-24.

White, F. R. 1961. The relationship between underfeeding and tumor formation, transplantation, and growth in rats and mice. Cancer Res. 21:281-290.

White, F. R., J. White, G. B. Mider, M. G. Kelly, W. E. Heston, and P. W. David. 1944. Effect of caloric restriction on mammary-tumor formation in strain C3H mice and on the response of strain dba to painting with methylcholanthrene. J. Natl. Cancer Inst. 5:43-48.

Wicha, M. S., L. A. Liotta, and W. R. Kidwell. 1979. Effects of free fatty acids on the growth of normal and neoplastic rat mammary epithelial cells. Cancer Res. 39:426-435.

Wieland, H., and E. Dane. 1933. [In German.] Untersuchungen über die Konstitution der Gallensäuren. LII. Mitteilung über die Haftstelle der Seitenkette. Hoppe Seylers Z. Physiol. Chem. 219:240-245.

Williams, R. R., P. D. Sorlie, M. Feinleib, P. M. McNamara, W. B. Kannel, and T. R. Dawber. 1981. Cancer incidence by levels of cholesterol. J. Am. Med. Assoc. 245:247-252.

Williamson, R. C. N., F. L. R. Bauer, J. S. Ross, J. B. Watkins, and R. A. Malt. 1979. Enhanced colonic carcinogenesis with azoxymethane in rats after pancreaticobiliary diversion at mid small bowel. Gastroenterology 76:1388-1392.

6 Protein

Dietary protein has often been associated with cancers of the breast, endometrium, prostate, colorectum, pancreas, and kidney. However, since the major dietary sources of protein (such as meat) contain a variety of other nutrients and nonnutritive components, the association of protein with cancer at these sites may not be direct but, rather, could reflect the action of another constituent concurrently present in protein-rich foods.

EPIDEMIOLOGICAL EVIDENCE

Armstrong and Doll (1975) examined incidence rates for 27 cancers in 23 countries and mortality rates for 14 cancers in 32 countries and correlated them with the per capita intake of a wide range of dietary constituents and other environmental factors. These investigators reported relationships between many of these variables. For example, the correlations of total protein and animal protein with total fat were 0.70 and 0.93, respectively, whereas correlations with the gross national product were 0.32 and 0.65. In a study that analyzed diet histories of more than 4,000 subjects, Kolonel et al. (1981) observed that the correlation between total protein and total fat consumption was 0.7.

Breast Cancer

In the study by Armstrong and Doll (1975) mentioned above, per capita intakes of total protein and animal protein were significantly correlated with the incidence of and mortality from breast cancer. In a similar study, Knox (1977) compared per capita intakes of individual foods and nutrients with the chief causes of mortality in 20 different countries: Canada, the United States, Japan, and 17 European countries. His results also indicated that there was a strong correlation between the per capita intake of animal protein and mortality from breast cancer. Armstrong and Doll (1975) found that there was a stronger association for animal protein than for total protein, and in both of these studies, the correlations of breast cancer with per capita total fat intake were generally as strong or stronger than those for animal protein.

Hems (1978) correlated 1970-1971 mortality rates for breast cancer in 41 countries with per capita food intake for 1964-1966. He found a direct correlation with intake of protein, total fat, and calories from animal products, independent of other components of the diet. However, time-trend data for breast cancer mortality and per capita food intake

in England and Wales supported the association with fat more strongly
than the association with protein (Hems, 1980). Gray et al. (1979)
analyzed international incidence and mortality rates for breast cancer
in relation to per capita intake of animal protein. They found a
direct correlation, even after controlling for height, weight, and age
at menarche.

Gaskill et al. (1979) examined age-adjusted breast cancer mortality
in relation to per capita intake for certain foods by state within the
United States. Although they found a direct correlation between breast
cancer mortality and per capita protein intake, this finding was not
statistically significant after controlling for age at first marriage
(as an indicator of age at first pregnancy). Kolonel et al. (1981)
found a direct correlation between consumption of animal protein and
the incidence of breast cancer in five different ethnic groups in
Hawaii based on diet histories obtained by interview.

Of three case-control studies of diet and breast cancer, significant direct associations with dietary fat only were found in two
(Miller et al., 1978; Phillips, 1975), whereas direct associations
with both animal fat and protein were found in the third (Lubin et
al., 1981).

Large Bowel Cancer

Gregor et al. (1969) reported a direct correlation between per
capita intake of animal protein and mortality from intestinal cancer
in 28 countries. Armstrong and Doll (1975) observed that per capita
intake of total protein, animal protein, and total fat were all strongly correlated with the incidence of and mortality from colon and rectal
cancer for both sexes. Their findings for cancer at these sites were
similar to those for breast cancer (i.e., there were stronger correlations for total fat and for animal protein than for total protein).
These authors also reported a strong association between the intake
of eggs and cancer of the colon and rectum. This association was
greater than that for total protein. In contrast to these direct
correlations, Bingham et al. (1979) found no significant association
for intakes of animal protein in a study correlating the average
intakes of foods, nutrients, and fiber in different regions of Great
Britian with the regional pattern of mortality from colon and rectal
cancers.

Jain et al. (1980) reported the only case-control study of large
bowel cancer in which protein was specifically examined. Although
these investigators found a direct association between consumption of
high levels of protein and risk of both colon and rectal cancer, they
found a stronger association for saturated fat.

The relationship of meat intake to risk of colorectal cancer has
been examined in a number of studies, but protein intake per se was not

estimated in most of them. However, because meat is a major source
of protein in the Western diet, findings in these studies may reflect
associations with protein. Berg and Howell (1974) and Howell (1975)
correlated international mortality rates for colon cancer with per
capita intake data and found the strongest correlations for meat,
especially beef. In a study by Armstrong and Doll (1975), the correlations were stronger for meat than for total protein and animal protein. In studies of the relationship between certain foods and cancer
of the large intestine, Knox (1977) reported the strongest correlations
for eggs, followed by beef, sugar, beer, and pork. In contrast, time-
trend data for per capita beef intake and colorectal cancer incidence
and mortality in the United States showed no clear association (Enstrom,
1975).

Haenszel et al. (1973) studied cases of large bowel cancer and
hospital controls among Japanese in Hawaii. They found an association between cancer at this site and consumption of legumes, starches,
and meats. The association was strongest for beef. A similar study
among Japanese in Japan (Haenszel et al., 1980) did not reproduce these
findings, nor did parallel case-control studies conducted in Norway and
Minnesota (Bjelke, 1978) and at the Roswell Park Memorial Institute
(Graham et al., 1978). All four of these case-control studies relied
solely on frequency of consumption data for their assessments of
dietary intake.

A somewhat contradictory observation was reported by Hirayama
(1981), whose large-scale cohort study in Japan indicated that there
was a decrease in overall risk for cancer, including intestinal cancer,
in association with daily intake of meat.

Pancreatic Cancer

Lea (1967) examined the relationship between per capita intake of
foods and nutrients and cancer mortality resulting from up to 22 different types of neoplasms in each of 33 countries. One of the findings
was a strong direct correlation between intake of animal protein and
pancreatic cancer. This result was reproduced by Armstrong and Doll
(1975). No case-control or cohort studies have confirmed this association specifically; however, a study of pancreatic cancer cases and
controls in Japan (Ishii et al., 1968), based on responses to a mailed
questionnaire completed mostly by relatives of deceased cases, showed
an association of the disease with consumption of high-meat diets
by men. Hirayama (1977) reported a relative risk of 2.5 for daily meat
intake and pancreatic cancer incidence in Japan in a cohort of 265,118
subjects followed prospectively. Since meat is a major source of
protein in the diet, these findings offer tentative support for the
results of correlation studies.

Other Cancers

Armstrong and Doll (1975) found a strong correlation (correlation coefficient = 0.8) between animal protein and the incidence of renal cancer. However, in a subsequent case-control study, Armstrong et al. (1976) found no clear association between renal cancer and consumption frequencies for several foods containing animal protein (e.g., meat, poultry, seafood, eggs, milk, and cheese).

The incidence of prostate cancer was significantly correlated with consumption of total and animal protein in the study by Kolonel et al. (1981), whereas mortality from, but not the incidence of, prostate cancer was similarly correlated in the study by Armstrong and Doll (1975). As noted in Chapter 5, Hirayama (1977) reported a sharp increase in the intake of animal protein in Japan since 1950. During this period, the incidence of prostate cancer in that country increased correspondingly. The intake of meat, especially beef, has also been correlated with mortality from prostate cancer (Armstrong and Doll, 1975; Howell, 1974).

The incidence of endometrial cancer has also been significantly correlated with the intake of total protein (Armstrong and Doll, 1975; Kolonel et al., 1981). This finding may simply reflect the high correlation between the occurrence of endometrial cancer and breast cancer, since the latter has also been associated with protein intake (see Chapter 16). No case-control studies have been conducted to examine this association.

EXPERIMENTAL EVIDENCE

There is much less literature on results of laboratory studies to determine the relationship between cancer and dietary protein than has been published for certain other nutrients (e.g., fat). However, an inhibitory effect of selected amino acid deficiencies on tumor responses in laboratory animals was claimed as early as 1936 (Voegtlin and Maver, 1936; Voegtlin and Thompson, 1936). During the subsequent 30 years, further studies concentrated primarily on the effect of protein intake on experimental animal models. From the end of that period to the present, attention became increasingly focused on epidemiological studies.

In general, animals fed minimum amounts of protein required for optimum growth have developed fewer tumors than comparable groups fed 2 to 3 times the minimum requirements. Unfortunately, a number of these earlier studies in animals are difficult to interpret for several reasons: several factors were being varied at the same time (Engel and Copeland, 1952a; Gilbert et al., 1958; Ross and Bras, 1965); dietary levels of the carcinogen were different in the high and low dietary protein groups (Harris, 1947); the total intake of food was less for animals fed very high levels of protein (Gilbert et al., 1958;

Tannenbaum and Silverstone, 1949), and tumor growth is known to be inhibited at lower food (and lower calorie) intake (Ross et al., 1970; Tannenbaum, 1945a,b); and a high dietary level of fat, which may have a tumor-enhancing effect, was present in the experimental diet (Ross and Bras, 1973). Nonetheless, several of the earlier reports have provided useful information either because they were well controlled or because they have been confirmed by other studies.

When considering the effect of dietary protein, it is important to determine whether such an effect is specific for a particular amino acid or is a general effect of protein. In a well-controlled study, Silverstone and Tannenbaum (1951) reported that the spontaneous hepatomas in C3H mice were less frequent (measured as percent of tumor-bearing animals) in animals fed a 9% casein diet than in animals fed 18% or 45% casein diets. No significant difference in hepatomas was observed for the latter two dietary groups. All three diets were isocaloric and were fed to the mice at equivalent time intervals. In additional experiments, this effect of protein was still marked when the animals were fed diets that maintained their individual body weights. Therefore, the investigators concluded that the effect of protein was neither confounded with total food or caloric intake nor related to the change in body weight. Adding 9% gelatin to the 9% casein diet had little effect, whereas supplementation of that diet with methionine and cystine (which is present in relatively low levels in gelatin) increased the incidence of hepatomas to the level observed for the mice fed the 18% casein diet. Therefore, it is the excess of total protein or its adequacy as indicated by amino acid balance that generates the increased tumor response. The addition of gelatin may have resulted in extra total protein, but it did not compensate for the growth-limiting sulfur amino acids. In one experiment, the effects of an animal protein (casein) and a plant protein (isolated soy protein) were compared, but no significant difference in tumor incidence was noted (Carroll, 1975).

In earlier studies, Larsen and Heston (1945) found that cystine added to a low casein diet given to Strain A male mice increased the incidence of spontaneous pulmonary tumors from 28% to 54%. White and Andervont (1943) observed that female C3H mice fed a cystine-deficient casein diet exhibited no mammary gland tumors after 22 months, but almost all the animals quickly developed tumors after their diets were supplemented with cystine. Similarly, White and White (1944) observed that mammary tumors occurred in only 25% of C3H mice fed a lysine-deficient gliadin diet but in nearly all of the mice when the diet was supplemented with lysine. White et al. (1947) later showed that only cystine (but not lysine and tryptophan) was able to enhance the incidence of 3-methylcholanthrene-induced leukemia in casein-fed mice. Thus, it appears that tumor enhancement by dietary protein occurs only when there is amino acid balance, suggesting that the effect is not due to specific amino acids or to amino acid imbalance.

The effect of dietary protein on tumor incidence has been observed both with and without pretreatment with chemical carcinogens. That is, both "spontaneous" and chemically induced tumor responses may be influenced by the level of dietary protein. These two kinds of responses may not be distinct, since certain so-called spontaneous tumors may be related to the prior ingestion of, or other exposure to, some unknown initiator of carcinogenicity. For example, Newberne et al. (1966) speculated that the occasional high incidence of liver tumors observed in earlier studies may have been caused by aflatoxin contamination of peanut meal fed to animals. Because it is now known that corn products may be similarly contaminated, results of earlier studies using degerminated corn grit diets should also be reevaluated, especially when an unexpectedly high incidence of liver tumors has been observed, as in the study of Engel and Copeland (1951). Similarly, the appearance of some presumably spontaneous tumors may be due to the very potent mutagens produced in heated or cooked foods (Sugimura, 1979).

Spontaneous Tumors

Ross and coworkers conducted extensive studies with large numbers of rats in order to examine the effects of diet on mortality patterns and lifespan (Ross and Bras, 1965, 1973; Ross et al., 1970). They focused on the influence of total food, caloric, and protein intake on the appearance of a variety of tumors of unknown etiology. The total incidence of various types of tumors was directly related to the intake of calories, and the tumors appeared sooner when the caloric intake was high (Ross and Bras, 1965).

Because the rats developed many types of tumors, the investigators could not compare the effect of diet on specific types of tumors. The highest number of any tumor type for any one diet was 11--the number of fibrosarcomas observed among the 210 animals in the 30% casein diet group. The authors did note, however, that in two groups with identical caloric intake, there were more tumors in the group with the higher protein intake. In these studies, only two of the four treatment groups differed in only one dietary variable--the ratio of casein to sucrose. The diet with the higher ratio contained 30% casein; the one with the lower ratio contained 8% casein. All other comparisons among the treatment groups were confounded by two or more simultaneous variables.

In a later study, Ross et al. (1970) reported that the prevalence of chromophobe adenomas of the anterior pituitary gland of male rats was directly related to the level of dietary protein (10%, 22%, or 51% casein). However, the tumor prevalence was 2.4% or less in each treatment group, which would seem to invalidate any such conclusion. Moreover, the simple composition of the diet used in these studies is now believed to be inadequate for studies of this type (Anonymous, 1977). In their most recent study, Ross and Bras (1973) examined the effect of

10%, 22%, and 51% casein on the development of 58 types of tumors, none of which involved more than 10% of the rats. They found that protein had no effect on animals fed ad libitum, but that there were fewer tumor-bearing animals in groups fed the lower protein diets if the daily food intake was restricted to 6 g.

In addition to the studies by Silverstone and Tannenbaum (1951) and White and Andervont (1943) described above, other reports that dietary protein affects "spontaneous" tumors are those of Slonaker (1931), White and White (1944), and Tannenbaum and Silverstone (1949). Although Ross and Bras (1973) have interpreted the work of Slonaker (1931) as having demonstrated an inverse relationship between protein intake and tumor incidence (mammary gland and ovarian tumors in female rats and skin tumors in male rats), further inspection of Slonaker's report is necessary. Slonaker (1931) stated that the diets contained 10%, 14%, 18%, 22%, and 26% protein, but he did not describe the composition of the diets. Moreover, the numbers of tumor-bearing female animals were 5/20, 6/19, 5/17, 2/16, and 4/21 for the low to high protein groups, and the author, without providing histological evidence, concluded that the tumors "became cancer-like in appearance." For the males, skin cancers were found in 1/22, 1/21, 1/17, 0/14, and 0/13 animals for the low to high protein groups. Therefore, no firm conclusions can be drawn concerning the association of protein intake with tumor appearance.

Tannenbaum and Silverstone (1949) described a study in which diets containing from 9% to 45% protein were fed ad libitum to an inbred strain of mice. The incidence of spontaneous hepatomas in the animals fed 9% casein diets was 11/44; in the animals fed 18% casein diets, it was 28/46. However, no significant effect on either the incidence or the average time of appearance was observed for the spontaneous mammary tumors.

Chemically Induced Tumors

More studies have been conducted to determine the relationship of dietary protein to chemically induced tumors than to spontaneous tumors.

When aflatoxin is fed with varying levels of protein, the incidence of liver tumors is depressed at lower protein intakes. Madhavan and Gopalan (1968) intubated weanling or young rats with aflatoxin and then fed them either 5% or 20% casein diets for 1 year. They observed that the incidence of hepatomas in the two groups was 0/12 and 15/30, respectively. These data summarize results from experiments that used different protocols. Wells et al. (1976) fed diets containing 8%, 22%, or 30% casein with 1.7 mg/kg aflatoxin B_1 (AFB_1) to male weanling rats for 3 months, then the same diets without AFB_1 for as long as 1 year. Hepatomas were found in 0/16, 6/9, and 8/10 rats, respectively. This finding confirmed the results

of Madhavan and Gopalan (1968). Similarly, Temcharoen et al. (1978)
fed male rats an equal mixture of aflatoxin B_1 and G_1 along with
diets containing either 5% casein or 20% casein for 33 weeks. They
found 4/47 hepatoma-bearing animals in the low protein group and 7/49
in the higher protein group, which is not in accord with their conclusion that "in animals fed a low-protein diet, aflatoxin induced
extensive . . . carcinogenic effects." In contrast to the incidence
of hepatomas, the incidence of cystic lesions, cholangiofibrosis,
cirrhosis, and hyperplastic nodules was higher among the animals fed
the low protein diets. This appears to be in agreement with the observations of other investigators that the effect of the level of
dietary protein on aflatoxin-induced hepatotoxicity is the opposite of
its effect on aflatoxin-induced carcinogenesis (Madhavan and Gopalan,
1965, 1968).

The effect of dietary protein on the emergence of precancerous
lesions is not clear from these studies. Madhavan and Gopalan (1968)
reported fewer "preneoplastic lesions" in the animals fed the low protein diet. But Temcharoen et al. (1978) observed more "hyperplastic
nodules" and other lesions in the low protein groups, suggesting that
their study might have been confounded by the simultaneous appearance
of toxic and carcinogenic lesions. Madhavan and Gopalan (1968)
administered aflatoxin early in their studies and then discontinued
further administration; Temcharoen et al. (1978) appeared to have
administered the toxin throughout the study, although this was not
explicitly stated. Part of the confusion about the association of low
protein intake and the hepatocarcinogenicity of aflatoxin results from
the use of the terms hepatotoxicity and hepatocarcinogenesis. These
effects are different, and have been used without definition in some
reports. Each of the studies cited above (i.e., Madhavan and Gopalan,
1968; Temcharoen et al., 1978; Wells et al., 1976) is singularly
inconclusive, but collectively they support the hypothesis that a high
protein diet enhances aflatoxin-induced hepatocarcinogenesis.

Morris et al. (1948) found that more tumors of a greater variety
appeared in rats treated with N-acetyl-2-aminofluorene (2-AAF) and fed
synthetic diets containing 18% and 24% casein than in similarly treated
animals fed diets containing 12% casein. Engel and Copeland (1952b)
observed that dietary protein did not affect 2-AAF-induced tumors in
rats fed ad libitum with diets containing 9% to 27% casein. There was,
however, a highly significant reduction in the incidence of mammary
tumors in rats fed diets containing 40% to 60% casein. When the 9% and
60% protein diets were pair-fed, i.e., fed to two matched groups, the
incidence of mammary tumors was 80% and 12%, respectively. Ad libitum
feeding of the 60% protein diet, however, overcame some of the inhibition (77% incidence), indicating inhibition of tumorigenesis by very
high protein diets can be overcome by increasing food intake. Harris
(1947) concluded that protein had no effect on carcinogenesis induced
either by 2-AAF or by aminofluorene (AF), which was applied to the

skin. In the 2-AAF-treated rats, reduction in the total incidence of tumors from 65% to 45% in males and from 80% to 70% in females resulted from a modest reduction in dietary casein from 20% to 13%. In animals receiving the low protein diet, the incidence of liver tumors was depressed from 50% to 30% in males and from 20% to 0 in females.

Walters and Roe (1964) injected mice within 24 hours of birth with 9,10-dimethyl-1,2-benzanthracene (DMBA) and then fed them diets containing either 25% or between 10% and 15% casein. The animals fed the higher level of casein developed significantly more lung tumors. In contrast, other reports showed that a reduction of the protein content of the diet enhanced the formation of DMBA-induced hepatomas (Elson, 1958; Miller et al., 1941; Silverstone, 1948) and mammary tumors (Clinton et al., 1979) in rats. Clinton et al. (1979) studied the effect of dietary protein levels on the incidence of DMBA-induced mammary tumors in rats and observed that the effect of protein depended on whether the dietary treatment occurred before or after the administration of the carcinogen.

Topping and Visek (1976) studied the effect of dietary protein on the induction of adenocarcinomas of the small and large intestines of rats by 1,2-dimethylhydrazine. They observed that the tumors were larger and more numerous in the rats fed diets containing 15% and 22.5% protein than in those given 7.5% protein diets. Moreover, the 22.5% protein diets also caused an earlier appearance of keratin-producing papillomas of the sebaceous glands of the external ear.

Shay et al. (1964) studied the effect of dietary protein on tumorigenesis induced by 3-methylcholanthrene. They observed an increase in mammary adenocarcinomas in pretreated rats fed high levels of protein (27% to 64% casein). In an earlier study, White et al. (1947) reported that a high protein diet enhanced 3-methylcholanthrene-induced leukemia in mice.

Extensive studies have been undertaken to determine the mechanism by which dietary protein alters AFB_1-induced tumorigenesis. A low protein intake depresses the mixed-function oxygenase (Mgbodile and Campbell, 1972) responsible for AFB_1 metabolism as well as the in vivo formation of AFB_1-DNA covalent adducts (Preston et al., 1976). Although Campbell (1979) suggested that modification of AFB_1 metabolism was responsible for the effect of dietary protein on AFB_1 tumorigenicity, more recent studies indicate that the effect of dietary protein on events occurring after initiation may be more important. For example, the development of γ-glutamyl transpeptidase hepatocellulular foci, which is an excellent early indicator of hepatocarcinogenesis (Tsuda et al., 1980), is greatly depressed in rats fed a 5% casein diet compared to rats fed a 20% casein diet, both given after the administration of AFB_1 is completed (Appleton and Campbell, 1981). This postinitiation effect of the low protein diet was even capable of overcoming the potential carcinogenic effects of a higher AFB_1-DNA adduct level, which had been established by feeding high levels of protein during AFB_1 administration.

Tumor Transplantation Studies

Low protein diets have also been associated with the general inhibition of the growth of transplanted tumors. Haley and Williamson (1960) implanted HAD-1 tumors into rats fed a diet with no protein and rats fed a 20% casein control diet. They observed that the resultant tumors were smaller in the no protein diet group. Earlier, Babson (1954) had found that increasing dietary casein from 0 to 18% increased tumor growth rates in rats implanted either with the Sarcoma R-1 tumor or the Flexner-Jobling carcinosarcoma. According to Devik et al. (1950), there was a prolonged inflammatory reaction to the implantation of the Walker carcinosarcoma 256 and incomplete connective tissue encapsulation in animals fed 5% casein diets, compared to animals fed 20% casein diets.

White and Belkin (1945) studied the effect of low protein diets on the "take" of implanted mammary carcinoma 15091a. Although the number of takes was higher (16/31) in the protein-deficient group than in the adequate dietary protein group (10/31), the growth rate at 3 weeks was only 74% of the rate for the higher protein diet. These tumor implantation studies were later summarized by White (1961).

The mechanism for the inhibition of tumor growth by low protein diets is not known. Jose and Good (1973) have proposed that the cellular immune response may be involved. This response is enhanced through a deficiency of blocking serum antibody production at low levels of protein intake.

An Evaluation of the Data from Animal Studies

The relationship of dietary protein to the carcinogenic process does not appear to be straightforward. Levels of protein ranging from those somewhat below the minimum required for optimum growth (approximately 5% of the diet) up to those generally consumed by mammals (15% to 20%) have been studied most extensively. In many studies in animals, diets with low protein (near or below the requirement for optimum growth) have generally been shown to suppress the carcinogenic process and the subsequent growth and development of tumors. The only apparent exception to this effect is the increase in DMBA-induced tumor yield in animals fed low protein diets. Although there is generally a tumor-enhancing effect from 20% to 25% dietary protein, higher levels appear either to produce no further enhancement or, in fact, to inhibit tumorigenesis (Appleton and Campbell, 1981; Engel and Copeland, 1952b; Ross and Bras, 1973; Ross et al., 1970; Saxton et al., 1948; Tannenbaum and Silverstone, 1949; Topping and Visek, 1976; Wells et al., 1976). It is not clear whether the general inhibition or the absence of effect on tumorigenesis at very high levels of dietary protein is due to a reduced intake of food and total calories or whether it is due to other adverse effects, e.g., renal toxicity due to high levels of protein.

SUMMARY

Epidemiological Evidence

Epidemiological studies have suggested possible associations between high levels of dietary protein and increased risk of cancers at a number of different sites. However, the literature on protein is much more limited than the literature concerning fats and cancer. In addition, because of the very high correlation between fat and protein intake in Western diets, and the more consistent and often stronger association of these cancers with fat intake, it seems more likely that dietary fat is the more active component. Nevertheless, the evidence does not completely preclude an independent effect of protein.

Experimental Evidence

In laboratory experiments, the relationship of dietary protein to carcinogenesis appears to depend upon the level of protein intake. In most studies, carcinogenesis was suppressed by diets containing levels of protein at or below the minimum required for optimum growth. Chemically induced carcinogenesis appears to be enhanced as protein intake is increased up to 2 or 3 times the normal requirement; however, higher levels of protein begin to inhibit carcinogenesis. There is some evidence to suggest that protein may affect the initiation phase of carcinogenesis and/or the subsequent growth and development of the tumor.

CONCLUSION

Thus, evidence from both epidemiological and laboratory studies suggests that protein intake may be associated with an increased risk of cancers of certain sites. Because of the relative paucity of data on protein compared to fat, and the strong correlation between intakes of fat and protein in the Western diet, the committee is unable to arrive at a firm conclusion about an independent effect of protein.

Anonymous. 1977. Report of the American Institute of Nutrition, Ad Hoc Committee on Standards for Nutritional Studies. J. Nutr. 107:1340-1348.

Appleton, B. S., and T. C. Campbell. 1981. Effects of dietary protein level and phenobarbital (PB) on aflatoxin (AFB_1)-induced hepatic γ-glutamyl transpeptidase (GGT) in the rat. Fed. Proc. Fed. Am. Soc. Exp. Biol. 40:842. Abstract 3477.

Armstrong, B., and R. Doll. 1975. Environmental factors and cancer incidence and mortality in different countries, with special reference to dietary practices. Int. J. Cancer 15:617-631.

Armstrong, B., A. Garrod, and R. Doll. 1976. A retrospective study of renal cancer with special reference to coffee and animal protein consumption. Br. J. Cancer 33:127-136.

Babson, A. L. 1954. Some host-tumor relationships with respect to nitrogen. Cancer Res. 14:89-93.

Berg, J. W., and M. A. Howell. 1974. The geographic pathology of bowel cancer. Cancer 34:805-814.

Bingham, S., D. R. R. Williams, T. J. Cole, and W. P. T. James. 1979. Dietary fibre and regional large-bowel cancer mortality in Britain. Br. J. Cancer 40:456-463.

Bjelke, E. 1978. Dietary factors and the epidemiology of cancer of the stomach and large bowel. Aktuel. Ernaehrungsmed. Klin. Prax. Suppl. 2:10-17.

Campbell, T. C. 1979. Influence of nutrition on metabolism of carcinogens. Adv. Nutr. Res. 2:29-55.

Carroll, K. K. 1975. Experimental evidence of dietary factors and hormone-dependent cancers. Cancer Res. 35:3374-3383.

Clinton, S. K., C. R. Truex, and W. J. Visek. 1979. Dietary protein, aryl hydrocarbon hydroxylase and chemical carcinogenesis in rats. J. Nutr. 109:55-62.

Devik, F., L. A. Elson, P. C. Koller, and L. F. Lamerton. 1950. Influence of diet on Walker rat carcinoma 256, and its response to X-radiation--Cytological and histological investigations. Br. J. Cancer 4:298-314.

Elson, L. A. 1958. Some dynamic aspects of chemical carcinogenesis. Br. Med. Bull. 14:161-164.

Engel, R. W., and D. H. Copeland. 1951. Influence of diet on the relative incidence of eye, mammary, ear-duct, and liver tumors in rats fed 2-acetylaminofluorene. Cancer Res. 11:180-183.

Engel, R. W., and D. H. Copeland. 1952a. Protective action of stock diets against the cancer-inducing action of 2-acetylaminofluorene in rats. Cancer Res. 12:211-215.

Engel, R. W., and D. H. Copeland. 1952b. The influence of dietary casein level on tumor induction with 2-acetylaminofluorene. Cancer Res. 12:905-908.

Enstrom, J. E. 1975. Colorectal cancer and consumption of beef and fat. Br. J. Cancer 32:432-439.

Gaskill, S. P., W. L. McGuire, C. K. Osborne, and M. P. Stern. 1979. Breast cancer mortality and diet in the United States. Cancer Res. 39:3628-3637.

Gilbert, C., J. Gillman, P. Loustalot, and W. Lutz. 1958. The modifying influence of diet and the physical environment on spontaneous tumour frequency in rats. Br. J. Cancer 12:565-593.

Graham, S., H. Dayal, M. Swanson, A. Mittelman, and G. Wilkinson. 1978. Diet in the epidemiology of cancer of the colon and rectum. J. Natl. Cancer Inst. 61:709-714.

Gray, G. E., M. C. Pike, and B. E. Henderson. 1979. Breast-cancer incidence and mortality rates in different countries in relation to known risk factors and dietary practices. Br. J. Cancer 39:1-7.

Gregor, O., R. Toman, and F. Prušová. 1969. Gastrointestinal cancer and nutrition. Gut 10:1031-1034.

Haenszel, W., J. W. Berg, M. Segi, M. Kurihara, and F. B. Locke. 1973. Large-bowel cancer in Hawaiian Japanese. J. Natl. Cancer Inst. 51:1765-1779.

Haenszel, W., F. B. Locke, and M. Segi. 1980. A case-control study of large bowel cancer in Japan. J. Natl. Cancer Inst. 64:17-22.

Haley, H. B., and M. B. Williamson. 1960. Growth of tumors in experimental wounds. Proc. Am. Assoc. Cancer Res. 3:116. Abstract 99.

Harris, P. N. 1947. Production of tumors in rats by 2-aminofluorene and 2-acetylaminofluorene: Failure of liver extract and of dietary protein level to influence liver tumor production. Cancer Res. 7:88-94.

Hems, G. 1978. The contributions of diet and childbearing to breast-cancer rates. Br. J. Cancer 37:974–982.

Hems, G. 1980. Associations between breast-cancer mortality rates, child-bearing and diet in the United Kingdom. Br. J. Cancer 41:429–437.

Hirayama, T. 1977. Changing patterns of cancer in Japan with special reference to the decrease in stomach cancer mortality. Pp. 55–75 in H. H. Hiatt, J. D. Watson, and J. A. Winsten, eds. Origins of Human Cancer, Book A: Incidence of Cancer in Humans. Cold Spring Harbor Laboratory, Cold Spring Harbor, N.Y.

Hirayama, T. 1981. A large-scale cohort study on the relationship between diet and selected cancers of the digestive organs. Pp. 409–429 in W. R. Bruce, P. Correa, M. Lipkin, S. R. Tannenbaum, and T. D. Wilkins, eds. Gastrointestinal Cancer, Endogenous Factors; Banbury Report 7. Cold Spring Harbor Laboratory, Cold Spring Harbor, N.Y.

Howell, M. A. 1974. Factor analysis of international cancer mortality data and per capita food consumption. Br. J. Cancer 29:328–336.

Howell, M. A. 1975. Diet as an etiological factor in the development of cancers of the colon and rectum. J. Chronic Dis. 28:67–80.

Ishii, K., K. Nakamura, H. Ozaki, N. Yamada, and T. Takeuchi. 1968. [In Japanese.] [Epidemiological problems of pancreas cancer.] Jpn. J. Clin. Med. 26:1839–1842.

Jain, M., G. M. Cook, F. G. Davis, M. G. Grace, G. R. Howe, and A. B Miller. 1980. A case-control study of diet and colorectal cancer. Int. J. Cancer 26:757–768.

Jose, D. G., and R. A. Good. 1973. Quantitative effects of nutritional essential amino acid deficiency upon immune responses to tumors in mice. J. Exp. Med. 137:1–9.

Knox, E. G. 1977. Foods and diseases. Br. J. Prev. Soc. Med. 31:71–80.

Kolonel, L. N., J. H. Hankin, J. Lee, S. Y. Chu, A. M. Y. Nomura, and M. W. Hinds. 1981. Nutrient intakes in relation to cancer incidence in Hawaii. Br. J. Cancer 44:332–339.

Larsen, C. D., and W. E. Heston. 1945. Effects of cystine and calorie restriction on the incidence of spontaneous pulmonary tumors in strain A mice. J. Natl. Cancer Inst. 6(1):31–40.

Lea, A. J. 1967. Neoplasms and environmental factors. Ann. R. Coll. Surg. Engl. 41:432-438.

Lubin, J. H., W. J. Blot, and P. E. Burns. 1981. Breast cancer following high dietary fat and protein consumption. Am. J. Epidemiol. 114:422. Abstract.

Madhavan, T. V., and C. Gopalan. 1965. Effect of dietary protein on aflatoxin liver injury in weanling rats. Arch. Pathol. 80:123-126.

Madhavan, T. V., and C. Gopalan. 1968. The effect of dietary protein on carcinogenesis of aflatoxin. Arch. Pathol. 85:133-137.

Mgbodile, M. U. K., and T. C. Campbell. 1972. Effect of protein deprivation of male weanling rats on the kinetics of hepatic microsomal enzyme activity. J. Nutr. 102:53-60.

Miller, A. B., A. Kelly, N. W. Choi, V. Matthews, R. W. Morgan, L. Munan, J. D. Burch, J. Feather, G. R. Howe, and M. Jain. 1978. A study of diet and breast cancer. Am. J. Epidemiol. 107:499-509.

Miller, J. A., D. L. Miner, H. P. Rusch, and C. A. Baumann. 1941. Diet and hepatic tumor formation. Cancer Res. 1:699-708.

Morris, H. P., B. B. Westfall, C. S. Dubnik, and T. B. Dunn. 1948. Some observations on carcinogenicity, distribution and metabolism of $\underline{N}$-acetyl-2-aminofluorene in the rat. Cancer Res. 8:390. Abstract.

Newberne, P. M., D. H. Harrington, and G. N. Wogan. 1966. Effects of cirrhosis and other liver insults on the induction of liver tumors by aflatoxin in rats. Lab. Invest. 15:962-969.

Phillips, R. L. 1975. Role of life-style and dietary habits in risk of cancer among Seventh-Day Adventists. Cancer Res. 35:3513-3522.

Preston, R. S., J. R. Hayes, and T. C. Campbell. 1976. The effect of protein deficiency on the $\underline{in\ vivo}$ binding of aflatoxin B_1 to rat liver macromolecules. Life Sci. 19:1191-1197.

Ross, M. H., and G. Bras. 1965. Tumor incidence patterns and nutrition in the rat. J. Nutr. 87:245-260.

Ross, M. H., and G. Bras. 1973. Influence of protein under- and overnutrition on spontaneous tumor prevalence in the rat. J. Nutr. 103:944-963.

Ross, M. H., G. Bras, and M. S. Ragbeer. 1970. Influence of protein and caloric intake upon spontaneous tumor incidence of the anterior pituitary gland of the rat. J. Nutr. 100:177-189.

Saxton, J. A., Jr., G. A. Sperling, L. L. Barnes, and C. M. McCay. 1948. The influence of nutrition upon the incidence of spontaneous tumors of the albino rat. Acta Unio Int. Cancrum 6:423-431.

Shay, H., M. Gruenstein, and M. B. Shimkin. 1964. Effect of casein, lactalbumin, and ovalbumin on 3-methylcholanthrene-induced mammary carcinoma in rats. J. Natl. Cancer Inst. 33:243-253.

Silverstone, H. 1948. The levels of carcinogenic azo dyes in the livers of rats fed various diets containing p-dimethylamino-azobenzene: Relationship to the formation of hepatomas. Cancer Res. 8:301-308.

Silverstone, H., and A. Tannenbaum. 1951. Proportion of dietary protein and the formation of spontaneous hepatomas in the mouse. Cancer Res. 11:442-446.

Slonaker, J. R. 1931. The effect of different per cents of protein in the diet. VII. Life span and cause of death. Am. J. Physiol. 98:266-275.

Sugimura, T. 1979. Naturally occurring genotoxic carcinogens. Pp. 241-261 in E. C. Miller, J. A. Miller, I. Hirono, T. Sugimura, and S. Takayama, eds. Naturally Occurring Carcinogens-Mutagens and Modulators of Carcinogenesis. Japan Scientific Societies Press, Tokyo; University Park Press, Baltimore, Md.

Tannenbaum, A. 1945a. The dependence of tumor formation on the degree of caloric restriction. Cancer Res. 5:609-615.

Tannenbaum, A. 1945b. The dependence of tumor formation on the composition of the calorie-restricted diet as well as on the degree of restriction. Cancer Res. 5:616-625.

Tannenbaum, A., and H. Silverstone. 1949. The genesis and growth of tumors. IV. Effects of varying the proportion of protein (casein) in the diet. Cancer Res. 9:162-173.

Temcharoen, P., T. Anukarahanonta, and N. Bhamarapravati. 1978. Influence of dietary protein and vitamin B_{12} on the toxicity and carcinogenicity of aflatoxins in rat liver. Cancer Res. 38:2185-2190.

Topping, D. C., and W. J. Visek. 1976. Nitrogen intake and tumori-genesis in rats injected with 1,2-dimethylhydrazine. J. Nutr. 106:1583-1590.

Tsuda, H., G. Lee, and E. Farber. 1980. Induction of resistant hepatocytes as a new principle for a possible short-term in vivo test for carcinogens. Cancer Res. 40:1157-1164.

Voegtlin, C., and M. E. Maver. 1936. Lysine and malignant growth. II. The effect on malignant growth of a gliadin diet. Public Health Rep. 51:1436-1444.

Voegtlin, C., and J. W. Thompson. 1936. Lysine and malignant growth. I. The amino acid lysine as a factor controlling the growth rate of a typical neoplasm. Public Health Rep. 51:1429-1436.

Walters, M. A., and F. J. C. Roe. 1964. The effect of dietary casein on the induction of lung tumours by the injection of 9,10-dimethyl-1,2-benzanthracene (DMBA) into newborn mice. Br. J. Cancer 18:312-316.

Wells, P., L. Alftergood, and R. B. Alfin-Slater. 1976. Effect of varying levels of dietary protein on tumor development and lipid metabolism in rats exposed to aflatoxin. J. Am. Oil Chem. Soc. 53:559-562.

White, F. R. 1961. The relationship between underfeeding and tumor formation, transplantation, and growth in rats and mice. Cancer Res. 21:281-290.

White, F. R., and M. Belkin. 1945. Source of tumor proteins. I. Effect of low-nitrogen diet on the establishment and growth of a transplanted tumor. J. Natl. Cancer Inst. 5:261-263.

White, F. R., and J. White. 1944. Effect of a low lysine diet on mammary-tumor formation in strain C3H mice. J. Natl. Cancer Inst. 5:41-42.

White, J., and H. B. Andervont. 1943. Effect of a diet relatively low in cystine on the production of spontaneous mammary-gland tumors in strain C3H female mice. J. Natl. Cancer Inst. 3:449-451.

White, J., F. R. White, and G. B. Mider. 1947. Effect of diets deficient in certain amino acids on the induction of leukemia in dba mice. J. Natl. Cancer Inst. 7:199-202.

7 Carbohydrates

In contrast to lipids and protein, which are the other two macronutrients in the diet, very little attention has been directed toward the
study of carbohydrate intake and the occurrence of cancer. The principal
carbohydrates in foods are sugars, starches, and cellulose. Evidence pertaining to sugars and starches is evaluated in this chapter. The data on
cellulose are discussed under dietary fiber (Chapter 8).

EPIDEMIOLOGICAL EVIDENCE

There is little epidemiological evidence to support a role for
carbohydrates per se in the etiology of cancer. Fiber as a separate
dietary component is discussed in Chapter 8.

Armstrong and Doll (1975) correlated per capita intake of foods and
specific nutrients with cancer incidence and mortality in 23 and 32
countries, respectively. They found a significant direct correlation
between sugar intake and pancreatic cancer mortality (but not incidence)
in women only. They also reported a weak association between liver
cancer incidence and the intake of potatoes--a starch-rich vegetable.
There are no reports of case-control studies that support either of these
findings.

Hems (1978) reported a study concerning the relationship of diet and
breast cancer among women in 41 countries. He found that a high intake
of refined sugar was one of the dietary components associated with
increased incidence of breast cancer. This finding is consistent with
findings in laboratory experiments. However, in an earlier study, Hems
and Stuart (1975) found an inverse relationship between breast cancer
incidence and another dietary carbohydrate--starch.

Hakama and Saxén (1967) analyzed age- and sex-adjusted mortality
rates for stomach cancer in 16 countries. They found a strong correlation (r = 0.75) with the per capita intake of cereal used as flour
from 1934 to 1938. In a study of per capita food intake and cancer risk
in 37 countries, Drasar and Irving (1973) observed a direct correlation
between breast cancer and the intake of simple sugars.

In a case-control study of gastric cancer, Modan et al. (1974)
observed that high starch foods were consumed more frequently by cases
than by controls. This finding has not been reported in other studies of
gastric cancer. De Jong et al. (1974) studied cases of esophageal cancer
and hospital controls in Singapore. Among their findings was a direct
association between consumption of bread and potatoes (major sources of

123

dietary carbohydrates) and risk of esophageal cancer. Once again, other investigators who have studied cancer at this site have not observed a similar association.

EXPERIMENTAL EVIDENCE

There have also been only a few laboratory experiments to study the relationship between carbohydrates and cancer. These studies have generally been conducted by varying the concentration of the test substance, e.g., starch, sucrose, dextrin, or glucose, in a basal diet. Often, little attention has been given to the differences in the caloric content of the control and experimental diets. Furthermore, the variation in carbohydrate content, resulting from attempts to "balance" diets on a weight basis, has generally been disregarded. A few recent studies have focused on the effects of long-term carbohydrate feeding on tumorigenesis.

Sucrose

The effects of long-term (more than 1 year) feeding or systemic administration of sucrose on spontaneously occurring tumors have been studied in both mice and rats. Roe et al. (1970) fed sucrose to mice at 10% by weight of the diet (∿15 g/kg body weight [bw]), and Friedman et al. (1972) fed rats sucrose at 77% by weight of the diet (∿40 g/kg bw). In neither study was there an increase in the incidence of tumors. Intraperitoneal or subcutaneous injections of sucrose given over various lengths of time (Nonaka, 1938; Takizawa, 1939; Zarattini, 1940) or systemic administration of 20% sucrose twice weekly for 2 years produced no evidence of carcinogenesis in either rats or mice (Hueper, 1965).

Hunter et al. (1978a) fed CFLP mice 20% sucrose in the diet for 2 years. The females, but not the males, exhibited a higher incidence of hepatocellular tumors. Parallel feeding studies by the same investigators in which 20% sucrose diets were fed to male and female Sprague-Dawley (CD) rats for up to 1 year and to male and female beagle dogs for up to 2 years did not provide any evidence that sucrose contributed to tumorigenesis. This study has not been repeated.

Hoehn and Carroll (1978) evaluated the effect of dietary carbohydrates on chemically induced tumors in rats. After breast tumors were induced with 7,12-dimethylbenz[a]anthracene, rats were fed diets containing either refined sugar or complex starches. Significantly more breast tumors were observed in rats fed refined sugar than in those fed starch.

Much more experimental work is required before a conclusion can be drawn about the relationship between sucrose and carcinogenesis.

Lactose

Gershoff and McGandy (1981) studied the interaction of dietary lactose (49%) or sucrose (43%-55% total weight) with vitamin A deficiency in the production of primary urinary bladder calculi in male Charles River rats. A small percentage of rats fed lactose in a diet with sufficient vitamin A developed vesicle stones. Approximately 60% of the rats fed lactose in vitamin-A-deficient diets developed bladder calculi. The bladder walls in most of the affected rats were grossly hypertrophic and had focal areas of transitional cell hyperplasia. Histological changes consistent with grade I to II transitional cell carcinomas were observed in approximately 30% of the stone-containing bladders. It was not possible to discern whether the deficiency of vitamin A contributed directly to bladder tumors or indirectly via stone formation and subsequent physical irritation of the bladder. Sucrose-fed rats with or without superimposed vitamin A deficiency did not exhibit calculi or histological changes of the bladder. The authors remarked that this was the first study to demonstrate the production of tumors by diet without an exogenous source of a carcinogen in animals not genetically predisposed to tumor formation.

Glucose

A preliminary report by Ingram and Castleden (1981) implicated dietary glucose in the development of carcinogen-induced tumors in the large bowel. In this study, male Wistar rats were fed Milne's Standard Laboratory Diet and given drinking water ad libitum either with or without 1.6% glucose. Both groups were injected subcutaneously with 1,2-dimethylhydrazine to induce bowel tumors. There were no differences in the number of small bowel tumors observed in the two groups; however, the rats given the glucose solution developed approximately twice the number of large bowel tumors observed in those given the drinking water alone. These results are difficult to interpret because approximately 35% of the Milne Standard Laboratory Diet is composed of carbohydrates, and this diet was fed to both groups of animals. The contribution of this diet to blood glucose levels is considerably greater than that supplied by the 1.6% glucose-water drinking solution. Thus, there is a possibility that the observed results were an indirect effect of the glucose-water solution rather than a direct effect of glucose.

Xylitol

Xylitol is present in many natural foods (Washüttl et al., 1973). Its sweetness is approximately equal to that of sucrose.

In a 2-year feeding study, CFLP male and female mice were fed 0, 2%, 10%, or 20% xylitol in the diet for as long as 106 weeks (Hunter et al.,

1978b). In the mice fed the 10% or 20% xylitol diets, there was a reduction in spontaneous hepatocellular tumors in the males, but not in the
females. However, the males in these dietary groups had more crystalline
bladder calculi and an associated increase in hyperplasia, metaplasia,
and neoplasia of the transitional epithelium of the bladder than did the
females fed similar diets, the control mice, or the mice fed 2% xylitol.

Sprague-Dawley CD male and female rats were fed 2%, 5%, 10%, or 20%
xylitol in the diet for 26 weeks without evidence of increased renal
calculi or hepatocellular abnormalities at autopsy. However, the incidence of adrenal medullary hyperplasia was greater in rats fed 5%, 10%,
or 20% xylitol than in the controls (Hunter et al., 1978b). In male and
female beagle dogs fed 10% or 20% xylitol in their diets for 52 weeks,
the single remarkable pathologic change was an increased liver weight at
autopsy. This slight hepatomegaly was associated with hepatocyte enlargement and altered hepatocyte appearance in the periportal areas of
the animals.

The quantity of xylitol in the 20% diet approaches the LD_{50} for
xylitol in mice (Kieckebuch et al., 1961). In rats, ingestion of 20%
xylitol may exceed the maximum metabolic turnover rate as calculated
from rates observed in humans (Bickel and Halmágyi, 1976).

SUMMARY

Epidemiological Evidence

The evidence concerning the role of carbohydrates in the development
of cancer in humans is extremely limited. In one study, the intake of
sugar was correlated with increased mortality from pancreatic cancer in
women only, and the intake of potatoes was correlated with increased
mortality from liver cancer in both sexes. In other studies, a high
intake of refined sugar and a low intake of starch have been associated
with an increased incidence of breast cancer. Frequent consumption of
starch has been associated with a high incidence of gastric cancer in one
case-control study and with esophageal cancer in another. However, the
evidence is insufficient to permit any firm conclusions to be drawn.

Experimental Evidence

The data from the few laboratory experiments designed to study the
role of carbohydrates in carcinogenesis are difficult to interpret
because of generally poor experimental designs and because there is
uncertainty about the actual carbohydrate content of the foods used in
the test diets.

A few recent studies suggest that dietary lactose combined with
vitamin A deprivation and long-term feeding of high levels of sucrose and

xylitol may contribute to carcinogenesis. These observations require further study.

CONCLUSION

Thus, the evidence from both epidemiological and laboratory studies is too sparse to suggest a direct role for carbohydrates (possibly exclusive of fiber) in carcinogenesis. However, excessive carbohydrate consumption contributes to caloric excess, which in turn has been implicated as a modifier of carcinogenesis.

REFERENCES

Armstrong, B., and R. Doll. 1975. Environmental factors and cancer incidence and mortality in different countries, with special reference to dietary practice. Int. J. Cancer 15:617–631.

Bickel, H., and M. Halmágyi. 1976. Requirement and utilization of carbohydrates and alcohol. Pp. 66–79 in F. W. Ahnefeld, C. Burri, W. Dick, and M. Halmágyi, eds. Parenteral Nutrition. Springer-Verlag, Berlin, Heidelberg, and New York.

de Jong, U. W., N. Breslow, J. G. E. Hong, M. Sridharan, and K. Shanmugaratnam. 1974. Aetiological factors in oesophageal cancer in Singapore Chinese. Int. J. Cancer 13:291–303.

Drasar, B., and D. Irving. 1973. Environmental factors and cancer of the colon and breast. Br. J. Cancer 27:167–172.

Friedman, L., H. L. Richardson, M. E. Richardson, E. J. Lethco, W. C. Wallace, and F. M. Sauro. 1972. Toxic response of rats to cyclamates in chow and semisynthetic diets. J. Natl. Cancer Inst. 49:751–764.

Gershoff, S. N., and R. B. McGandy. 1981. The effects of vitamin A-deficient diets containing lactose in producing bladder calculi and tumors in rats. Am. J. Clin. Nutr. 34:483–489.

Hakama, M., and E. A. Saxén. 1967. Cereal consumption and gastric cancer. Int. J. Cancer 2:265–268.

Hems, G. 1978. The contribution of diet and childbearing to breast-cancer rates. Br. J. Cancer 37:974–982.

Hems, G., and A. Stuart. 1975. Breast cancer rates in populations of single women. Br. J. Cancer 31:118–123.

Hoehn, S. K., and K. K. Carroll. 1978. Effects of dietary carbohydrate on the incidence of mammary tumors induced in rats by 7,12-dimethylbenz(a)anthracene. Nutr. Cancer 1:27–30.

Hueper, W. C. 1965. Are sugars carcinogens? An experimental study. Cancer Res. 25:440–443.

Hunter, B., C. Graham, R. Heywood, D. E. Prentice, F. J. C. Roe, and D. N. Noakes. 1978a. Tumorigenicity and Carcinogenicity Study with Xylitol in Long-Term Dietary Administration to Mice (Final report). Huntingdon Research Centre, Huntingdon, Cambridgeshire, England. Volumes 20–23 of Xylitol. F. Hoffman La Roche Company, Ltd., Basel, Switzerland. 1500 pp.

Hunter, B., J. Colley, A. E. Street, R. Heywood, D. E. Prentice, and
G. Magnusson. 1978b. Xylitol Tumorigenicity and Toxicity Study in
Long-Term Dietary Administration to Rats (Final Report). Huntingdon
Research Centre, Huntingdon, Cambridgeshire, England. Volumes 11-14
of Xylitol. F. Hoffman La Roche Company, Ltd., Basel, Switzerland.
2225 pp.

Ingram, D. M., and W. M. Castleden. 1981. Glucose increases experimentally induced colorectal cancer: A preliminary report. Nutr.
Cancer 2:150-152.

Kieckebuch, W., W. Gzeim, and K. Lang. 1961. [In German.] Die
Verwertbarkeit von Xylit als Nahrungskohlenhydrat und seine
Verträglichkeit. Klin. Wochenschr. 39:447-448.

Modan, B., F. Lubin, V. Barrell, R. A. Greenberg, M. Modan, and S.
Graham. 1974. The role of starches in the etiology of gastric
cancer. Cancer 34:2087-2092.

Nonaka, T. 1938. [In Japanese; English Title.] The occurrence of subcutaneous sarcomas in the rat after repeated injections of glucose
solution. Gann 32:234-235.

Roe, F. J. C., L. S. Levy, and R. L. Carter. 1970. Feeding studies on
sodium cyclamate, saccharin and sucrose for carcinogenic and tumour-
promoting activity. Food Cosmet. Toxicol. 8:135-145.

Takizawa, N. 1939. [In Japanese; German Title.] Über die Erzeugung
des Maussarkoms durch die subcutane Injektion der konzentrierten
Zuckerlösung. (II. Mitteilung.) Gann 33:193-195.

Washüttl, J., D. Reiderer, and E. Bancher. 1973. A qualitative and
quantitative study of sugar-alcohols in several foods. J. Food
Sci. 38:1262-1263.

Zarattini, A. 1940. [In Italian.] Sulla produzione sperimentale del
sarcoma nei ratti mediante somministrazione paraenterale di glucosio.
Tumori 26:77-84.

8 Dietary Fiber

Recently, attention has been directed toward the physiological significance of dietary fiber, which generally includes indigestible carbohydrates and carbohydrate-like components of food such as cellulose, lignin, hemicelluloses, pentosans, gums, and pectins. The principal characteristic of these indigestible substances is their provision of bulk in the diet. The major categories of foods that provide dietary fiber are vegetables, fruits, and whole grain cereals.

Because of the complex composition of dietary fiber, the physiological functions and metabolic activity of its individual components have not been adequately studied. Most earlier analyses focused on the intake of so-called "crude fiber." Therefore, they generally underestimated the fiber content since crude fiber only determines cellulose and lignin. Consequently, early reports provided incomplete data on the amount and type of fiber consumed.

During the past few decades, the consumption of dietary fiber has decreased in many parts of the Western world (National Academy of Sciences, 1980). On the basis of observations concerning the relationship of diet and the incidence of disease, Burkitt and Trowell (1975) hypothesized that many chronic diseases including cancer are associated with a low intake of dietary fiber.

EPIDEMIOLOGICAL EVIDENCE

The epidemiological data on fiber are related primarily to its possible role in protection against large bowel cancer. Several different mechanisms have been proposed for this protective effect: Fiber can dilute carcinogens present in the large bowel; it can decrease transit time, thereby decreasing contact time between carcinogen and tissue; it can affect the production of putative carcinogens or procarcinogens in the stool such as the bile acids; or, by influencing the composition and metabolic activity of the fecal flora, it can alter the spectrum of fecal bile acids and their derivatives that are present in the stool. Most data on the fiber content of foods are incomplete, because they pertain only to crude fiber. Since any effect associated with dietary fiber may be restricted to selected components, epidemiological studies of dietary fiber will have limited value until detailed information on each of its constituents becomes available.

Attempts to correlate the fiber content of diets with colorectal cancer risk have yielded mixed results. Malhotra (1977) suggested that the differences in colon cancer incidence among northern and southern

130

populations in India might be explained by the high levels of roughage, cellulose, and vegetable fiber in the northern Indian diet and the very low levels in the southern Indian diet. There was a virtual absence of the disease in the Punjabis from the north. He also found that vegetable fibers were abundant in the stools of Indians from the north, but completely absent in samples obtained from inhabitants of the southern regions. MacLennan et al. (1978) observed similar differences after comparing the diets of adult men from Copenhagen, Denmark (high risk group for colon cancer) and from Kuopio, Finland (low risk group). The Danes consumed less fiber and their stools weighed less than those of the Finns. These findings lend support to the hypothesis that dietary fiber plays a protective role in carcinogenesis. Bingham et al. (1979) calculated the average fiber intake by populations in different regions of Great Britain. They found no significant correlation between total fiber intake and corresponding mortality rates for colon and rectal cancers. However, the mean intakes of the pentosan fraction of total dietary fiber and of vegetables other than potatoes were inversely correlated with mortality from colon cancer. This finding suggested the importance of examining the specific components of fiber rather than crude or total fiber in studies of large bowel cancer.

Other correlation analyses have not supported the hypothesis that fiber intake is inversely associated with the risk of colon cancer. Liu et al. (1979) examined mortality from colon cancer in 20 industralized countries between 1967 and 1973 and compared the rates to per capita food intake for these same areas from 1954 to 1965. Although fiber intake was inversely correlated with colon cancer mortality, this relationship was no longer significant in a partial correlation analysis controlling for cholesterol intake. The authors concluded that cholesterol, not fiber, was an important risk factor for colon cancer. In other studies, Drasar and Irving (1973) failed to find a correlation between colon cancer incidence in 37 countries and per capita intake of various fiber-containing foods, and Lyon and Sorenson (1978) found little difference in fiber intake between the population of Utah (low risk) and the population of the United States as a whole.

In a number of case-control studies, investigators have attempted to examine the relationship between dietary fiber and risk of large bowel cancer, again with inconsistent results. Modan et al. (1975) assessed the frequency with which certain food items were consumed by colon and rectal cancer cases and both hospital and neighborhood controls. They found that the consumption of high-fiber foods by colon cancer cases was significantly lower than that of both groups of controls, but there was no such difference between rectal cancer cases and controls. Using a similar approach, Bjelke (1978) observed that the consumption of dietary fiber by colorectal cancer cases was lower than that of controls in parallel studies conducted in Minnesota and Norway.

Dales et al. (1978) studied cases of colorectal cancer in U.S. blacks. Controls were selected from two hospitals and a multiphasic health check-up clinic. By assessing the frequency of consumption of selected food items, they found that the cases consumed fewer fiber-containing foods than did the controls, and that there was a consistent dose-response relationship. Significantly more cases than controls reported the consumption of a diet that was high in saturated fat but low in fiber.

In a case-control study of diet and colorectal cancer in Canada, Jain et al. (1980) attempted to compute consumption of dietary fiber based on the actual fiber content of food rather than on a simple grouping of food items as other investigators had done. They found an elevated risk associated with increased consumption of calories, total fat, total protein, saturated fat, oleic acid, and cholesterol, but no association with the consumption of crude fiber, vitamin C, or linoleic acid. Unfortunately, data on the specific components of fiber were not available for their analysis.

A direct association between fiber consumption and large bowel cancer was reported by Martínez et al. (1979), who conducted a case-control study in Puerto Rico. Based on frequency-of-consumption dietary histories, they found higher consumption of fiber and total residue in cases than in controls. They provided no explanation for this unusual finding, which, however, is consistent with the observation of Hill et al. (1979) that the highest socioeconomic group studied in Hong Kong had the highest incidence of colon cancer and a high intake of fiber and calories, whereas the middle and lowest socioeconomic groups had correspondingly lower incidence rates and intakes.

Glober et al. (1974, 1977), compared bowel transit-times in men from three different populations: Japanese in Japan (low risk for colon cancer), Japanese in Hawaii (high risk for colon cancer), and Caucasians in Hawaii (also high risk for colon cancer). They found that bowel transit-times were similar in both Japanese populations, and were shorter than in the Caucasians. Mean stool weight, however, was similar in the two high-risk populations and was notably less than that for the Japanese in Japan. Thus, their data did not support the hypothesis that dietary fiber protects against colon cancer by decreasing transit time in the bowel, thereby decreasing the contact time between carcinogens and tissues.

Dietary fiber can also affect the amount of bile acids excreted into the lumen of the intestine. However, since dietary fat influences bile acid excretion as well, the relative effects of both of these dietary components need further study. Studies of the composition of bile acids in the feces of humans are reviewed in Chapter 5.

EXPERIMENTAL EVIDENCE

A variety of chemical carcinogens cause colon cancer in rats. Among these are 1,2-dimethylhydrazine (DMH), azoxymethane (AOM), methyl-azoxymethanol (MAM) acetate, 3,2'-dimethyl-4-aminobiphenyl (DAB), and

nitrosomethylurea (NMU). Colon cancer can be induced in these laboratory animals by parenteral administration of DMH, AOM, MAM, and DAB; by
feeding DMH; and by intrarectal instillation of NMU. Bran protects rats
against DMH-induced colon cancer, regardless of whether the carcinogen is
administered orally or subcutaneously (Barbolt and Abraham, 1978; Chen et
al., 1978; Wilson et al., 1977). However, it has no effect on the
incidence or number of tumors in the duodenum or cecum. Cellulose has
been found to protect rats against DMH-induced tumors (Freeman et al.,
1978, 1980), but pectin does not (Freeman et al., 1980). Cellulose does
not appear to protect against tumors induced by AOM or NMU (Ward et al.,
1973; Watanabe et al., 1978).

Fleiszer et al. (1980) have studied the effects of different levels
of fiber on DMH-induced colon cancer in rats. Four diets were used:
very high fiber (28%) supplied as bran cereal; high fiber (15%) supplied
as a special rat chow; low fiber (5%) supplied as standard rat chow; and
a fiber-free, semipurified diet. Fewer cancers occurred in the rats fed
the very high fiber and high fiber diets, than in those given the low
fiber diet. Because the basal diet for the fiber-free group was considerably different, the response of these animals cannot be reasonably
compared with those of the other animals.

Although components of dietary fiber generally appear to exert a
protective effect against DMH-induced carcinogenesis, Glauert et al.
(1981) recently reported that dietary agar (a fiber-rich component of
the diet) enhanced DMH-induced colon cancer in mice.

The effects of dietary fiber have been compared in rats treated with
AOM or NMU (Watanabe et al., 1979). The substances tested were alfalfa,
pectin, and wheat bran fed as 15% of a diet that also contained 5% cellulose. When the carcinogen was given parenterally, pectin exerted a
protective effect but alfalfa and bran were ineffective. When the carcinogen was given by intrarectal instillation, alfalfa enhanced carcinogenesis, but pectin and bran were not protective.

Alfalfa has a relatively strong ability to bind bile acids (Story and
Kritchevsky, 1976). Cassidy et al. (1981) demonstrated that substances
with this binding capacity disrupt the topography of the colonic mucosa.
The denuded epithelium would then be susceptible to the action of a
locally administered carcinogen.

Although some data suggest that some types of fiber (e.g., bran and
cellulose) can protect rats from the action of certain chemical carcinogens, the collated data from different experiments are difficult to compare or interpret, primarily because of the lack of uniform experimental
protocols. The strains of rats, their diets, age, the carcinogens used,
and routes of administration all differ. The animal model is useful to
study the effects of fiber on carcinogenesis in the large bowel, but the
lack of standardization must be borne in mind when assessing or comparing
data.

SUMMARY

Epidemiological Evidence

Both correlation and case-control studies have yielded results that either support or contradict the hypothesis that dietary fiber protects against colorectal cancer. In both types of studies, most analyses have been based on total fiber consumption estimated by grouping foods (such as fruits, vegetables, and cereals) according to their fiber content. However, in the only case-control study and the only correlation study in which the total fiber consumption was quantified rather than estimated from the fiber-rich foods in the diet, no association was found between total fiber consumption and the risk of colon cancer. Thus, the epidemiological evidence suggesting an inverse relationship between total fiber intake and the occurrence of colon cancer is not yet compelling.

In the only study in which the effects of individual components of fiber were assessed, there was an inverse correlation between the incidence of colon cancer and the consumption of the pentosan fraction of fiber (found in whole wheat products). Thus, it seems likely that further epidemiological study of fiber will be productive only if the relationship of cancer to specific components of fiber can be analyzed.

Experimental Evidence

A few laboratory studies have also shown that some types of high fiber ingredients (e.g., cellulose and bran) depress the tumorigenicity of certain chemical carcinogens. However, the data are inconsistent-- especially with respect to the type of fiber or specific chemical carcinogen. Moreover, they are difficult to equate with the results of epidemiological studies because most laboratory experiments have examined specific fibers or their individual components, whereas most epidemiological studies have focused on fiber-containing foods whose exact composition has not been determined. Further information is needed on the basic chemistry and biological effects of fiber and its components to pursue experimental studies that will produce meaningful results.

CONCLUSION

The committee found no conclusive evidence to indicate that dietary fiber (such as that present in fruits, vegetables, grains, and cereals) exerts a protective effect against colorectal cancer in humans. Both epidemiological and laboratory reports suggest that if there is such an effect, specific components of fiber, rather than total dietary fiber, are more likely to be responsible.

REFERENCES

Barbolt, T. A., and R. Abraham. 1978. The effect of bran on dimethyl-hydrazine-induced colon carcinogenesis in the rat. Proc. Soc. Exp. Biol. Med. 157:656-659.

Bingham, S., D. R. R. Williams, T. J. Cole, and W. P. T. James. 1979. Dietary fibre and regional large-bowel cancer mortality in Britain. Br. J. Cancer 40:456-463.

Bjelke, E. 1978. Dietary factors and the epidemiology of cancer of the stomach and large bowel. Aktuel. Ernaehrungsmed. Klin. Prax. Suppl. 2:10-17.

Burkitt, D. P., and H. C. Trowell. 1975. Refined Carbohydrate Foods and Disease. Some Implications of Dietary Fibre. Academic Press, London, New York, and San Francisco. 356 pp.

Cassidy, M. M., F. G. Lightfoot, L. E. Grau, J. A. Story, D. Kritchevsky, and G. V. Vahouny. 1981. Effect of chronic intake of dietary fibers on the ultrastructural topography of rat jejunum and colon: A scanning electron microscopy study. Am. J. Clin. Nutr. 34:218-228.

Chen, W.-F., A. S. Patchefsky, and H. S. Goldsmith. 1978. Colonic protection from dimethylhydrazine by a high fiber diet. Surg. Gynecol. Obstet. 147:503-506.

Dales, L. G., G. D. Friedman, H. K. Ury, S. Grossman, and S. R. Williams. 1978. A case-control study of relationships of diet and other traits to colorectal cancer in American blacks. Am. J. Epidemiol. 109:132-144.

Drasar, B. S., and D. Irving. 1973. Environmental factors and cancer of the colon and breast. Br. J. Cancer 27:167-172.

Fleiszer, D. M., D. Murray, G. K. Richards, and R. A. Brown. 1980. Effects of diet on chemically induced bowel cancer. Can. J. Surg. 23:67-73.

Freeman, H. J., G. A. Spiller, and Y. S. Kim. 1978. A double-blind study on the effect of purified cellulose dietary fiber on 1,2-dimethylhydrazine-induced rat colonic neoplasia. Cancer Res. 38:2912-2917.

Freeman, H. J., G. A. Spiller, and Y. S. Kim. 1980. A double-blind study on the effects of differing purified cellulose and pectin fiber diets on 1,2-dimethylhydrazine-induced rat colonic neoplasia. Cancer Res. 40:2661-2665.

Glauert, H. P., M. R. Bennink, and C. H. Sander. 1981. Enhancement of 1,2-dimethylhydrazine-induced colon carcinogenesis in mice by dietary agar. Food Cosmet. Toxicol. 19:281-286.

Glober, G. A., K. L. Klein, J. O. Moore, and B. C. Abba. 1974. Bowel transit-times in two populations experiencing similar colon-cancer risks. Lancet 2:80-81.

Glober, G. A., A. Nomura, S. Kamiyama, A. Shimada, and B. C. Abba. 1977. Bowel transit-time and stool weight in populations with different colon-cancer risks. Lancet 2:110-111.

Hill, M., R. MacLennan, and K. Newcombe. 1979. Letter to the Editor: Diet and large-bowel cancer in three socioeconomic groups in Hong Kong. Lancet 1:436.

Jain, M., G. M. Cook, F. G. Davis, M. G. Grace, G. R. Howe, and A. B. Miller. 1980. A case-control study of diet and colo-rectal cancer. Int. J. Cancer 26:757-768.

Liu, K., J. Stamler, D. Moss, D. Garside, V. Persky, and I. Soltero. 1979. Dietary cholesterol, fat, and fibre, and colon-cancer mortality. Lancet 2:782-785.

Lyon, J. L., and A. W. Sorenson. 1978. Colon cancer in a low-risk population. Am. J. Clin. Nutr. 31:S227-S230.

MacLennan, R., O. M. Jensen, J. Mosbech, and H. Vuori. 1978. Diet, transit time, stool weight, and colon cancer in two Scandinavian populations. Am. J. Clin. Nutr. 31:S239-S242.

Malhotra, S. L. 1977. Dietary factors in a study of cancer colon from cancer registry, with special reference to the role of saliva, milk and fermented milk products and vegetable fibre. Med. Hypotheses 3:122-126.

Martínez, I., R. Torres, Z. Frías, J. R. Colón, and M. Fernández. 1979. Factors associated with adenocarcinomas of the large bowel in Puerto Rico. Pp. 45-52 in J. M. Birch, ed. Advances in Medical Oncology, Research and Education. Volume 3: Epidemiology. Pergamon Press, Oxford, New York, Toronto, Sydney, Paris, and Frankfurt.

Modan, B., V. Barell, F. Lubin, M. Modan, R. A. Greenberg, and S. Graham. 1975. Low-fiber intake as an etiologic factor in cancer of the colon. J. Natl. Cancer Inst. 55:15-18.

National Academy of Sciences. 1980. Recommended Dietary Allowances, 9th Edition. Committee on Dietary Allowances, Food and Nutrition Board, National Academy of Sciences, Washington, D.C. 187 pp.

Story, J. A., and D. Kritchevsky. 1976. Comparison of the binding of various bile acids and bile salts in vitro by several types of fiber. J. Nutr. 106:1292-1294.

Ward, J. M., R. S. Yamamoto, and J. H. Weisburger. 1973. Cellulose dietary bulk and azoxymethane-induced intestinal cancer. J. Natl. Cancer Inst. 51:713-715.

Watanabe, K., B. S. Reddy, C. Q. Wong, and J. H. Weisburger. 1978. Effect of dietary undegraded carrageenin on colon carcinogenesis in F344 rats treated with azoxymethane or methylnitrosourea. Cancer Res. 38:4427-4430.

Watanabe, K., B. S. Reddy, J. H. Weisburger, and D. Kritchevsky. 1979. Effect of dietary alfalfa, pectin, and wheat bran on azoxymethane- or methylnitrosourea-induced colon carcinogenesis in F344 rats. J. Natl. Cancer Inst. 63:141-145.

Wilson, R. B., D. P. Hutcheson, and L. Wideman. 1977. Dimethyl-hydrazine-induced colon tumors in rats fed diets containing beef fat or corn oil with and without wheat bran. Am. J. Clin. Nutr. 30:176-181.

9 Vitamins

In recent years, there has been considerable interest in the role of vitamins A, C, and E in the genesis and prevention of cancer. In contrast, little attention has been paid to the B vitamins and others such as vitamin K. The evidence concerning vitamins A, C, E, and selected B vitamins is discussed below.

VITAMIN A

Of the entire collection of chemically diverse substances classi- fied as vitamins, those subsumed under the general term "vitamin A" are of the greatest current interest in terms of their possible association with the process of carcinogenesis. The only well-understood function of vitamin A is its role in the visual cycle. The involvement of this vitamin in cell differentiation, although less well documented, pro- vides a rational basis for examining its relationship to cancer.

Ingested vitamin A is absorbed in the bloodstream and stored in the liver, and can reach toxic levels if large amounts are consumed. Blood levels of vitamin A are regulated by a feedback mechanism, but they do not usually reflect the amounts consumed in the diet or stored in the liver.

Epidemiological Evidence

The impact of vitamin A on carcinogenesis is of considerable interest. Several epidemiological investigations, mostly case-control studies, have indicated an inverse relationship between "vitamin A" intake and a variety of cancers. With few exceptions, the estimates of vitamin A were based on frequency of ingestion of a group of foods (e.g., green and yellow vegetables) known to be rich in β-carotene (a provitamin that may be enzymatically converted to vitamin A in vivo) and a few foods such as whole milk and liver containing preformed retinol (vitamin A). Thus, to a large extent, these studies have measured indirect indices of β-carotene intake. In this discussion the term vitamin A will also be used to include β-carotene, since the two components are not distinguished in most of the reports.

Lung. Bjelke (1975) was one of the first investigators to report epidemiological data suggesting that vitamin A plays a protective role against cancer. Using frequency data collected by a questionnaire

138

mailed to a cohort of Norwegian men, he derived a vitamin A index based on limited sources of the vitamin. He observed lower values for lung cancer cases than for controls after controlling for cigarette smoking. MacLennan et al. (1977) found an inverse association between consumption of green, leafy vegetables rich in "vitamin A" and lung cancer in a case-control study among Chinese females in Singapore.

In a case-control study conducted by Gregor et al. (1980), hospital outpatients, mostly from a rheumatology clinic, were used as controls. These investigators found that significantly less vitamin A had been consumed by male lung cancer cases than by controls, mainly because cases had consumed fewer vitamin A supplements and less liver. The few female cases had a different proportional distribution of tumor cell type than the males and showed an opposite (direct) overall association with vitamin A intake, although they also consumed fewer vitamin A supplements than the controls.

The use of vitamin A supplements was inversely associated with cancer, including lung cancer, in men (but not women) in a case-control study reported by Smith and Jick (1978). Mettlin et al. (1979) reported results of a case-control study in which an index of vitamin A consumption, based on frequency of consumption of a group of food items, was inversely associated with lung cancer in males, after controlling for cigarette smoking. In 28 patients with bronchial carcinoma, plasma levels of vitamin A were lower than those in a small group of controls (Basu et al., 1976; Sakula, 1976).

Shekelle et al. (1981) reported the findings of a 19-year follow-up study of 1,954 men in Chicago. Lung cancer incidence was inversely associated with carotene intake both with and without adjustment for cigarette smoking. There was no significant association of lung cancer with the intake of preformed vitamin A.

Larynx. Graham et al. (1981) studied male cases of laryngeal cancer and controls. After controlling for cigarette smoking and alcohol consumption, they found an inverse relationship (with a dose-response gradient) between cancer risk and indices of both vitamins A and C intake based on frequency of consumption of selected foods. They reported similar results for vegetable consumption in general, but not for cruciferous vegetables in particular.

Bladder. In a case-control study designed like the one conducted on lung cancer, Mettlin et al. (1979) reported a similar inverse association of a vitamin A consumption index with bladder cancer, after controlling for coffee consumption, smoking, and occupational exposure.

Esophagus. Wynder and Bross (1961) reported that frequencies of consumption of milk, and of green and yellow vegetables (sources of vitamin A and β-carotene, respectively) were lower for esophageal cancer cases than for controls. Mettlin et al. (1981) reported a similar inverse association and a dose-response gradient for frequency of consumption of fruits and vegetables in a study of male cases and controls, after controlling for cigarette smoking and alcohol consumption. Although they also found an inverse relationship for an index of vitamin A consumption based on selected foods, there was an even stronger inverse relationship for an index of vitamin C consumption. Also consistent with these findings were observations of populations in the Caspian littoral of Iran (a region of particularly high esophageal cancer incidence) indicating that consumption of green vegetables and fresh fruit and estimated vitamin A and C intake in high risk areas were lower than in areas of low risk (Hormozdiari et al., 1975; Joint Iran-International Agency for Research on Cancer Study Group, 1977). In a subsequent case-control study in this region, investigators also found that cases had consumed smaller amounts of uncooked vegetables (as well as fruits) than had controls (Cook-Mozaffari, 1979; Cook-Mozaffari et al., 1979).

Stomach. Among other findings, Hirayama (1967) reported an inverse association between daily consumption of milk (a vitamin A source) and stomach cancer in a case-control study in Japan. More recently, Hirayama (1977) reported a similar "protective" effect of milk based on data from a prospective cohort study involving 265,118 subjects. There was also a lower risk for stomach cancer among non-smokers who consumed green and yellow vegetables.

Graham et al. (1972) reported higher consumption of uncooked vegetables (likely sources of β-carotene) by controls than by cases in a case-control study of gastric cancer in New York State. A similar inverse association with consumption of raw vegetables was noted by Haenszel et al. (1972) in a case-control study in Hawaii.

Colon/Rectum. In ongoing cohort studies in Norway and Minnesota, Bjelke (1978) has found that milk and several vegetables have been consumed with less frequency by colorectal cancer cases than by controls. An index of vitamin A intake (which was highly correlated with consumption of vegetables) showed the same inverse relationship.

Prostate. In a study on prostate cancer, Schuman et al. (1982) found that foods rich in vitamin A (e.g., liver) and β-carotene (e.g., carrots) were consumed less frequently by cases than by controls.

General. In three recent reports based on data from cohort studies in the United States and England, the investigators observed that there was an inverse relationship between serum levels of vitamin A and subsequent risk of cancer in general (Cambien et al., 1980; Kark et al., 1980; Wald et al., 1980). The relationship between dietary intake of vitamin A and its level in serum (which is under homeostatic control) is not yet clear in populations such as these, which are generally not deficient in this nutrient.

Experimental Evidence

In the following discussion, the term "vitamin A" is used to include: vitamin A itself, synthetic analogues of vitamin A called retinoids, and naturally occurring plant constituents, the carotenoids, which can be converted to vitamin A in vivo.

Vitamin A is necessary for normal differentiation of epithelial cells in many tissues. A deficiency of this vitamin results in metaplasia, a pathological condition in which a keratinizing squamous epithelium replaces the form of epithelium that is normal to various tissues (Wolbach and Howe, 1925). In the bronchial mucosa, for example, the mucus-secreting columnar epithelium is replaced by a stratified squamous epithelium. Of relevance to the relationship between vitamin A and cancer is the occurrence of metaplasia, early in the evolution of many neoplasms. In the tissue undergoing malignant transformation, the normal differentiation pattern is lost and a new form of epithelium appears.

Vitamin A Deficiency. Since the appearance of metaplasia is common to both vitamin A deficiency and early neoplasia, a deficiency of this vitamin might enhance the neoplastic response to chemical carcinogens. In vitro experiments in organ cultures have supported this concept. In an organ culture of mouse prostatic tissue, vitamin A was shown to prevent the induction of metaplasia induced either by a culture medium deficient in vitamin A or by carcinogenic polycyclic aromatic hydrocarbons (Lasnitzki, 1963). In organ cultures of hamster tracheas, vitamin A inhibited the induction of squamous cell metaplasia and proliferative epithelial lesions by benzo[a]pyrene (Crocker and Sanders, 1970).

Some in vivo experiments have produced similar results. For example, Nettesheim and Williams (1976) reported that the induction of neoplastic lesions of the lungs by 3-methylcholanthrene was enhanced in rats deprived of vitamin A intake. This conclusion was based on observations of squamous nodules in the lungs, which have been demonstrated to be precursors of squamous cell carcinomas. Vitamin A deficiency also affects the mucosa of the urinary bladder, producing squamous cell metaplasia as well as a high incidence of cystitis, ureteritis, and pyelonephritis. The effects of vitamin A deficiency have been investigated in rats given $\underline{N}$-[4-(5-nitro-2-furyl)-2-thiazolyl]-formamide (FANFT), a compound that causes cancer of the bladder. In Sprague-Dawley rats maintained on a diet deficient in vitamin A, there was an acceleration in the neoplastic response to FANFT, resulting in an earlier appearance of urinary bladder tumors and the development of ureteral and pelvic carcinomas (Cohen et al., 1976).

Although squamous cell metaplasia in the mucosa of the large bowel does not occur with vitamin A deficiency, several studies have been conducted to determine the effect of such a deficiency on carcinogen-induced neoplasia of the large bowel in the rat (Narisawa et al., 1976; Newberne and Rogers, 1973; Rogers et al., 1973). Rogers et al. (1973) studied the effects of a low vitamin A intake on response of rats to intragastric administration of 1,2-dimethylhydrazine. They observed a slight increase in the incidence of tumors of the large bowel in the animals on the low vitamin A diet. Different results were obtained by Narisawa et al. (1976), who administered the carcinogen N-methyl-N'-nitro-N-nitrosoguanidine (MNNG) intrarectally to rats. In this study, animals fed a diet free of vitamin A developed fewer neoplastic lesions of the large bowel than those supplemented with vitamin A or fed a commercial chow diet with adequate vitamin A content.

An experiment of a somewhat different nature was conducted by Newberne and Rogers (1973). In this study, rats were exposed to the carcinogen aflatoxin and were fed diets containing various amounts of vitamin A. Animals deficient in vitamin A developed tumors of the large bowel, whereas rats fed a diet containing adequate amounts of vitamin A did not. Neoplasms of the liver developed in both groups of animals; however, there were fewer liver tumors in the group deficient in vitamin A. Thus, the overall effect was a shift in site of neoplasms rather than an overall change in tumor incidence (Newberne and Rogers, 1973).

In summary, studies in animals indicate that a deficiency of vitamin A can result in an increased susceptibility to carcinogen-induced neoplasia; however, there are exceptions.

Excess Intake of Vitamin A. Investigations have also been conducted to determine the effect of excess vitamin A on the occurrence of neoplasia in animals. Saffiotti et al. (1967) demonstrated that a high intake of vitamin A protected against benzo[a]pyrene-induced metaplasia and squamous cell neoplasms of the tracheobroncial tree in hamsters. Supporting data reported by Nettesheim and Williams (1976) indicated that vitamin A protects against 3-methylcholanthrene-induced squamous cell metaplasia and early neoplastic lesions of the lung in rats. In contrast, Smith et al. (1975) observed that an intake of high levels of vitamin A increases the incidence of respiratory tract tumors in hamsters. Retinyl acetate has also been shown to enhance hormone-induced mammary tumorigenesis in female GR/A mice (Welsch et al., 1981). In studies of other target sites, Chu and Malmgren (1965) and Shamberger (1971) observed that a high intake of vitamin A inhibited formation of tumors of the forestomach and cervix in hamsters and the skin of mice. Rogers et al. (1973) reported that the induction of neoplasia in the large bowel of rats by 1,2-dimethylhydrazine (DMH) was slightly enhanced by a high intake of the vitamin.

To summarize, studies in animals indicate that an increased intake of this vitamin has a protective effect against the induction of cancer by chemical carcinogens in most, but not all, instances.

Retinoids. Results from the studies of vitamin A have stimulated efforts to find analogues with a greater inhibitory effect on neoplasia, less toxicity, and a capability of reaching target tissues in concentrations higher than those of the naturally occurring vitamin. Many such compounds, the retinoids, have been synthesized, but are not normal constituents of the diet. Experiments to study the inhibition of carcinogen-induced neoplasia of the breast, urinary bladder, skin, and lung by these analogues have produced impressive results (see review by Sporn and Newton, 1979, 1981; Sporn et al., 1976). These compounds have also been responsible for regression of skin papillomas in mice (Bollag, 1971). The effects of these compounds buttress observations from studies of naturally occurring vitamin A.

Carotenoids. In plants there is a group of compounds, the carotenoids, that can be converted into vitamin A in vivo. These compounds can also be absorbed unchanged from the gastrointestinal tract and exist in tissues in their original form. In a recent review of epidemiological data on vitamin A and related compounds, Peto et al. (1981) considered the possibility that β-carotene itself rather than its derivative, vitamin A, may have the capacity to inhibit carcinogenesis in epithelial cells. Only a few studies have been conducted to investigate the effects of carotenoids on neoplasia in laboratory animals. Recently, Mathews-Roth et al. (1977) observed that β-carotene, canthaxanthin (4-4'-diketo-β-carotene), and phytoene can produce a significant protective effect against the development of UV-induced skin tumors in hairless mice. Since canthaxanthin and phytoene are carotenoids that do not have vitamin A activity, the protective effect appears to reside in the carotenoid structure per se. In an earlier study, Shamberger (1971) reported experiments in which β-carotene applied to the skin of mice concomitantly with croton oil increased the formation of epidermal tumors previously initiated by 7,12-dimethylbenz-[a]anthracene (DMBA). Considerable further research is necessary to evaluate the effects of carotenoids on carcinogenesis in laboratory animals.

Summary

Epidemiological Evidence. A growing accumulation of epidemiological evidence indicates that there is an inverse relationship between the risk of cancer and the consumption of foods containing vitamin A (e.g., liver) or its precursors (e.g., some carotenoids in dark green and deep yellow vegetables). Most of the data, however, do not show whether the effects are due to carotenoids, to vitamin A itself, or to some other constituents of these foods. In these studies, investigators found an inverse association between estimates of "vitamin A" intake and carcinoma at several sites, e.g., the lung, the urinary bladder, and the larynx. All these cancers involve epithelial cells.

Experimental Evidence. Studies in animals indicate that vitamin A deficiency generally increases susceptibility to chemically induced

neoplasia, and that an increased intake of the vitamin appears to protect against carcinogenesis in most, but not all, cases. Because high
doses of vitamin A are toxic, many of these studies have been conducted
with its synthetic analogues, retinoids, which lack some of the toxic
effects of the vitamin. These analogues have been shown to inhibit
chemically induced neoplasia of the breast, urinary bladder, skin, and
lung.

Conclusion

The committee concluded that the laboratory evidence shows that
vitamin A itself and many of the retinoids are able to suppress chemically induced tumors. The epidemiological evidence is sufficient to
suggest that foods rich in carotenes or vitamin A are associated with a
reduced risk of cancer. The toxicity of vitamin A in doses exceeding
those required for optimum nutrition, and the difficulty of epidemiological studies to distinguish the effects of carotenes from those of
vitamin A, argue against increasing vitamin A intake by the use of
supplements.

VITAMIN C (ASCORBIC ACID)

Epidemiological Evidence

The associations of vitamin C with cancer in epidemiological studies are mostly indirect since they are based on the consumption of
foods known to contain high concentrations of the vitamin. In general,
the data suggest that vitamin C may lower the risk of cancer, particularly in the esophagus and stomach.

In 1964, Meinsma noted that the consumption of citrus fruits by
cases of gastric cancer was lower than that by controls. Similar
inverse associations between fresh fruit consumption or vitamin C
intake and gastric cancer have been reported by Higginson (1966),
Haenszel and Correa (1975), Bjelke (1978), and Kolonel et al. (1981).
These observations are consistent with the hypothesis that vitamin C
protects against gastric cancer by blocking the reaction of secondary
and higher amines with nitrite to form nitrosamines (Correa et al.,
1975).

As noted in the discussion of vitamin A, Mettlin et al. (1981)
found inverse associations of indices of both vitamin A and vitamin
C consumption with esophageal cancer, based on frequency of consumption of selected food items by male cases and controls. The relationship was stronger for vitamin C than for vitamin A, however, and
only the association with vitamin C was statistically significant
after controlling for smoking and alcohol use. In studies of human
populations on the Caspian littoral of Iran, inverse associations have

been found between esophageal cancer and consumption of fresh fruits and estimated intake of vitamin C, based on correlational and case-control data (Cook-Mozaffari, 1979; Cook-Mozaffari et al., 1979; Hormozdiari et al., 1975; Joint Iran-International Agency for Research on Cancer Study Group, 1977).

A protective role for vitamin C in laryngeal cancer was also inferred in a case-control study conducted by Graham et al. (1981). These investigators found an inverse relationship between cancer risk and indices of both vitamins C and A, after controlling for cigarette smoking and alcohol consumption. There was a similar relationship for vegetable consumption in general, but not for cruciferous vegetables in particular.

Wassertheil-Smoller et al. (1981) recently reported a similar inverse association between vitamin C consumption (calculated from analysis of 3-day records of foods and a 24-hour recall) and uterine cervical dysplasia in a case-control study of women in New York. The findings persisted after the investigators controlled for age and sexual activity in the analysis.

In contrast, Jain et al. (1980) found no association between vitamin C consumption and colon cancer in a case-control study based on quantitative data obtained from dietary histories.

Experimental Evidence

Vitamin C has also been studied for its effects on cancer under a variety of experimental conditions. The simplest studies are those that have demonstrated that ascorbic acid can prevent the reaction of nitrites with amines or amides to form carcinogenic nitroso compounds. Ascorbic acid effectively competes for the nitrite, thereby inhibiting the formation of the carcinogenic nitroso compounds (Ivankovic et al., 1975; Mirvish, 1981; Mirvish et al., 1972, 1975). Investigations of this phenomenon in vitro and in vivo have been published by a number of scientists. In a prototype in vitro study, Mirvish et al. (1972) demonstrated that ascorbic acid inhibited formation of nitroso compounds resulting from the reaction of nitrites with oxytetracycline, morpholine, piperazine, N-methylaniline, methylurea, and dimethylamine. In subsequent in vivo studies, they showed that ascorbic acid inhibits formation of nitroso carcinogens in mice (Mirvish et al., 1975). In their experimental model, Swiss and Strain A mice were fed amines or amides in the diet and were given nitrite in their drinking water. Under these conditions, pulmonary tumors developed. The addition of ascorbic acid to the diet resulted in a marked inhibition of these tumors. Ascorbic acid also consistently produced an inhibitory effect in other in vivo studies when nitrite and amino compounds were administered by the same routes (Ivankovic et al., 1975; Mirvish, 1981; Rustia, 1975).

The effect of vitamin C on carcinogenesis resulting from exposures to already formed carcinogens is not clearly understood. Experiments to study this are complicated by the fact that the guinea pig is the only laboratory animal that, like primates, does not synthesize vitamin C. Moreover, the endogenous synthesis of vitamin C responds easily to various stimuli, e.g., exposures to certain xenobiotic compounds. Data presented in two abstracts indicate that ascorbic acid inhibited neoplasia of the large bowel in rats given 1,2-dimethylhydrazine (Logue and Frommer, 1980; Reddy and Hirota, 1979). Kallistratos and Fasske (1980) reported that administration of a high dose of ascorbic acid in the diet of rats inhibited the induction of sarcoma by benzo[a]pyrene. Only a few animals were used in this investigation. Soloway et al. (1975) reported that ascorbic acid had no effect on the occurrence of neoplasia in the rat bladder after administration of FANFT. Overall, the reported protective effects of ascorbic acid on neoplasia are not impressive, except for those brought about through an indirect mechanism, i.e., the prevention of the formation of carcinogenic N-nitroso compounds. In only two instances have investigators reported inhibition of carcinogenesis in the same tissue, i.e., the large bowel (Logue and Frommer, 1980; Reddy and Hirota, 1979). However, since these studies were reported only in abstract form, their results warrant further investigation.

In a study with a small number of guinea pigs, a high dietary intake of ascorbic acid had a slight enhancing effect on the induction of sarcoma by 3-methylcholanthrene (Banic, 1981). Russell et al. (1952) also studied the induction of sarcoma by the same compound in three groups of guinea pigs: a group deficient in vitamin C, a group receiving vitamin C but on a food-restricted diet, and a group fed ad libitum. The number of animals developing tumors was similar in all three groups, but the latent period was slightly shorter in the vitamin-C-deficient group, indicating that the response produced by vitamin C deficiency was very slight or nonexistent.

Recently, observations on the effects of vitamin C on cells in culture have indicated that ascorbic acid can affect cellular manifestations of malignancy. When C3H/10T1/2 mouse embryo cells are exposed to 3-methylcholanthrene, morphological transformation occurs. However, the transformation is prevented if ascorbic acid is added to the culture medium. Addition of the ascorbic acid as late as 23 days after the treatment with 3-methylcholanthrene still completely inhibits transformation. Under some circumstances, it is possible to cause reversion of chemically transformed cells to normal-appearing morphological phenotypes by adding ascorbic acid to the culture medium (Benedict et al., 1980). The mechanism for inhibition and reversion is presently unknown.

The effects of ascorbic acid on human leukemia cells in culture have also been studied. Low concentrations of ascorbic acid were found to suppress growth of human leukemia cells from patients with acute nonlymphocytic leukemia under conditions in which growth of normal myeloid colonies was not suppressed (Park et al., 1980).

Summary

Epidemiological Evidence. The epidemiological data pertaining to the effect of vitamin C on the occurrence of cancer are not extensive. Furthermore, they provide mostly indirect evidence since they are based on the consumption of foods, especially fresh fruits and vegetables, known to contain high concentrations of the vitamin, rather than on actual measurements of vitamin C intake. The results of several case-control studies and a few correlation studies suggest that the consumption of vitamin-C-containing foods is associated with a lower risk for certain cancers, particularly gastric and esophageal cancer.

Experimental Evidence. In the laboratory, ascorbic acid can inhibit the formation of carcinogenic N-nitroso compounds, both in vitro and in vivo. On the other hand, studies of its inhibitory effect on the action of preformed carcinogens have not provided conclusive results. In recent studies, the addition of ascorbic acid to cells grown in culture prevented the chemically induced transformation of these cells and, in some cases, caused reversion of transformed cells.

Conclusion

The limited evidence suggests that vitamin C can inhibit the formation of some carcinogens and that the consumption of vitamin-C-containing foods is associated with a lower risk of cancers of the stomach and esophagus.

VITAMIN E (α-Tocopherol)

Epidemiological Evidence

There are as yet no epidemiological data associating vitamin E with cancer risk, and such data may prove difficult to obtain for several reasons. First, vitamin E is present in a wide variety of foods (e.g., vegetable oils, whole grain cereal products, and eggs), which makes it difficult to identify groups of people with substantially different levels of intake. In addition, a clear-cut deficiency has not been established in humans. Vitamin E is also relatively unstable during storage, and its concentration can vary greatly within individual foodstuffs.

Experimental Evidence

Of the various tocopherols, vitamin E (α-tocopherol) is most widely distributed among different foods and has the greatest biological activity (Harris et al., 1972). The vast majority of studies of the relationship of the tocopherols and cancer have been conducted with α-tocopherol. Like vitamin C, α-tocopherol competes for available nitrite, thereby blocking the formation of carcinogenic nitroso compounds from reactions between nitrite and nitrosatable substrates such as amines or amides (Fiddler et al., 1978; Mergens et al., 1978, 1979). An important difference between these vitamins is their solubility. Ascorbic acid is water soluble, whereas α-tocopherol is soluble in lipids. Thus, the inhibitory effects of α-tocopherol would take place largely in a lipid milieu.

There have been no in vivo studies to determine the effects on neoplasia resulting from α-tocopherol-induced inhibition of nitroso compound formation. However, Kamm et al. (1977) have reported that the in vivo formation of nitrosamines from precursor compounds resulted in hepatotoxicity. In this study, rats were intubated with a solution containing sodium nitrite and aminopyrene. This was followed by oral administration of α-tocopherol or vehicle. Animals receiving the vehicle had elevated SGPT (serum glutamic-pyruvic transaminase), indicating liver damage. Rats receiving α-tocopherol had either a lower elevation of SGPT or no elevation at all, depending on the dose of α-tocopherol administered. These investigators also reported that the rats receiving α-tocopherol had a markedly lower level of nitrosamines in their serum than did the corresponding controls.

Efforts to inhibit neoplasia by administering increased amounts of vitamin E have a long history. In one of the earliest studies, Jaffe (1946) reported that the number of mixed tumors resulting from intraperitoneal injection of 3-methylcholanthrene was lower in rats receiving a diet with added wheat germ oil than in rats on a control diet. Subsequently, Haber and Wissler (1962) studied the effect of α-tocopherol supplements on subcutaneous sarcomas induced by injecting mice with 3-methylcholanthrene. Their data suggested that α-tocopherol inhibited the occurrence of these sarcomas. In studies by Epstein et al. (1967), α-tocopherol and a number of other phenolic antioxidants did not suppress the formation of subcutaneous sarcomas induced in mice by injections of 3,4,9,10-dibenzpyrene. More recently, Wattenberg (1972) reported that addition of α-tocopherol to the diet prior to administration of the carcinogen failed to inhibit DMBA-induced neoplasia of the forestomach of mice.

Several investigators have studied the effects of α-tocopherol on DMBA-induced formation of mammary tumors. Wattenberg (1972) reported that ingestion of high levels of α-tocopherol only during the period before DMBA was administered did not inhibit the occurrence of mammary tumors. In a brief report, Harman (1969) presented data showing that a large vitamin E supplement in a semipurified diet fed from 11 days prior to DMBA administration until completion of the study decreased the number of tumor-bearing rats by slightly less than one-half. In another brief report, Lee and Chen (1979) indicated that rats fed diets either lacking α-tocopherol or containing one-half the minimum level recommended had an increased tumor incidence as compared to animals receiving a diet with adequate or excessive amounts of vitamin E.

The effects of vitamin E on epidermal neoplasia have also been studied. In one study, an increased intake of vitamin E was reported to have no inhibitory effect in mice (Wattenberg, 1972); in another, it was observed to produce a small degree of inhibition of mammary tumors in rats (Lee and Chen, 1979). Shamberger (1970) reported that addition of vitamin E to a solution containing tumor promoters (e.g., croton oil, croton resin, and phenol) inhibited formation of tumors in some instances, but this was not a consistent effect.

Cook and McNamara (1980) compared the effects of high and low doses of vitamin E on dimethylhydrazine-induced neoplasia in the large intestine of mice. The diet fed to the mice consisted of natural constituents fortified by vitamins and minerals, and contained 26% fat. Although the tumor incidence was similar in both groups, the average number of tumors per animal was less in the high vitamin E group than in the low vitamin E group.

Studies of the effects of vitamin E on carcinogenesis do not show severe or consistent inhibitory effects. It is possible that vitamin E can inhibit under certain conditions, but a reproducible experimental model in which vitamin E consistently inhibits neoplasia has not yet been found.

Summary and Conclusions

There are no reports of epidemiological studies concerning vitamin E intake and the risk of cancer.

Vitamin E (α-tocopherol), like ascorbic acid, inhibits the formation of nitrosamines *in vivo* and *in vitro*. However, there are no reports on the effect of this vitamin on nitrosoamine-induced neoplasia. There is limited evidence suggesting that vitamin E may inhibit tumorigenesis in several model systems.

The data are not sufficient to permit any firm conclusion to be drawn about the effect of vitamin E on cancer in humans.

CHOLINE AND SELECTED B VITAMINS

Since the B vitamins are essential components of any adequate diet and are necessary for the continued maintenance of cellular integrity and metabolic function, severe deficiencies in any of them will clearly reduce the growth rate of tumor cells and interfere with the normal functioning of the organism (Young and Newberne, 1981). However, only a few of these vitamins, such as thiamine, riboflavin, pyridoxine, vitamin B_{12}, and folic acid, are discussed in this chapter because data for others are inadequate. Choline, although not a vitamin by strict definition, is generally included in the vitamin B complex. To consider the roles of choline and the B vitamins in carcinogenesis, one must recognize the complex interrelationships of these vitamins with each other and with other components of diet, such as dietary protein and total calories. For example, secondary changes in protein, nucleic acid, carbohydrate, fat, and/or mineral metabolism can account for many of the effects observed with specific vitamins. Thus, although certain models have defined the roles of several of these vitamins at the molecular level, their overall contribution to modulation of carcinogenesis is difficult to assess.

Epidemiological Studies

No epidemiological studies have been conducted on the role of the B vitamins in carcinogenesis.

Experimental Studies

In much of the work demonstrating effects of specific B vitamins on carcinogenesis in model systems, there has been no control for intake of other dietary constituents, notably protein and calories. Thus, many results of such efforts are not useful since these two major components have considerable effect on the overall outcome of carcinogenesis. Notable early exceptions are studies by Tannenbaum and by Boutwell. These studies show that intake of B vitamins has either no effect, or at most a minimal effect, on carcinogenesis. Tannenbaum and Silverstone (1952) reported that there were no significant differences in the incidence of tumors among groups of animals fed minimal, moderate, or high levels of the B vitamins. In three of four experiments, however, the rate of tumor development was faster in mice ingesting moderate amounts of vitamins than in mice ingesting either high or low amounts. Boutwell et al. (1949) detected no effects of specific components, although when intake of all B vitamins was low, the incidence of tumors in mice was decreased.

Enzymatic activation or deactivation of procarcinogens involves competing pathways. These metabolic pathways can be modulated by dietary constituents such as vitamins and other nutrients, which in turn modulate carcinogenesis. For example, Kensler et al. (1941) demonstrated that riboflavin provided partial protection against hepatic cancer caused by orally administered dimethylaminoazobenzene in rats by enhancing the detoxification of that carcinogen by a flavin-dependent enzyme system (Miller and Miller, 1953; Miller et al., 1952). It seems likely that the opposite effect, i.e., enhancement of carcinogenic potential, might be observed if vitamin B_2 (riboflavin) were required for activation to the ultimate carcinogen. The cumulative effect of riboflavin-supplemented diets on hepatocarcinogenesis caused by other compounds and on tumorigenesis at other sites has not been adequately assessed. Thus, despite the existence of one clearly defined effect, which has a molecular basis, it is difficult to generalize about the role of vitamin B_2 in carcinogenesis.

The complex interrelationships between the B vitamins and other dietary components have been thoroughly examined in studies of diets deficient in lipotropes (e.g., methionine, choline, and folate) and high in fat content (Rogers and Newberne, 1980). Although the major lipotropes are choline and methionine, folate (and to some extent vitamin B_{12}) can also exert lipotropic action. Modulation of carcinogenesis by other vitamins, such as inositol and vitamin B_6, may contribute to the overall lipotropic activity of these diets. Individual B vitamins may have enhancing effects on carcinogenesis, depending on experimental conditions. Thus, only carefully controlled experiments can shed light on the specific contribution of each of the B vitamins. The overall results clearly demonstrate that the effects of B vitamins on carcinogenesis depend on the specific chemical carcinogen, the target organ, and the strain and sex of the animal. The relative importance of the individual dietary components may vary, depending on experimental conditions.

The relationship of the results of the short-term tests to those from in vivo studies for carcinogenicity of chemicals in animals adds a further complication. These differences in the findings from these two types of studies have been reviewed for various compounds including aflatoxin B_1 (Rogers and Newberne, 1969), N-nitrosodiethylamine (Rogers, 1977), N-nitrosodibutylamine, N-nitrosodimethylamine, N-2-fluorenylacetamide, 7,12-dimethylbenzanthracene, 1,2-dimethylhydrazine, and 3,3-diphenyl-3-dimethylcarbamyl-1-propine (Rogers and Newberne, 1980). Rogers and Newberne (1980) observed that the most consistent results obtained with lipotrope-deficient diets in rats were enhancement of hepatocarcinogenesis and, to a lesser extent, of colon carcinogenesis. These diets do not have a consistent effect on tumor induction in target organs other than the liver and colon (Rogers, 1977). In many cases, abnormalities in the metabolism of carcinogens can be demonstrated; however, their effects on tumor incidence cannot always be predicted.

Recently, considerable effort has been expended to determine whether or not the metabolism and transport of vitamins or the binding of the appropriate coenzyme forms to apoenzymes are altered in tumor cells (Thanassi et al., 1981; Tryfiates, 1981). For instance, in Morris hepatoma cells, the transport and phosphorylation of pyridoxine appear to be severely impaired (Thanassi et al., 1981). Effects on the metabolism of riboflavin have also been reported (Rivlin, 1973), but it is not known whether the observed alterations have any influence on the modulation of carcinogenesis. The alterations in vitamin B_6 metabolism may be due to secondary changes in the metabolism of amino acids, especially tryptophan (Bell, 1980; Bell et al., 1972; Byar and Blackard, 1977).

The effects on carcinogenesis by the B vitamins cannot be ascribed solely to effects modulating the stages of initiation or promotion

(Pitot and Sirica, 1980). These vitamins may also modulate other processes such as immunosurveillance, which may affect the ultimate outcome of carcinogenesis. Impairment of the immune function has been demonstrated in pyridoxine-deficient animals (Axelrod and Trakatellis, 1964), and it seems likely that major disruption of energy or carbohydrate metabolism by deficiencies of riboflavin or thiamine, as well as disruption of normal cell replication by deficiencies in folate or vitamin B_{12}, would affect immune surveillance. Because of the interrelationships among the B vitamins and their relationships with other major dietary components, it is difficult to explain specifically the effects on promotional events (Diamond et al., 1980).

The modulation of carcinogenesis by the B vitamins under conditions of normal dietary intake is probably minimal. However, a change of intake of a specific B vitamin may be warranted when a specific chemical carcinogen is present.

Summary and Conclusions

The relationship of dietary B vitamins to the occurrence of cancer has not been studied epidemiologically. There have been a few inadequate laboratory investigations to determine whether there is a relationship between the various B vitamins and the occurrence of cancer. Therefore, no conclusions can be drawn.

REFERENCES

Axelrod, A. E., and A. C. Trakatellis. 1964. Relationship of pyridoxine to immunological phenomena. Vitam. Horm. (N.Y.) 22:591-607.

Banic, S. 1981. Vitamin C acts as a cocarcinogen to methylcholanthrene in guinea-pigs. Cancer Lett. 11:239-242.

Basu, T. K., D. Donaldson, M. Jenner, D. C. Williams, and A. Sakula. 1976. Plasma vitamin A in patients with bronchial carcinoma. Br. J. Cancer 33:119-121.

Bell, E. 1980. Letter to the Editor: The excretion of a vitamin B6 metabolite and the probability of recurrence of early breast cancer. Eur. J. Cancer 16:297-298.

Bell, E. D., D. Tong, W. I. P. Mainwaring, J. L. Hayward, and R. D. Bulbrook. 1972. Tryptophan metabolism and recurrence rates after mastectomy in patients with breast cancer. Clin. Chim. Acta 42:445-447.

Benedict, W. F., W. L. Wheatley, and P. A. Jones. 1980. Inhibition of chemically induced morphological transformation and reversion of the transformed phenotype by ascorbic acid in C3H/10T-1/2 cells. Cancer Res. 40:2796-2801.

Bjelke, E. 1975. Dietary vitamin A and human lung cancer. Int. J. Cancer 15:561-565.

Bjelke, E. 1978. Dietary factors and the epidemiology of cancer of the stomach and large bowel. Aktuel. Ernaehrungsmed. Klin. Prax. Suppl. 2:10-17.

Bollag, W. 1971. Therapy of chemically induced skin tumors of mice with vitamin A palmitate and vitamin A acid. Experientia 27:90-92.

Boutwell, R. K., M. K. Brush, and H. P. Rusch. 1949. The influence of vitamins of the B complex on the induction of epithelial tumors in mice. Cancer Res. 9:747-752.

Byar, D., and C. Blackard. 1977. Comparisons of placebo, pyridoxine, and topical thiotepa in preventing recurrence of stage I bladder cancer. Urology 10:556-561.

Cambien, F., P. Ducimetiere, and J. Richard. 1980. Total serum cholesterol and cancer mortality in a middle-aged population. Am. J. Epidemiol. 112:388-394.

Chu, E. W., and R. A. Malmgren. 1965. An inhibitory effect of vitamin A on the induction of tumors of forestomach and cervix in the Syrian hamster by carcinogenic polycyclic hydrocarbons. Cancer Res. 25:884-895.

Cohen, S. M., J. F. Wittenberg, and G. T. Bryan. 1976. Effect of avitaminosis A and hypervitaminosis A on urinary bladder carcinogenicity of N-[4-(5-nitro-2-furyl)-2-thiazolyl]formamide. Cancer Res. 36:2334-2339.

Cook, M. G., and P. McNamara. 1980. Effect of dietary vitamin E on dimethylhydrazine-induced colonic tumors in mice. Cancer Res. 40:1329-1331.

Cook-Mozaffari, P. 1979. The epidemiology of cancer of the oesophagus. Nutr. Cancer 1(2):51-60.

Cook-Mozaffari, P. J., F. Azordegan, N. E. Day, A. Ressicand, C. Sabai, and B. Aramesh. 1979. Oesophageal cancer studies in the Caspian littoral of Iran: Results of a case-control study. Br. J. Cancer 39:293-309.

Correa, P., W. Haenszel, C. Cuello, S. Tannenbaum, and M. Archer. 1975. A model for gastric cancer epidemiology. Lancet 2:58-60.

Crocker, T. T., and L. L. Sanders. 1970. Influence of vitamin A and 3,7-dimethyl-2,6-octadienal (citral) on the effect of benzo(a)-pyrene on hamster trachea in organ culture. Cancer Res. 30:1312-1318.

Diamond, L., T. G. O'Brien, and W. M. Baird. 1980. Tumor promoters and the mechanism of tumor promotion. Adv. Cancer Res. 32:1-74.

Epstein, S. S., S. Joshi, J. Andrea, J. Forsyth, and N. Mantel. 1967. The null effect of antioxidants on the carcinogenicity of 3,4,9,10-dibenzpyrene to mice. Life Sci. 6:225-233.

Fiddler, W., J. W. Pensabene, E. G. Piotrowski, J. G. Phillips, J. Keating, W. J. Mergens, and H. L. Newmark. 1978. Inhibition of formation of volatile nitrosamines in fried bacon by the use of cure-solubilized α-tocopherol. J. Agric. Food Chem. 26:653-656.

Graham, S., W. Schotz, and P. Martino. 1972. Alimentary factors in the epidemiology of gastric cancer. Cancer 30:927-938.

Graham, S., C. Mettlin, J. Marshall, R. Priore, T. Rzepka, and D. Shedd. 1981. Dietary factors in the epidemiology of cancer of the larynx. Am. J. Epidemiol. 113:675-680.

Gregor, A., P. N. Lee, F. J. C. Roe, M. J. Wilson, and A. Melton. 1980. Comparison of dietary histories in lung cancer cases and controls with special reference to vitamin A. Nutr. Cancer 2:93-97.

Haber, S. L., and R. W. Wissler. 1962. Effect of vitamin E on carcinogenicity of methylcholanthrene. Proc. Soc. Exp. Biol. Med. 111:774-775.

Haenszel, W., and P. Correa. 1975. Developments in the epidemiology of stomach cancer over the past decade. Cancer Res. 35:3452-3459.

Haenszel, W., M. Kurihara, M. Segi, and R. K. C. Lee. 1972. Stomach cancer among Japanese in Hawaii. J. Natl. Cancer Inst. 49:969-988.

Harman, D. 1969. Dimethylbenzanthracene induced cancer: Inhibiting effect of dietary vitamin E. Clin. Res. 17:125. Abstract.

Harris, R. S., P. Schudel, H. Mayer, O. Isler, S. R. Ames, G. Brubacher, O. Wiss, J. Green, K. E. Mason, and M. K. Horwitt. 1972. Tocopherols. Pp. 165-317 in The Vitamins: Chemistry, Physiology, Pathology, Methods, Volume 5, 2nd Edition. Academic Press, New York and London.

Higginson, J. 1966. Etiological factors in gastro-intestinal cancer in man. J. Natl. Cancer Inst. 37:527-545.

Hirayama, T. 1967. The epidemiology of cancer of the stomach in Japan with special reference to the role of diet. Pp. 37-48 in R. J. C. Harris, ed. Proceedings of the 9th International Cancer Congress. UICC Monograph Series Volume 10. Springer-Verlag, Berlin, Heidelberg, and New York.

Hirayama, T. 1977. Changing patterns of cancer in Japan with special reference to the decrease in stomach cancer mortality. Pp. 55-75 in H. H. Hiatt, J. D. Watson, and J. A. Winsten, eds. Origins of Human Cancer, Book A: Incidence of Cancer in Humans. Cold Spring Harbor Laboratory, Cold Spring Harbor, N.Y.

Hormozdiari, H., N. E. Day, B. Aramesh, and E. Mahboubi. 1975. Dietary factors and esophageal cancer in the Caspian littoral of Iran. Cancer Res. 35:3493-3498.

Ivankovic, S., R. Preussmann, D. Schmähl, and J. W. Zeller. 1975. Prevention by ascorbic acid of in vivo formation of N-nitroso compounds. Pp. 101-102 in P. Bogovski and E. A. Walker, eds. N-Nitroso Compounds in the Environment. IARC Scientific Publications No. 9. International Agency for Research on Cancer, Lyon, France.

Jaffe, W. G. 1946. The influence of wheat germ oil on the production of tumors in rats by methylcholanthrene. Exp. Med. Surg. 4:278-282.

Jain, M., G. M. Cook, F. G. Davis, M. G. Grace, G. R. Howe, and A. B. Miller. 1980. A case-control study of diet and colo-rectal cancer. Int. J. Cancer 26:757-768.

Joint Iran-International Agency for Research on Cancer Study Group. 1977. Esophageal cancer studies in the Caspian littoral of Iran: Results of population studies--a prodrome. J. Natl. Cancer Inst. 59:1127-1138.

Kallistratos, G., and E. Fasske. 1980. Inhibition of benzo(a)-pyrene carcinogenesis in rats with vitamin C. J. Cancer Res. Clin. Oncol. 97:91-96.

Kamm, J. J., T. Dashman, H. Newmark, and W. J. Mergens. 1977. Inhibition of amine-nitrite hepatotoxicity by α-tocopherol. Toxicol. Appl. Pharmacol. 41:575-583.

Kark, J. D., A. H. Smith, and C. G. Hames. 1980. The relationship of serum cholesterol to the incidence of cancer in Evans County, Georgia. J. Chronic Dis. 33:311-322.

Kensler, C. J., K. Sugiura, N. F. Young, C. R. Halter, and C. P. Rhoads. 1941. Partial protection of rats by riboflavin with casein against liver cancer caused by dimethylaminoazobenzene. Science 93:308-310.

Kolonel, L. N., A. M. Y. Nomura, T. Hirohata, J. H. Hankin, and M. W. Hinds. 1981. Association of diet and place of birth with stomach cancer incidence in Hawaii Japanese and Caucasians. Am. J. Clin. Nutr. 34:2478-2485.

Lasnitzki, I. 1963. Growth pattern of the mouse prostate gland in organ culture and its response to sex hormones, vitamin A, and 3-methylcholanthrene. Natl. Cancer Inst. Monogr. 12:381-403.

Lee, C., and C. Chen. 1979. Enhancement of mammary tumorigenesis in rats by vitamin E deficiency. Proc. Am. Assoc. Cancer Res. Am. Soc. Clin. Oncol. 20:132. Abstract 531.

Logue, T., and D. Frommer. 1980. The influence of oral vitamin C supplements on experimental colorectal tumour induction. Austr. N. Z. J. Med. 10:588. Abstract.

MacLennan, R., J. Da Costa, N. E. Day, C. H. Law, Y. K. Ng, and K. Shanmugaratnam. 1977. Risk factors for lung cancer in Singapore Chinese, a population with high female incidence rates. Int. J. Cancer 20:854-860.

Mathews-Roth, M. M., M. A. Pathak, T. B. Fitzpatrick, L. H. Harber, and E. H. Kass. 1977. Beta carotene therapy for erythropoietic protoporphyria and other photosensitivity diseases. Arch. Dermatol. 113:1229-1232.

Meinsma, L. 1964. [In Dutch; English Summary.] Nutrition and Cancer. Voeding 25:357-365.

Mergens, W. J., J. J. Kamm, H. L. Newmark, W. Fiddler, and J. Pensabene. 1978. Alpha-tocopherol: Uses in preventing nitrosamine formation. Pp. 199-212 in E. A. Walker, M. Castegnaro, L. Griciute, and R. E. Lyle, eds. Environmental Aspects of N-Nitroso Compounds. IARC Scientific Publications No. 19. International Agency for Research on Cancer, Lyon, France.

Mergens, W. J., F. M. Vane, S. R. Tannenbaum, L. Green, and P. L. Skipper. 1979. In vitro nitrosation of methapyrilene. J. Pharm. Sci. 68:827-832.

Mettlin, C., S. Graham, and M. Swanson. 1979. Vitamin A and lung cancer. J. Natl. Cancer Inst. 62:1435-1438.

Mettlin, C., S. Graham, R. Priore, J. Marshall, and M. Swanson. 1981. Diet and cancer of the esophagus. Nutr. Cancer 2:143-147.

Miller, E. C., A. M. Plescia, J. A. Miller, and C. Heidelberger. 1952. The metabolism of methylated aminoazo dyes. I. The demethylation of 3'-methyl-4-dimethyl-C[14]-aminoazobenzene in vivo. J. Biol. Chem. 196:863-874.

Miller, J. A., and E. C. Miller. 1953. The carcinogenic aminoazo dyes. Adv. Cancer Res. 1:339-396.

Mirvish, S. S. 1981. Inhibition of the formation of carcinogenic N-nitroso compounds by ascorbic acid and other compounds. Pp. 557-587 in J. H. Burchenal and H. F. Oettgen, eds. Cancer: Achievements, Challenges, and Prospects for the 1980s, Volume 1. Grune and Stratton, New York, London, Toronto, Sydney, and San Francisco.

Mirvish, S. S., L. Wallcave, M. Eagen, and P. Shubik. 1972. Ascorbate-nitrite reaction: Possible means of blocking the formation of carcinogenic N-nitroso compounds. Science 177:65-68.

Mirvish, S. S., A. Cardesa, L. Wallcave, and P. Shubik. 1975. Induction of mouse lung adenomas by amines or ureas plus nitrite and by N-nitroso compounds: Effect of ascorbate, gallic acid, thiocyanate, and caffeine. J. Natl. Cancer Inst. 55:633-636.

Narisawa, T., B. S. Reddy, C.-Q. Wong, and J. H. Weisburger. 1976. Effect of vitamin A deficiency on rat colon carcinogenesis by N-methyl-N'-nitro-N-nitrosoguanidine. Cancer Res. 36:1379-1383.

Nettesheim, P., and M. L. Williams. 1976. The influence of vitamin A on the susceptibility of the rat lung to 3-methylcholanthrene. Int. J. Cancer 17:351-357.

Newberne, P. M., and A. E. Rogers. 1973. Rat colon carcinomas associated with aflatoxin and marginal vitamin A. J. Natl. Cancer Inst. 50:439-448.

Park, C. H., M. Amare, M. A. Savin, and B. Hoogstraten. 1980. Growth suppression of human leukemic cells in vitro by L-ascorbic acid. Cancer Res. 40:1062-1065.

Peto, R., R. Doll, J. D. Buckley, and M. B. Sporn. 1981. Can dietary beta-carotene materially reduce human cancer rates? Nature 290:201-208.

Pitot, H. C., and A. E. Sirica. 1980. The stages of initiation and promotion in hepatocarcinogenesis. Biochim. Biophys. Acta 605:191-215.

Reddy, B. S., and N. Hirota. 1979. Effect of dietary ascorbic acid on 1,2-dimethylhydrazine-induced colon cancer in rats. Fed. Proc. Fed. Am. Soc. Exp. Biol. 38:714. Abstract 2565.

Rivlin, R. S. 1973. Riboflavin and cancer: A review. Cancer Res. 33:1977-1986.

Rogers, A. E. 1977. Reduction of N-nitrosodiethylamine carcinogenesis in rats by lipotrope or amino acid supplementation of a marginally deficient diet. Cancer Res. 37:194-199.

Rogers, A. E., and P. M. Newberne. 1969. Aflatoxin B_1 carcinogenesis in lipotrope-deficient rats. Cancer Res. 29:1965-1972.

Rogers, A. E., and P. M. Newberne. 1980. Lipotrope deficiency in experimental carcinogenesis. Nutr. Cancer 2:104-112.

Rogers, A. E., B. J. Herndon, and P. M. Newberne. 1973. Induction by dimethylhydrazine of intestinal carcinoma in normal rats and rats fed high or low levels of vitamin A. Cancer Res. 33:1003-1009.

Russell, W. O., L. R. Ortega, and E. S. Wynne. 1952. Studies on methylcholanthrene induction of tumors in scorbutic guinea pigs. Cancer Res. 12:216-218.

Rustia, M. 1975. Inhibitory effect of sodium ascorbate on ethyl-urea and sodium nitrite carcinogenesis and negative findings in progeny after intestinal inoculation of precursors into pregnant hamsters. J. Natl. Cancer Inst. 55:1389-1394.

Saffiotti, U., R. Montesano, A. R. Sellakumar, and S. A. Borg. 1967. Experimental cancer of the lung: Inhibition by vitamin A of the induction of tracheobronchial squamous metaplasia and squamous cell tumors. Cancer 20:857-864.

Sakula, A. 1976. Letter to the Editor: Vitamin A and lung cancer. Br. Med. J. 2:298.

Schuman, L. M., J. S. Mandell, A. Radke, U. Seal, and F. Halberg. 1982. Some selected features of the epidemiology of prostatic cancer: Minneapolis-St. Paul, Minnesota case-control study, 1976-1979. Pp. 345-354 in K. Magnus, ed. Trends in Cancer Incidence: Causes and Practical Implications. Hemisphere Publishing Corp., Washington, New York, and London.

Shamberger, R. J. 1970. Relationship of selenium to cancer. I. Inhibitory effect of selenium on carcinogenesis. J. Natl. Cancer Inst. 44:931-936.

Shamberger, R. J. 1971. Inhibitory effect of vitamin A on carcinogenesis. J. Natl. Cancer Inst. 47:667-673.

Shekelle, R. B., S. Liu, W. J. Raynor, Jr., M. Lepper, C. Maliza, and A. H. Rossof. 1981. Dietary vitamin A and risk of cancer in the Western Electric Study. Lancet 2:1185-1189.

Smith, D. M., A. E. Rogers, B. J. Herndon, and P. M. Newberne. 1975. Vitamin A (retinyl acetate) and benzo(a)pyrene-induced respiratory tract carcinogenesis in hamsters fed a commercial diet. Cancer Res. 35:11-16.

Smith, P. G., and H. Jick. 1978. Cancers among users of preparations containing vitamin A. Cancer 42:808-811.

Soloway, M. S., S. M. Cohen, J. B. Dekernion, and L. Persky. 1975. Failure of ascorbic acid to inhibit FANFT-induced bladder cancer. J. Urol. 113:483-486.

Sporn, M. B., and D. L. Newton. 1979. Chemoprevention of cancer with retinoids. Fed. Proc. Fed. Am. Soc. Exp. Biol. 38:2528-2534.

Sporn, M. B., and D. L. Newton. 1981. Recent advances in the use of retinoids for cancer prevention. Pp. 541-548 in J. H. Burchenal and H. F. Oettgen, eds. Cancer: Achievements, Challenges and Prospects for the 1980's, Volume 1. Grune and Stratton, New York, London, Toronto, Sydney, and San Francisco.

Sporn, M. B., N. M. Dunlop, D. L. Newton, and J. M. Smith. 1976. Prevention of chemical carcinogenesis by vitamin A and its synthetic analogs (retinoids). Fed. Proc. Fed. Am. Soc. Exp. Biol. 35:1332-1338.

Tannenbaum, A., and H. Silverstone. 1952. The genesis and growth of tumors. V. Effects of varying the level of B vitamins in the diet. Cancer Res. 12:744-749.

Thanassi, J. W., L. M. Nutter, N. T. Meisler, P. Commers, and J.-F. Chiu. 1981. Vitamin B_6 metabolism in Morris hepatomas. J. Biol. Chem. 256:3370-3375.

Tryfiates, G. P. 1981. Effects of pyridoxine on serum protein expression in hepatoma-bearing rats. J. Natl. Cancer Inst. 66:339-344.

Wald, N., M. Idle, J. Boreham, and A. Bailey. 1980. Low serum-vitamin A and subsequent risk of cancer--Preliminary results of a prospective study. Lancet 2:813-815.

Wassertheil-Smoller, S., S. L. Romney, J. Wylie-Rosett, S. Slagle, G. Miller, D. Lucido, C. Duttagupta, and P. R. Palan. 1981. Dietary vitamin C and uterine cervical dysplasia. Am. J. Epidemiol. 114:714-724.

Wattenberg, L. W. 1972. Inhibition of carcinogenic and toxic effects of polycyclic hydrocarbons by phenolic antioxidants and ethoxy-quin. J. Natl. Cancer Inst. 48:1425-1430.

Welsch, C. W., M. Goodrich-Smith, C. K. Brown, and N. Crowe. 1981. Enhancement by retinyl acetate of hormone-induced mammary tumorigenesis in female GR/A mice. J. Natl. Cancer Inst. 67:935-938.

Wolbach, S. B., and P. R. Howe. 1925. Tissue changes following deprivation of fat-soluble A vitamin. J. Exp. Med. 42:753-777.

Wynder, E. L., and I. J. Bross. 1961. A study of etiological factors in cancer of the esophagus. Cancer 14:389-413.

Young, V. R., and P. M. Newberne. 1981. Vitamins and cancer prevention: Issues and dilemmas. Cancer 47:1226-1240.

10 Minerals

Very few epidemiological studies have been conducted to determine
the relationship between minerals and the incidence of cancer in humans.
This is due partly to the difficulty of identifying populations with
significantly different intakes of the various minerals. In contrast,
there have been numerous studies in laboratory animals. In these investigations, the carcinogenic effects of many metals, administered at
high doses to the animals parenterally, have been well established and
have been reviewed extensively (Furst, 1979; Sunderman, 1977). However,
the results of these studies have shed little light on the potential
carcinogenic risk posed by trace elements in the amounts occurring
naturally in the diet of humans.

Very few feeding studies have been conducted to test the carcinogenicity of trace elements in animals. The carcinogenic action of these
elements is difficult to test in animals because some of them are toxic
at levels that exceed dietary requirements, and because it is difficult to control synergistic interactions of the element under investigation with other elements that may contaminate air, diet, and drinking
water. This chapter contains an evaluation of a few of those trace
elements that are nutritionally significant and suspected of playing a
role in carcinogenesis. The committee sought evidence primarily from
those experiments in which the element was fed to the animal or from
epidemiological reports of exposure through diet. Results obtained from
laboratory experiments using other routes of exposure, or evidence from
occupational exposure of humans, are described briefly when sufficient
information about dietary exposure could not be found. The effects of
both the deficiencies as well as excessive intakes of minerals are also
discussed in this chapter.

Schroeder and his associates investigated the carcinogenicity of
trace elements in a series of large experiments extending over 15 years
(Kanisawa and Schroeder, 1967; Schroeder and Mitchener, 1971a,b, 1972;
Schroeder et al., 1964, 1965, 1968, 1970). Animals were raised in an
environment that permitted maximum control of trace element contamination; they were fed one diet of known composition; and they were observed
for their lifetime. The following elements were studied in at least 50
mice and/or rats per treatment: fluorine, titanium, vanadium, chromium,
nickel, gallium, germanium, arsenic, selenium, yttrium, zirconium, niobium, rhodium, palladium, cadmium, indium, tin, antimony, tellurium, and
lead. These elements were added to the drinking water at levels of 5
mg/liter, except for selenium (3 mg/liter) and tellurium (2 mg/liter).
These levels (approximately 100 times greater than the concentrations
present naturally in the diet) did not significantly affect growth and
survival of the animals. The interpretation of these findings of no

effects or minimally significant effects must be cautious, in view of the small number of animals used. Only rhodium and palladium (tested in mice only) showed any signs of carcinogenicity, but as Schroeder and Michener (1971a) stated, "The results were at a minimally significant level of confidence." Further studies are needed to confirm these findings. Schroeder also reported that selenate, but not selenite, increased the incidence of spontaneous malignant mammary and subcutaneous tumors in rats after lifetime exposure (11 in 75 controls vs 20 in 73 selenate-fed animals). These results were not confirmed in similar studies in mice. (The effects of selenium on carcinogenesis are discussed in further detail below.) None of the remaining elements examined increased tumor incidence. A significant reduction in tumor incidence was observed in mice fed arsenic and cadmium and in mice and rats fed lead.

SELENIUM

Signs of chronic selenium toxicity in animals have been recognized for almost 700 years, but selenium was not identified as the responsible agent until the 1930's. Twenty years later, the economic importance of selenosis and selenium deficiency for animal producers became apparent. This discovery stimulated the mapping of selenium distribution in the soils, forages, and tissues of humans in several continents. Extreme differences of exposure were delineated, even within individual countries. This knowledge enabled investigators to make epidemiological correlations of diseases, including cancer, in humans and animals and to conduct laboratory experiments to test the resulting hypotheses (National Academy of Sciences, 1971).

Epidemiological Evidence

Selenium has been reported as having a possible protective effect against cancer. Shamberger and colleagues correlated selenium levels in forage crops (grouped into high, medium, and low categories) with cancer mortality by state in the United States (Shamberger and Frost, 1969; Shamberger and Willis, 1971; Shamberger et al., 1976). They found an inverse relationship in both males and females, especially for cancers of the gastrointestinal and genitourinary tracts. In other studies, Schrauzer and coworkers correlated per capita intake with cancer mortality rates in more than 20 countries (Schrauzer, 1976; Schrauzer et al., 1977a,b). The consumption estimates were based on international food disappearance data for major food sources (e.g., cereals, meat, and seafoods) to which the investigators attributed plausible mean selenium values. They found an inverse relationship between selenium intake and leukemia as well as with cancers of the colon, rectum, pancreas, breast, ovary, prostate, bladder, lung (males), and skin. Using pooled blood samples from healthy donors in 19 U.S. states and 22 countries, they also correlated blood levels of selenium with corresponding cancer mortality rates. They found significant inverse relationships for most of these same sites.

10-2

Shamberger et al. (1973) compared the blood selenium levels in more than 100 cancer patients with those in 48 normal subjects attending a clinic. The levels in patients with gastrointestinal cancers and Hodgkin's disease were significantly lower than those in the normal subjects, but there were no differences between the normal subjects and patients with cancers at other sites, such as the breast. It is not clear from this study whether the observed difference in the selenium levels was the result or the cause of the cancers.

Jansson et al. (1975, 1978) examined cancer mortality rates in the United States by county. They compared the rates in the northeastern part of the country with corresponding levels of selenium in the water supply. In contrast to other investigators, they reported a direct correlation between mortality from colorectal cancer and selenium levels in the drinking water.

Experimental Evidence

Carcinogenicity. During the past 40 years selenium has been alternately described as a carcinogen and an anticarcinogen, on the basis of experiments on animals. Because studies conducted during the 1940's showed that high levels of selenium induced or enhanced tumor formation, the Food and Drug Administration until recently prohibited the enrichment of animal feeds with selenium, even in areas with established selenium deficiency. In contrast to the results of the earlier investigations, more recent studies by several independent investigators have established that dietary selenium has a protective effect against tumors induced by a variety of chemical carcinogens or at least one viral agent.

A critical review of the experimental conditions suggests that the earlier studies demonstrating carcinogenic or promoting properties of selenium can be faulted on the basis of experimental design. Nelson et al. (1943) fed a 12% protein diet to 18 control rats and to 126 rats whose diet was enriched with selenium (5, 7, and 10 μg/g) as seleniferous grain or selenides. Fifty-three of the test animals and 14 of the controls survived to an age of 1.5 to 2 years. The livers of the control rats were normal, but all animals fed the high selenium diet had liver cirrhosis. Of these, 11 had developed nonmetastasizing adenomas and the rest showed hyperplasia. These findings can be attributed to a combination of two insults: the near toxic levels of selenium and the marginal protein content of the diet.

Harr et al. (1967) investigated the effect of selenium on tumor formation in 1,437 rats fed a range of selenium levels for as long as 30 months. Eighty-eight rats were also fed 2-acetylaminofluorene (2-AAF) along with selenium. The experimental design also included a repetition of the earlier experiment by Nelson et al. (1943), i.e., a marginal protein diet was supplemented with selenium as selenate at 0.5, 2.4, or 8 μg/g. As expected, diets containing selenium in concentrations

higher than 8 µg/g were toxic and killed the rats within the first
month. The rats fed the two lower levels survived for more than a year.
Autopsies and histological examinations performed on 1,123 of the rats on
various dietary treatments provided no evidence for a carcinogenic effect
of selenium. Forty-three tumors occurred in 88 of the rats fed 50 or
100 µg/g of AAF diet without added selenium; the rest of the autopsied
animals exibited 20 neoplasms, randomly distributed, regardless of the
level of dietary selenium. Although there were no hepatic tumors in any
autopsied animals that did not receive the carcinogen, approximately half
of the selenium-supplemented rats that survived for more than 9 months
had hyperplastic lesions in the liver, whereas none occurred in the
controls.

In another series of studies, Volgarev and Tscherkes (1967) measured
the effect of selenium in 200 rats, but they did not use a selenium-
free control group. In the first experiment, 40 rats were fed selenium
as selenate at 4.3 to 8.6 µg/g of diet. All animals developed liver cirrhosis, 10 had neoplastic tumors, 4 had precancerous lesions, and 9 were
unaffected. In a second experiment, only 5 neoplasms were observed among
60 rats. The third experiment failed to produce any tumors in 100
animals.

Schroeder and Mitchener (1971b, 1972) studied the effect of selenium supplementation (2 to 3 mg/liter in drinking water as selenate
or selenite) in lifetime experiments with rats and mice. Neither form
of selenium affected the incidence of tumors in mice, and selenite had
no effect in rats. Specifically, no hepatic cirrhosis was observed.
However, following an epidemic of pneumonia in the rat colonies, there
were 30 tumors in 73 animals in the selenate group, but only 20 in 75
animals in the controls.

Antitumorigenic Effects. A large accumulation of evidence indicates
that supplementation of the diet or drinking water with selenium protects
against tumors induced by a variety of chemical carcinogens and at least
one viral agent (Table 10-1). Although most investigators found that
tumor incidence in the selenium-supplemented animals was approximately
one-half that of the control animals, Schrauzer et al. (1978) reported
that spontaneous breast tumors in female C3H mice were reduced from 82%
in controls to 10% in the selenium-supplemented animals. In all but two
of the experiments, comparisons were made between controls receiving
diets with nutritionally adequate selenium levels and test animals fed
diets supplemented with selenium levels 20 to 50 times higher than the
animal's requirements. In the remaining two experiments, Harr et al.
(1972) and Ip and Sinha (1981) used selenium-deficient diets and demonstrated beneficial effects of selenium supplementation at levels close to
the physiological requirement. Of special nutritional importance is
their finding that the incidence of tumors induced by 7,12-dimethyl-
benz[a]anthracene (DMBA) was enhanced by diets high in polyunsaturated
fatty acids and by dietary deficiency of selenium. Supplementation with
physiological levels of selenium (0.1 µg/g diet) resulted in protection
against tumor formation (Ip and Sinha, 1981).

10-4

TABLE 10-1

Effect of Selenium on Tumor Incidence

Carcinogen or Tumor Type	Method of Application	Dose of Selenium (μg/g Diet)	Effect	References
3'-Methyl-4-dimethylamino-azobenzene (3'-MeDAB)	In diet for 2 weeks, then selenium in diet for 4 weeks	5	50% reduction in tumor incidence	Clayton and Baumann, 1949
7,12-Dimethylbenz[a]an-thracene (DMBA)	In diet	1.0	Reduced incidence of skin papilloma	Shamberger, 1970
2-Acetylaminofluorene (2-AAF)	In selenium-deficient diet for 200 days	0.5, 2.5	Reduced incidence of hepatic and mammary neoplasia	Harr et al., 1972
1,2-Dimethylhydrazine (DMH)	Weekly injection	4	50% reduction in incidence of colon cancer	Griffin, 1979
Methylazoxymethanol (MAM)	Weekly injection	4	No effect	Griffin, 1979
3'-MeDAB	In diet for 8 weeks	6	Reduced incidence of liver tumors	Griffin, 1979
3'-MeDAB	In diet for 9 weeks	2, 4	Reduced incidence of liver tumors even when selenium was given during final stage of study	Griffin, 1979
Spontaneous mammary tumor	Virally transmitted	2	Decreased tumor in-cidence; no effect on transplanted tumor	Schrauzer et al., 1978
Mammary tumor	Virally transmitted	2, 6	Decreased tumor in-cidence; no effect on transplanted tumor	Medina and Shepherd, 1980
N-Nitrosomethylurea (NMU)	One intraperitoneal injection	5 days after injection of carcinogen	Reduction of cancers per rat	Thompson and Becci, 1980
Ascites tumor cells	One intraperitoneal injection	2 μg/g body wt.; 9 injections in 3 weeks	Reduction of tumor growth	Greeder and Milner, 1980

Although these data indicate that selenium has an antitumorigenic effect, they provide no information on the mechanism of action or on the stage of tumor development during which selenium might exert its protective action. In at least two studies, selenium was introduced only after the carcinogen was applied and led to a reduction in tumor incidence. Schrauzer et al. (1978) stated that the selenium levels in the recipient animals do not influence the fate of transplanted tumor cells; others observed a strong reduction in the growth of inoculated Ehrlich ascites cells in recipient animals injected with high doses of selenium compounds for 3 weeks after the inoculation (Greeder and Milner, 1980).

Mutagenicity. In vitro studies have not shed much light on the mechanisms of action of selenium. On the one hand, selenium concentrations from 0.1 to 40 mM exert antimutagenic effects against a variety of mutagens in vitro, including the naturally occurring mutagen malonaldehyde (Jacobs et al., 1977; Shamberger et al., 1978). On the other hand, similar concentrations of selenium have been reported to increase DNA fragmentation and chromosome aberrations in human and microbial cell cultures (Lo et al., 1978; Nakamuro et al., 1976). These contrasting reports cannot be reconciled.

Potential Mechanisms of Action. There are data suggesting that selenium in vitro and in vivo may decrease the activity of hydroxylating enzymes that activate procarcinogens and may increase a detoxifying enzyme—glucuronyl transferase (Griffin, 1979). These results suggest that selenium acts during the early stages of initiation.

The best known functions of selenium at nutritionally adequate, but not at excessive, levels are its role as a part of the enzyme glutathione peroxidase and its interaction with heavy metals. Glutathione peroxidase destroys hydroperoxides and lipoperoxides, thereby protecting the constituents of the cells against free radical damage. Ip and Sinha (1981) have shown that selenium, through its function in glutathione peroxidase, could well be involved in protecting against cancer induced by high intakes of fat, especially polyunsaturated fatty acids. Glutathione peroxidase activity in human blood increases with increasing selenium intakes, but reaches a plateau at intakes well below those customary in the United States (Thomson and Robinson, 1980). Thus, if the antitumorigenic effect of selenium is mediated through its function in glutathione peroxidase, attempts to increase the enzyme activity by selenium supplementation, superimposed on an adequate diet in the United States, would not be successful.

The second function of selenium is to protect against acute and chronic toxicity of certain heavy metals. Although selenium is known to interact with cadmium and mercury, the mechanism of action is not known. Selenium does not cause an increased elimination of the toxic elements, but, rather, an increased accumulation in some nontoxic form (National Academy of Sciences, 1971). It is conceivable that carcinogenic effects of these, and perhaps other heavy metals, could be counteracted by selenium, in a manner similar to its protection against their general toxicity.

Summary

Epidemiological Evidence. The epidemiological evidence pertaining to the relationship between selenium and cancer is derived from a limited number of geographical correlation studies in which the risk of cancer was correlated with estimates of per capita selenium intake, with the selenium levels in blood specimens, or with selenium concentrations in water supplies. Although these studies generally demonstrated an inverse relationship between the level of selenium and the risk of cancer, it is not clear whether this relationship applies to all cancer sites or only to specific cancer sites, such as those in the gastrointestinal tract. There are as yet no data from case-control or cohort studies.

Experimental Studies. Numerous experiments in animals have demonstrated an antitumorigenic effect of selenium. The relevance of most of these studies to the risk of cancer for humans is not apparent since the levels of selenium used far exceeded dietary requirements and often bordered on levels that might be toxic. However, one experiment has demonstrated increased susceptibility to DMBA-induced tumors when selenium deficiency was aggravated by high dietary levels of polyunsaturated fatty acids, and protection by a physiological supplement of selenium (0.1 µg/g) to the diet (Ip and Sinha, 1981). The interpretation of these results is further complicated because of the varied protocols used in these experiments and the knowledge that selenium interacts with many other nutrients, such as heavy metals in the diet.

The minimum requirement for selenium in mammalian species is 0.05 µg/g of diet, one-hundredth of the levels used in many studies of carcinogenesis. A level of 4 or 5 µg/g may not be acutely or even chronically toxic when fed along with a well-balanced, nutritious diet, but it becomes chronically toxic when the quality of the diet is lowered, for example when the protein content is reduced. At least two experiments have demonstrated that selenium deficiency enhances carcinogenesis and that physiological amounts of selenium have a significant protective effect. The effectiveness of doses in the wide range between the nutritionally adequate and the higher, effective level used in many antitumorigenic studies has not yet been adequately investigated. The data on the mutagenicity of selenium compounds are also contradictory. However, these experiments provide sufficient evidence to suggest that the antitumorigenic effect of selenium should be investigated further. Recent data do not support the earlier reports that selenium per se is carcinogenic.

Conclusion

Both the epidemiological and laboratory studies suggest that selenium may offer some protection against the risk of cancer. However, firm conclusions cannot be drawn on the basis of the present limited evidence. Increasing the selenium intake to more than 200 µg/day (the

upper limit of the range of Safe and Adequate Daily Dietary Intakes
published in the Recommended Dietary Allowances [National Academy of
Sciences, 1980b]) by the use of supplements has not been shown to confer health benefits exceeding those derived from the consumption of a
balanced diet.

ZINC

Zinc is an essential constituent of more than 100 enzymes and is
essential for life. Through its function in nucleic acid polymerases,
zinc plays a predominant role in nucleic acid metabolism, cell replication, tissue repair, and growth (Prasad, 1978). Severe zinc deficiency
in humans has been known for 20 years; more moderate forms have been
linked to protein-energy malnutrition. Marginal zinc deficiency is
suspected to occur in a substantial number of infants and older children
in the United States (Prasad, 1978).

Pronounced zinc deficiency in animals and humans results in depressed
immune functions. Both tissue-mediated and humoral responses are
affected. Golden et al. (1978) have observed that impairment of delayed
hypersensitivity reactions to Candida albicans antigen in malnourished
children can be normalized by topically applied zinc preparations, but it
is not known whether or to what degree immunocompetence is impaired
by marginal zinc deficiency.

Epidemiological Evidence

There have been few epidemiological studies of the relationship
between exposure to zinc and risk of cancer. Stocks and Davies (1964)
correlated cancer mortality with the zinc and copper content of soil in
12 districts of England and Wales. They found higher zinc levels and
higher ratios of zinc to copper in the soil of vegetable gardens near
houses in which a death from gastric cancer had occurred than in the soil
of gardens near houses in which there was a death attributed to another
cause. The levels near houses with deaths from "other cancers" did not
differ from those of the noncancer households. These analyses were made
only when the deceased had resided in the same house for 10 or more
years. Since the copper levels in soil varied little, the differences
could be attributed to zinc.

Schrauzer et al. (1977a,b) examined per capita food intake data in 27
countries. They found a direct correlation between estimated zinc intake
and age-adjusted mortality from leukemia and cancers of the intestine,
breast, prostate, and skin. Based on these findings and the inverse
correlation between zinc and selenium concentrations in blood, they
suggested that zinc increases cancer risk by its antagonism of selenium.

Van Rensburg (1981) observed that wheat and corn are the primary
dietary staples in many populations at high risk for esophageal cancer

around the world. In contrast, the staples in low-risk populations include millet, cassava, yams, and peanuts. Since diets based on wheat and corn generally contain low concentrations of zinc, magnesium, nicotinic acid, and possibly riboflavin, he suggested that a deficiency of one or more of these micronutrients might be etiologically related to esophageal cancer.

A number of investigators have examined the relationship between cancer and levels of zinc in blood and other body tissues. Schrauzer et al. (1977b) found that mean zinc concentrations in pooled blood from healthy donors in 19 U.S. collection sites correlated directly with corresponding mortality rates from cancers of the large bowel, breast, ovary, lung, bladder, and oral cavity. Zinc and selenium levels in the blood were inversely correlated with each other. Strain et al. (1972) compared zinc and copper levels in the serum of patients with broncho-genic carcinoma and the levels in the serum of controls. Although zinc levels did not differ between the two groups, the copper levels were lower in the controls, resulting in higher ratios of zinc to copper in the cancer patients. On the other hand, Davies et al. (1968) reported that zinc levels in the plasma of bronchogenic carcinoma patients were lower than those of other cancer patients and lower than normal labora-tory values.

Lin et al. (1977) examined serum, hair, and tissues from Chinese men in Hong Kong for levels of zinc and other minerals. They found that levels of zinc in serum and diseased esophageal tissue from esophageal cancer patients were much lower than those in other cancer patients and in normal subjects. Zinc levels in hair were lower in both cancer groups than in normal subjects. The serum of esophageal cancer patients also contained slightly elevated copper levels and much lower iron levels than the serum of normal subjects. Györkey et al. (1967) reported that zinc concentrations in malignant prostatic tissue were lower than those in normal tissue, whereas benign hypertrophied prostatic tissue contained higher zinc levels. In all of these studies, the altered zinc levels may have followed, rather than preceded, the onset of the cancers.

Experimental Evidence

Experiments in animals have demonstrated both enhancing and retarding effects of zinc on tumor growth. Several reports suggest that a zinc deficiency strongly inhibits the growth of transplanted tumors in animals and prolongs survival time. The studies by Petering et al. (1967) with transplanted Walker 256 carcinoma in rats were confirmed by DeWys et al. (1970) and extended to other types of tumors, such as leukemias, Lewis lung carcinoma (DeWys and Pories, 1972), Ehrlich ascites tumor (Barr and Harris, 1973), P388 leukemia (Minkel et al., 1979), and plasmacy-toma TEPC-183 (Fenton et al., 1980). The results of these studies are consistent with the knowledge that rapidly growing tumor cells require zinc for growth; however, they do not suggest zinc deficiency as a therapeutic modality because zinc deficiency by itself, with or with-out concomitant malignancies, results in death of the animals.

The results of these studies contradict reports indicating that zinc deficiency enhances chemically induced carcinogenesis. For example, Fong et al. (1978) observed that the incidence of esophageal tumors induced by nitrosomethylbenzylamine (NMBA) was significantly higher in zinc-deficient rats than in control rats. The intragastric intubation of NMBA in a dose of 48 μg/g body weight resulted in a 15% incidence of carcinoma in control rats fed ad libitum and a 43% incidence in rats maintained on zinc-deficient diets. In two consecutive experiments, lowering the dose of NMBA to 34 μg/g body weight produced no cancer in the control rats, but 83% and 33% in the zinc-deficient animals. In contrast, some studies have indicated that zinc intake greatly exceeding nutritional requirements suppresses carcinogenesis induced by DMBA in Syrian hamsters (Poswillo and Cohen, 1971) or by azo dyes in rats (Duncan and Dreosti, 1975). But Schrauzer (1979) demonstrated that high concentrations of zinc (200 mg/liter) in the drinking water of C3H mice countered the protective effect of selenium against spontaneous mammary carcinoma and resulted in a significant increase in tumor growth.

These contradictory reports are not easily reconciled. Perhaps there are two different mechanisms of action by which zinc influences two different phases of carcinogenesis: Zinc, perhaps through its effect on the immune system, may be protective during the early phases of transformation, whereas the demonstrated role of zinc in cell proliferation may explain the protective effect of zinc deficiency against the growth of established tumors. Furthermore, numerous interactions of zinc with other trace elements, such as selenium, are incompletely understood. Thus, the evidence is insufficient to determine the answer to an important question: Does marginal zinc deficiency, believed to be widespread, especially among children, present a risk for or provide protection against carcinogenesis?

Summary

Epidemiological Evidence. There are few epidemiological data concerning dietary zinc and cancer. Some studies have suggested that higher levels of dietary zinc are associated with an increase in the incidence of cancer at several different sites, including the breast and stomach, and other studies have reported lower levels of zinc in the serum and tissue of patients with esophageal, bronchogenic, and other cancers, compared to corresponding levels in controls. However, the possibility that the lower serum and tissue levels resulted from the cancer itself has not been ruled out.

Experimental Evidence. Experiments in animals have shown that zinc can either enhance or retard the growth of tumors. Zinc deficiency appears to retard the growth of transplanted tumors, whereas it enhances the incidence of some chemically induced cancers. In some experiments, dietary zinc exceeding nutritional requirements has been shown to suppress chemically induced tumors in rats and hamsters, but when given in drinking water it counteracts the protective effect of selenium in mice. These data are insufficient to explain the effects of zinc and of interactions between zinc and other minerals on tumorigenesis.

Conclusion

The epidemiological evidence concerning zinc is too sparse and the results of laboratory experiments too contradictory to permit any conclusion to be drawn. In view of the important nutritional role of zinc and of its many interactions with other minerals involved in carcinogenesis, additional research is warranted to resolve the contradictory results.

IRON

Epidemiological Evidence

Iron deficiency has been associated with cancers of the upper alimentary tract including the esophagus and stomach. In epidemiological studies conducted in Sweden, iron deficiency was associated with Plummer-Vinson (Paterson-Kelly) syndrome, which in turn was associated with increased risk for cancer of the upper alimentary tract (Larsson et al., 1975; Wynder et al., 1957). Improved nutrition, especially with regard to iron and vitamins in the diet, has been associated with the virtual elimination of new cases of Plummer-Vinson disease in areas of Sweden where it had formerly been highly endemic (Larsson et al., 1975).

Broitman et al. (1981) studied iron-deficient patients with antecedent lesions of gastric carcinoma in an area of Colombia with high risk for this cancer. They found that hypochlorhydria and achlorhydria, which are associated with chronic atrophic gastritis resulting from iron deficiency, permitted bacterial colonization of the stomach. The investigators postulated that these bacteria could reduce ingested nitrate to nitrite, leading to the formation of nitrosamines that are carcinogenic in the stomach of laboratory animals, and are suspected of being carcinogenic in humans. A similar mechanism was suggested by Ruddell et al. (1978) to explain the increased risk of gastric cancer in patients with pernicious anemia.

There have been no epidemiological reports of cancer associated with increased dietary intake of iron, although heavy inhalation exposure to high levels of iron oxide has been related to increased risk for lung and laryngeal cancers in miners of iron ore, metal workers, and workers in iron foundries (Cole and Goldman, 1975). In addition, sarcomata have developed in patients at sites of injection of iron-dextran solutions (MacKinnon and Bancewicz, 1973; Robinson et al., 1960), and many clinical reports have associated hemochromatosis with an increased risk for hepatomas and possibly other hepatic and extrahepatic cancers (Armann et al., 1980; Scott and Theologides, 1974; Steinherz et al., 1976; Sussman et al., 1974).

Experimental Evidence

Mild iron deficiency appeared to protect mice from the hepatocellular and porphyric toxicity due to 2,3,7,8-tetrachlorodibenzo-p-dioxin (TCDD) (Sweeney et al., 1979). It is not known if such protection might extend to the teratogenic or possible carcinogenic action of TCDD. Rats made severely deficient in iron through manipulation of their diet became anemic and developed fatty livers (Vitale et al., 1978), but they were devoid of any neoplastic lesions. However, in the same study, iron-deficient rats given 1,2-dimethylhydrazine developed neoplastic lesions in their livers within 4 months, as compared to 6 months in the iron-sufficient group. The authors concluded that severe lack of iron appeared to function as a cocarcinogen (Vitale et al., 1978).

Brusick et al. (1976) found that Fe(II) as iron sulfate induced reverse mutations in Salmonella typhimurium strains TA1537 and TA1538 with the S9 fraction of various species. Weak mutagenic activity was also observed in nonactivated suspensions.

Summary

Epidemiological Evidence. Iron deficiency has been related to an increase in the risk of Plummer-Vinson syndrome, which is associated with upper alimentary tract cancer. Some evidence suggests that iron deficiency may be related to gastric cancer, also through an indirect mechanism. Although epidemiological and clinical reports have suggested that heavy exposure to iron by inhalation increases the risk of cancer, there is no evidence pertaining to the effect of high levels of dietary iron on the risk of cancer in humans.

Experimental Evidence. The evidence from experiments in animals is limited. In one study, dietary deficiency of iron was associated with an earlier onset of chemically induced tumors in rats. These data are not sufficient to clarify the role of iron in carcinogenesis.

Conclusion

The data are not sufficient for a firm conclusion to be drawn about the role of iron in carcinogenesis.

COPPER

Copper is an essential nutrient that is widely distributed in foods. Public water supplies may be an additional source of copper. The intake of copper in 28 countries has been reported by Schrauzer et al. (1977b) to vary between 1.6 and 3.3 mg/day. However, more recent studies indicate that the average copper intake for U.S. adults is ∿1 mg/day (Holden et al., 1979; Klevay et al., 1979).

Epidemiological Evidence

Schrauzer et al. (1977b) used pooled blood samples from healthy donors in 19 U.S. states to correlate blood levels of copper with corresponding cancer mortality rates. They found weak direct associations for cancers of the intestine, breast, lung, and thyroid. From reported average concentrations of copper in major food items and international food disappearance data, they were also able to correlate per capita intake of copper with cancer mortality rates in 27 countries. In this portion of their study, they found direct associations for leukemia and cancers of the intestine, breast, and skin. These investigators proposed that the mechanism for the apparent carcinogenicity of copper might involve selenium antagonism, since large doses of copper produce symptoms of selenium deficiency in animals (Jensen, 1975).

The possibility that dietary exposure to copper, through the copper content of either foods or cookware, may play an etiologic role in gastric carcinogenesis is raised by the experiments of Endo et al. (1977), who found that the copper ion may be involved in conversion of creatine and creatinine to methylguanidine, a precursor of methylnitrosoguanidine. However, no epidemiological data on the relationship of gastric cancer and dietary copper have been reported.

In a number of clinical studies, levels of copper in the serum and tissues of cancer patients were found to be higher than normal laboratory values and higher than levels in healthy subjects or in noncancerous tissues (Schwartz, 1975). However, the possibility that these levels are the consequence, rather than the cause, of the disease cannot be ruled out. Indeed, many of these reports indicate that changes in copper levels may be effected by therapy or by different stages and activity of the disease.

Inhalation of copper has been suggested as a possible cause of hepatic angiosarcoma as well as pulmonary adenocarcinoma and alveolar cell carcinoma in workers who sprayed vineyards with a fungicide called the Bordeaux mixture (copper sulfate plus lime) (Pimentel and Menezes, 1977). An increased risk for bronchogenic carcinoma has also been reported for copper miners in cases where exposure to radiation was dismissed as a likely cause (Newman et al., 1976).

Thus, although some data suggest that copper is carcinogenic in humans, very little epidemiological evidence implicates dietary sources per se.

Experimental Evidence

Several independent studies have demonstrated that high levels of copper salts added to the diets of animals provided various degrees of protection against chemically induced liver tumors. The effects ranged from a prolongation of the induction time to partial or complete protection against tumor formation. These studies, in which a variety of different carcinogens were used, have been reviewed by Brada and Altman (1978). Since these effects were obtained with extremely high concentrations of copper (from 0.3% to 0.6% copper acetate in the diet) and since similar effects have been produced when manganese or nickel were substituted for copper (Yamane and Sakai, 1973), the action of copper may be pharmacologic, perhaps toxic in nature and nonspecific. There is no experimental evidence that the copper levels in animal tissues influence their susceptibility to carcinogens.

Summary

Epidemiological Evidence. Although there are some data from clinical and epidemiological studies concerning the association of copper with neoplasia in humans, there is little evidence pertaining to the role of dietary copper in the etiology of human cancer.

Experimental Evidence. Experiments in animals have indicated that pharmacological doses of copper appear to protect against chemically induced tumors, but there are no studies to indicate whether the nutritional copper status of animals influences their susceptibility to cancer.

Conclusion

The evidence does not permit any conclusion to be drawn about the role of dietary copper in carcinogenesis.

IODINE

Iodine is an essential micronutrient in the diet and is an integral component of thyroid hormones. Dietary deficiency of iodine is associated with enlargement of the thyroid gland and endemic goiter, but this does not occur commonly in the United States.

The mean daily intake of iodine in the United States is estimated to range from approximately 60 to 680 µg/day. Even the lower level is adequate to meet the minimum daily requirements of 50 µg, and many diets furnish iodine in excess of the Recommended Dietary Allowance of 150 µg (Fisher and Carr, 1974). The iodization of table salt, the use of iodine in disinfectants, and the addition of iodate to dough conditioners have contributed to the drastic reduction in iodine deficiency in the United States. Together, these sources can also result in high intakes of iodine, which are considered excessive by some nutritionists.

Epidemiological Evidence

Wahner et al. (1966) concluded that thyroid cancer occurred more frequently in Cali, Colombia (an area of endemic goiter) than in New York State or Puerto Rico. Their analysis was based on published data from the United States and on a large autopsy series conducted by the authors in Colombia. Although papillary carcinoma was the type of cancer found most frequently in their series, the relative proportion of follicular carcinomas was high compared with other areas of the world.

Williams et al. (1977) compared the incidence and histologic types of thyroid cancer in two contrasting populations: Icelanders with high iodide diets and Scots from northeast Scotland with normal levels of dietary iodide. Based on a pathological review of all surgical thyroid specimens in these areas, the investigators were able to determine the histology-specific incidence rates of thyroid cancer. Their results indicated that the incidence of papillary carcinoma and the ratio of papillary to follicular carcinomas were higher in Iceland than in Scotland. They concluded that high intake of iodide was associated only with the papillary type of thyroid cancer, and suggested that low levels of dietary iodide may increase the risk for follicular carcinoma of the thyroid.

In studies that have not distinguished histologic types of thyroid cancer, investigators have tended to find no associations with exposure to iodine. Clements (1954) found no difference between observed and expected deaths from thyroid cancer by state in Australia, despite the fact that iodine intakes varied and endemic goiter was particularly prevalent in Tasmania. Pendergrast et al. (1961) compared thyroid cancer mortality rates by state in the United States with corresponding prevalence rates of endemic goiter and found no association between the two diseases. They also examined secular trends in mortality from these two diseases and observed that there had been a decline in endemic goiter rates but not in thyroid cancer rates in the United States during the previous 30-year period. Mortality data, used in both of these studies, can be quite misleading for thyroid cancer and other cancers that have very high survival rates.

A second type of cancer associated with iodine deficiency is breast cancer in females. In an analysis similar to that of Pendergrast et al. (1961) for thyroid cancer, Bogardus and Finley (1961) compared mortality rates for this cancer by state in the United States with the prevalence of endemic goiter. They found a direct association between the two diseases. Commenting on this observation, Stadel (1976) noted that breast cancer in females is highly correlated with endometrial and ovarian cancers and hypothesized that low iodine intake may be etiologically related to all three cancers. However, the results of many other studies do not support this association. Edington (1976) reported conflicting data obtained in sub-Saharan Africa, where these three cancers are rare despite very low levels of dietary iodine. In Hawaii and Iceland, iodine intake is high, but there are also high incidence rates for breast cancer (Waterhouse et al., 1976).

Experimental Evidence

Eskin et al. (1967) and Aquino and Eskin (1972) reported that iodine deficiency produces hyperplastic changes in the breast tissue of female rats during puberty. Because of the epidemiological correlations indicating a higher incidence of mammary carcinoma in areas with endemic goiter, Eskin (1978) studied the influence of iodine deficiency, per se, on mammary tissue when the thyroid was maintained in a normal state. Deficiency resulted in dysplastic changes of the epithelium, which were aggravated by estrogen treatment and advanced to preneoplastic and neoplastic conditions. These changes were reversible by supplementation with inorganic iodine but not thyroxine which, in higher doses, increased the dysplastic changes. Eskin proposed that iodine deficiency itself rather than hypothyroidism was responsible for these effects and demonstrated similar changes by blocking iodine uptake with perchlorate. Upon termination of the blockade or dietary iodine supplementation, most but not all of the hyperplastic tissue changes returned to normal. The iodine-deficient prepubescent rats were also susceptible to earlier appearance of DMBA-induced mammary tumors, suggesting a cocarcinogenic effect of iodine deficiency.

Eskin et al. (1976) also demonstrated that the ratios of DNA to RNA in the breast of iodine-deficient rats were much higher than those for control rats. In addition, observed alterations in the estrogen receptor protein may suggest that mammary tumorigenesis may be stimulated in the presence of estrogen and higher physiological levels of its receptor, as observed in iodine deficiency. Exposure of iodine-deficient animals to a carcinogen such as 2-acetylaminofluorene (2-AAF) or to thyroid irradiation has been reported to result in increased yields of malignant thyroid tumors (Bielchowsky, 1944; Doniach, 1958).

Summary

Epidemiological Evidence. Although studies that focused on mortality from thyroid cancer showed no association of the disease with dietary iodine, a large series of autopsies from Colombia and a study of cancer incidence in Iceland and Scotland, based on histology-specific analyses, suggested that the risk of follicular thyroid carcinoma may be increased in iodine-deficient populations. In the Iceland/Scotland study, investigators also found a higher incidence of papillary carcinoma in the population with high dietary iodine intake. However, the relationship between iodine and thyroid cancer should be studied further before firm conclusions can be drawn. Epidemiological studies provide no clear evidence that the risk of cancers of the breast, ovary, and endometrium are related to dietary iodine deficiency.

Experimental Evidence. Experimentally induced iodine deficiency seems to predispose rats to the development of preneoplastic and neoplastic lesions in mammary tissue and to reduce the induction time of chemically induced mammary and thyroid tumors.

Conclusion

Although limited epidemiological and laboratory evidence suggests that iodine deficiency is associated with an increased risk for thyroid cancer in humans, the evidence is not conclusive.

MOLYBDENUM

Epidemiological Evidence

A few reports have indirectly implicated molybdenum deficiency in the etiology of cancer, especially cancer of the esophagus. In China, the Coordinating Group for Research on Etiology of Esophageal Cancer in North China (1975) and Yang (1980) reported that correlation analyses by county have shown an inverse association of esophageal cancer with the levels of molybdenum and a variety of other minerals in the soil. Molybdenum levels in hair were low in areas at high risk for this cancer. Low levels of molybdenum in the soil have also been observed in a region of Africa with high mortality rates from esophageal cancer (Burrell et al., 1966). Furthermore, low levels of molybdenum in water supplies have been correlated with excess esophageal cancer mortality in the United States (Berg et al., 1973).

In areas of China at high risk for esophageal cancer, supplementation of the soil with ammonium molybdate has been observed to increase the molybdenum and ascorbic acid content of locally produced grains and vegetables and to decrease their nitrate and nitrite concentration (Luo et al., 1981). The investigators have proposed that high ascorbic acid and decreased nitrate and nitrite content of vegetables and grains could decrease the high incidence of esophageal cancer in these areas.

Experimental Evidence

Luo et al. (1981) studied the effect of molybdenum supplementation on the induction of tumors by N-nitrososarcosine in the esophagus and forestomach of Sprague-Dawley rats. They observed that tumor incidence in the group supplemented with molybdenum (2 mg/liter drinking water) was lower than that in the control group, whose diet contained a molybdenum concentration of 26 μg/kg diet.

Molybdenum in the form of molybdenum oxide was shown to induce a significant increase in the number of lung adenomas in Strain A mice (Stoner et al., 1976). Molybdenum as potassium molybdate and ammonium molybdate was positive in Bacillus subtilus rec assay (Nishioka, 1975). Nishioka (1975) also noted the mutagenicity of ammonium molybdate in Escherchia coli.

Summary

Epidemiological Evidence. In a few studies, investigators have found an inverse correlation between molybdenum levels in the soil and water and the risk of esophageal cancer, especially in China. Supplementation of molybdenum-deficient soil in high risk areas of China has been observed to increase the ascorbic acid content and lower the nitrate content of locally grown plants and grains, and is therefore being considered as a means of reducing the risk of esophageal cancer.

Experimental Evidence. Data from one report of laboratory experiments suggest that molybdenum supplementation of the diet may reduce the incidence of nitrosamine-induced tumors of the esophagus and forestomach.

Conclusion

The epidemiological and laboratory evidence is too meager to assess the validity of the associations suggested by the studies summarized above.

CADMIUM

Regarded only as a toxic substance for many years, cadmium is now beginning to be recognized as an element with a possible physiological function (Schwarz, 1977). Market Basket Surveys conducted by the Food and Drug Administration indicate that the per capita intake of cadmium in the United States ranged from 26 to 61 µg/day during 1968-1974 (Mahaffey et al., 1975). The tolerable weekly intake for cadmium established by a FAO/WHO Expert Committee is from 400 to 500 µg/week (World Health Organization, 1972).

Epidemiological Evidence

In a correlation analysis based on cancer mortality by state and trace element content of the water supplies in 10 river basins of the United States, Berg and Burbank (1972) found direct associations between cadmium levels and mortality from myeloma, lymphoma, and cancers at several other sites, including the mouth and pharynx, the esophagus, the large intestine, the larynx, the lung, the breast (female), and the bladder. Four other trace elements (arsenic, beryllium, nickel, and lead) were also directly associated with cancer, but chromium, cobalt, and iron were not.

Schrauzer et al. (1977a,b) correlated estimated per capita cadmium intakes with cancer mortality rates in 27 countries. They found significant direct associations with leukemia and cancers of the intestine, female breast, uterus, prostate, and skin, and an inverse association with liver cancer. A similar analysis, based on the cadmium concentration in pooled blood samples and cancer mortality in 19 U.S. states, yielded significant direct correlations for uterine cancer and stomach cancer in females. Schrauzer and colleagues suggested that cadmium may act as a selenium antagonist to prevent its uptake and lower its physiological activity as an anticarcinogen.

Kolonel (1976) reported the results of a case-control study in which the combined exposure to cadmium from three sources (diet, cigarette smoking, and workplace) was associated with increased risk for renal cancer. In studies based on occupational exposure (Adams et al., 1969; Kipling and Waterhouse, 1967; Lemen et al., 1976; Potts, 1965), investigators have observed associations between exposure to cadmium and prostate cancer. However, the main source of exposure to cadmium for the general population is diet (Friberg et al., 1974), and a case-control study of prostate cancer that included dietary as well as occupational exposure (Kolonel and Winkelstein, 1977) failed to confirm this association between cadmium and prostate cancer.

Experimental Evidence

Carcinogenicity. Except for one long-term study in which Schroeder et al. (1964, 1965) observed no carcinogenic effect in mice given cadmium at 5 mg/liter drinking water, no studies have been conducted in laboratory animals to determine the effect of dietary cadmium on carcinogenicity.

Intramuscular injection of cadmium powder induced sarcomas in hooded rats (Heath et al., 1962). Subcutaneous injections of cadmium sulfide, cadmium oxide, cadmium sulfate, or cadmium chloride induced sarcomas and Leydig cell tumors in Wistar rats of the Chester Beatty strain (WI/Cbi) (Haddow et al., 1964; Kazantzis and Hanbury, 1966; Roe et al., 1964). Intratesticularly administered cadmium chloride also induced teratomas in White Leghorn cockerels (Guthrie, 1964) and sarcomas in Wistar rats and albino mice (Gunn et al., 1963, 1964, 1967).

Mutagenicity and Related Tests. Sirover and Loeb (1976) found that various salts of cadmium decreased the fidelity of avian myeloblastosis virus (AMV)/DNA polymerase for replication of synthetic polynucleotide templates. Cadmium salts were mutagenic to Escherichia coli (Yagi and Nishioka, 1977) and positive in rec assay in Bacillus subtilis (Nishioka, 1975). Shiraishi et al. (1972) found that in vitro treatment of human lymphocytes with cadmium sulfide induced chromosome aberrations. Casto et al. (1976) reported that cadmium (II) induced the formation of morphologically altered colonies in Syrian hamster fetal cells.

Summary

Epidemiological Evidence. The effect of dietary cadmium on cancer has been examined in only a few epidemiological studies. The results of three studies suggested that ingestion of cadmium in food or drinking water is associated with an increased risk of cancer, but another study did not confirm these findings. Occupational exposure to cadmium has been associated with an increase in the risk of renal and prostate cancer.

Experimental Evidence. Data from one laboratory experiment suggest that cadmium given in drinking water is not carcinogenic in mice, whereas intramuscular and subcutaneous injections of cadmium salts induce cancer in rats and mice. Some salts of cadmium induce mutations in bacteria and chromosome aberrations in human lymphocytes in culture. The implications of the latter findings for the effect of dietary exposure to cadmium are not clear.

Conclusion

The evidence from epidemiological and laboratory studies does not permit any firm conclusions to be drawn about the effects of dietary exposure to cadmium.

ARSENIC

Arsenic is considered to be an essential element for growth in animals (Schwarz, 1977). Small amounts of this element are widely distributed throughout the soils and waters of the world, and trace amounts occur in foods (especially seafood) and in some meats and vegetables. Arsenic may be present in food as a contaminant or as the unintentional residue of calcium arsenate or lead arsenate, which are used as insecticides, particularly on fruits and potatoes. A Market Basket Survey of 28 cities conducted by the Food and Drug Administration (FDA) during 1969-1970 revealed that arsenic levels in dairy products were less than 0.1 mg/kg, but ranged from 0.1 to 2.6 mg/kg in meat, fish, and poultry (Corneliussen, 1972). In the most recent published survey (for FY 1977), arsenic was detected in 45 of 300 (15%) food composites in amounts ranging between 0.02 and 0.83 mg/kg (U.S. Food and Drug Administration, 1980). In one study of selected trace elements in 727 samples of U.S. surface waters, the concentration of arsenic ranged from <10 to 1,100 µg/liter (Durum et al., 1971). In river waters, the median concentration of arsenic was less than 10 µg/liter. The daily intake of arsenic in the United States was reported to average 63 µg/day between 1965 and 1970, 10 µg/day in 1973, and 21 µg/day in 1974 (Mahaffey et al., 1975).

Because of the variations in individual susceptibility to the toxicity of arsenic and differences in toxicity of the various chemical forms of arsenic, it is difficult to estimate the average tolerable level for arsenic. No provisional tolerable daily intake has been established for arsenic by the World Health Organization.

Epidemiological Evidence

Most of the epidemiological evidence for the carcinogenicity of arsenic has been obtained in studies of lung cancer among workers occupationally exposed to inorganic arsenic by inhalation. In addition, several clinical reports have recorded observations of an unexpectedly high frequency of skin cancer among patients treated with inorganic arsenic drugs (e.g., Fowler's solution). Neither of these sources of exposure is dietary.

Water supplies may contain arsenic, and the consumption of contaminated water has also been associated with an increased risk for skin cancer in certain regions of the world. For example, studies in Taiwan have shown a direct relationship between the arsenic content of well water and the prevalence of skin cancer in the population drinking the water (Tseng, 1977; Tseng et al., 1968).

Epidemiological literature on cancer risk associated with occupational, medicinal, and drinking water sources of exposure to arsenic has been reviewed in publications by the International Agency for Research on Cancer (1973, 1980a) and the National Academy of Sciences (1977a,b; 1980a).

The occurrence of cancers of the skin, lung, and liver (hemangioendotheliomas) in association with clinical evidence of chronic arsenism has been reported among vineyard workers in the Federal Republic of Germany and in France (Galy et al., 1963; Latarjet et al., 1964; Roth, 1957a,b). The workers had been exposed to arsenic both from inhalation of arsenical pesticides and from ingestion of contaminated wine. These reports suggest the possibility that a carcinogenic risk resulted from the ingestion of the wine. On the other hand, Nelson et al. (1973) found no increased risk for total cancer mortality or for lung cancer specifically in a cohort of residents in the State of Washington who had consumed apples from orchards treated with lead arsenate sprays. (There was also no increase among the workers who applied the sprays.) Moreover, ingestion of arsenic-contaminated foods in Japan, including powdered milk and soy sauce, has not been associated with any increased occurrence of cancer (Tsuchiya, 1977).

Experimental Evidence

Carcinogenicity. Hueper and Payne (1962) exposed rats and C57BL mice from the age of 2 months to 15 months to a 0.0004% solution of arsenic in 12% aqueous ethanol through drinking water. The incidence of tumors in the treated group was no greater than that in the untreated controls. The tumor incidence in Swiss mice receiving 0.01% was similar to that of the control mice (Baroni et al., 1963). In another study, Rockland all-purpose mice fed potassium arsenite at 169 µg/g diet for 48 weeks and also exposed to this chemical by skin painting failed to develop more tumors than did the control animals (Boutwell, 1963).

In rats exposed daily to 10 mg of lead arsenate or calcium arsenate for 2 years, there was no increase in the incidence of tumors (Fairhall and Miller, 1941). Byron et al. (1967) similarly reported no evidence of carcinogenicity in a 2-year study in which Osborne-Mendel rats were fed sodium arsenite (which provided arsenic at 0-250 µg/g diet) or sodium arsenate (which provided arsenic at 0 to 440 µg/g diet). In dogs, sodium arsenite or sodium arsenate fed at levels of 5, 25, 50, and 125 µg/g diet for 2 years produced no increase in the incidence of tumors (Byron et al., 1967).

Cocarcinogenicity. Arsenic has also been evaluated as a cocarcinogen, but the results were negative when tested in combination with urethane, DMBA, and N-nitrosodiethylamine (Furst, 1977).

Mutagenicity. Rossman et al. (1977) reported that sodium arsenite significantly decreased the survival of wild type Escherichia coli (WP) after irradiation, suggesting that it inhibits one or more steps in the postreplication DNA repair pathways. Arsenic (III) yielded positive results in Bacillus subtilis rec assay (Nishioka, 1975). It has also been shown to transform Syrian hamster cells in vitro and to enhance the susceptibility of these cells to transformation by simian adenovirus (Casto et al., 1976).

Chromosome breakage in leukocytes of humans exposed to arsenic compounds was reported by Petres and Berger (1972) and Petres and Hundeiker (1968). Analysis of lymphocytes from exposed patients indicated that frequent chromosome aberrations occurred even decades after the last exposure (Petres et al., 1970, 1977). Paton and Allison (1972) reported that sodium arsenite and acetylarsan induced chromosome aberrations in diploid fibroblasts of humans.

Nordenson et al. (1978) reported that exposure to arsenic combined with cigarette smoking significantly enhanced the incidence of chromosome aberrations in the lymphocytes of smelter workers, compared to the incidence for nonsmoking smelter workers exposed to arsenic alone. The authors speculated that the chromosome aberrations may have been initiated by smoking or by some other agent in the workplace environment, and that exposure to arsenic may have inhibited their repair.

Summary and Conclusions

Arsenic is unique among the various agents covered in this report in that it has been associated with cancer in humans but not in laboratory animals.

Epidemiological Evidence. There is good evidence that drinking water heavily contaminated with arsenic increases the risk of skin cancer in humans in some parts of the world, and some evidence that the risk of lung cancer is increased by inhaling arsenic in occupational settings.

However, the reported epidemiological studies do not provide sufficient information to determine the effects of the normally low levels of dietary arsenic on cancer risk.

Experimental Evidence. Arsenic does not appear to induce tumors in laboratory animals despite extensive testing in animals of various species. It is possible that humans are more sensitive to the carcinogenic effects of arsenic and that the appropriate animal species, strain, dosage schedule, compound, or the route of exposure have not yet been identified.

LEAD

Although a requirement for trace amounts of lead (29 ng/g diet) has recently been demonstrated in rats for the maintenance of growth, reproduction, and hemopoiesis (Reichlmayr-Lais and Kirchgessner, 1981), it is not known to be essential to human nutrition. Humans are exposed to oxides and salts of lead through various environmental sources such as automobile exhausts, atmospheric dust, drinking water, food, and paint, all of which contribute to the total body burden of lead. The dietary intake of lead in the United States was estimated to be 60 µg/person/day in 1973 and 19 µg/day in 1974 (Mahaffey et al., 1975).

Epidemiological Evidence

Berg and Burbank (1972) correlated the levels of eight trace elements in the water supplies of 10 major river basins in the United States with corresponding cancer mortality rates for white and nonwhite males and females. There were significant correlations for five of the eight elements. Among these was lead, which was directly correlated with cancers of the stomach, small intestine, large intestine, ovary, and kidney, as well as with myeloma, all lymphomas, and all leukemias. Nelson et al. (1973) found no increased risk for cancer mortality in a population that consumed apples from orchards treated with lead arsenate spray; thus, neither lead nor arsenic in this form was implicated as a carcinogen.

Occupational exposure to lead has not been conclusively associated with any form of cancer. Most studies have shown no association (Dingwall-Fordyce and Lane, 1963; Robinson, 1976), although the results of the study by Cooper and Gaffey (1975) can be interpreted as either demonstrating or not demonstrating a relationship, depending on the method of analysis used (International Agency for Research on Cancer, 1980b; Kang et al., 1980).

Experimental Evidence

Carcinogenicity. The number of renal tumors that developed in Swiss mice fed 0.1% lead subacetate was significantly higher than that observed in untreated controls (Van Esch and Kroes, 1969). There were also significantly more renal tumors in Wistar rats fed lead acetate, as compared to controls (Mao and Molnar, 1967; Shakerin and Paloucek, 1965; Van Esch et al., 1962; Zawirska and Medras, 1968). Lead nitrate and lead powder were found not to be carcinogenic when fed to Long Evans and Fischer rats, respectively (Furst et al., 1976; Schroeder et al., 1970). In several other feeding studies, the majority of rats developed renal tumors; however, these studies did not include concurrent untreated control animals (Boyland et al., 1962; Hass et al., 1967; Ito, 1973; Ito et al., 1971).

Mutagenicity. Lead (II) reacted with phosphate groups of DNA bases to yield stable complexes (Venugopal and Luckey, 1978; Sissoëff et al., 1976). Sirover and Loeb (1976) reported that 4 mM lead chloride diminished the fidelity of DNA polymerase.

Lead acetate was found to be negative in the Ames test and E. coli pol A assay for DNA-modifying effects (Rosenkranz and Poirier, 1979); in the host-mediated assay in Swiss Webster mice with Ames Salmonella strains and Saccharomyces cerevisiae D3 as indicator organisms (Simmon et al., 1979); in the mitotic recombination assay with Saccharomyces cerevisiae D3 (Simmon, 1979); and in the Bacillus subtilis rec assay (Kada et al., 1980; Nishioka, 1975).

Bone marrow cells from rats treated with 1% lead acetate in drinking water had more chromatid gaps, fragments, deletions, and translocations than did the same cells from controls (Teodorescu and Calugăru, 1972).

Bauchinger and Schmid (1972) reported that there were more achromatic lesions in Chinese hamster ovary cells treated with 1 mM lead acetate than in untreated controls. Morphological transformations of Syrian hamster embryo cells were observed after exposure to lead acetate (1-2.5 g/liter medium), which produced fibrosarcomas in Syrian hamsters (DiPaolo et al., 1978).

Lead acetate (10^{-2} mM) induced achromatic lesions and chromatid and isochromatid breaks (Beek and Obe, 1974), but not sister chromatid exchanges in leukocytes from humans (Beek and Obe, 1975).

Summary

Epidemiological Evidence. There is very little epidemiological evidence linking dietary lead to the risk of cancer in humans. The only study that correlated lead levels in drinking water supplies and cancer mortality suggested that lead increased the risk of cancer. Exposure to lead in industrial settings has not been clearly associated with an increased risk for any form of cancer.

Experimental Evidence. The ingestion of high levels of lead compounds induces renal tumors in mice and rats.

Conclusion

On the basis of experiments in animals, it would seem that exposure to large amounts of some compounds of lead may pose a carcinogenic risk to humans. However, there is little direct epidemiological evidence to support this conclusion.

REFERENCES

Adams, R. G., J. F. Harrison, and P. Scott. 1969. The development of cadmium-induced proteinuria, impaired renal function, and osteomalacia in alkaline battery workers. Q. J. Med. 38:425-443.

Aquino, T. I., and B. A. Eskin. 1972. Rat breast structure in altered iodine metabolism. Arch. Pathol. 94:280-285.

Armann, R. W., E. Müller, J. Bansky, G. Schüler, and W. H. Häcki. 1980. High incidence of extrahepatic carcinomas in idiopathic hemochromatosis. Scand. J. Gastroenterol. 15:733-736.

Baroni, C., G. J. van Esch, and U. Saffiotti. 1963. Carcinogenesis tests of two inorganic arsenicals. Arch. Environ. Health 7:668-674.

Barr, D. H., and J. W. Harris. 1973. Growth of the P388 leukemia as an ascites tumor in zinc-deficient mice. Proc. Soc. Exp. Biol. Med. 144:284-287.

Bauchinger, M., and E. Schmid. 1972. [In German; English Summary.] Chromosomenanalysen in Zellkulturen des chinesischen Hamsters nach Applikation von Bleiacetat. Mutat. Res. 14:95-100.

Beek, B., and G. Obe. 1974. Effect of lead acetate on human leukocyte chromosomes in vitro. Experientia 30:1006-1007.

Beek, B., and G. Obe. 1975. The human leukocyte test system. VI. The use of sister chromatid exchanges as possible indicators for mutagenic activities. Humangenetik 29:127-134.

Berg, J. W., and F. Burbank. 1972. Correlations between carcinogenic trace metals in water supplies and cancer mortality. Ann. N.Y. Acad. Sci. 199:249-264.

Berg, J. W., W. Haenszel, and S. S. Devesa. 1973. Epidemiology of gastrointestinal cancer. Pp. 459-464 in Seventh National Cancer Conference Proceedings. J. B. Lippincott, Philadelphia.

Bielschowsky, F. 1944. Tumors of the thyroid produced by 2-acetylaminofluorene and allylthiourea. Br. J. Exp. Pathol. 25:90-94.

Bogardus, G. M., and J. W. Finley. 1961. Breast cancer and thyroid disease. Surgery 49:461-468.

Boutwell, R. K. 1963. A carcinogenicity evaluation of potassium arsenite and arsanilic acid. J. Agric. Food Chem. 11:381-385.

Boyland, E., C. E. Dukes, P. L. Grover, and B. C. V. Mitchley. 1962. The induction of renal tumours by feeding lead acetate to rats. Br. J. Cancer 16:283-288.

Brada, Z., and N. H. Altman. 1978. The inhibitory effect of copper on ethionine carcinogenesis. Adv. Exp. Med. Biol. 91:193-206.

Broitman, S. A., H. Velez, and J. J. Vitale. 1981. A possible role of iron deficiency in gastric cancer in Colombia. Adv. Exp. Med. Biol. 91:155-181.

Brusick, D., F. Gletten, D. R. Jagannath, and U. Weeks. 1976. The mutagenic activity of ferrous sulfate for Salmonella typhimurium. Mutat. Res. 38:386. Abstract 27.

Burrell, R. J. W., W. A. Roach, and A. Shadwell. 1966. Esophageal cancer in the Bantu of the Transkei associated with mineral deficiency in garden plants. J. Natl. Cancer Inst. 36:201-214.

Byron, W. R., G. W. Bierbower, J. B. Brouwer, and W. H. Hansen. 1967. Pathological changes in rats and dogs from two-year feeding of sodium arsenite or sodium arsenate. Toxicol. Appl. Pharmacol. 10: 132-147.

Casto, B. D., W. J. Pieczynski, R. L. Nelson, and J. A. DiPaolo. 1976. In vitro transformation and enhancement of viral transformation with metals. Proc. Am. Assoc. Cancer Res. Am. Soc. Clin. Oncol. 17:12. Abstract 46.

Clayton, C. C., and C. A. Baumann. 1949. Diet and azo dye tumors: Effect of diet during a period when the dye is not fed. Cancer Res. 9:575-582.

Clements, F. W. 1954. The relationship of thyrotoxicosis and carcinoma of the thyroid to endemic goitre. Med. J. Aust. 2:894-897.

Cole, P., and M. B. Goldman. 1975. Occupation. Pp. 167-183 in J. F. Fraumeni, Jr., ed. Persons at High Risk of Cancer: An Approach to Cancer Etiology and Control. Academic Press, New York, San Francisco, and London.

Cooper, W. C., and W. R. Gaffey. 1975. Mortality of lead workers. J. Occup. Med. 17:100-107.

Coordinating Group for Research on Etiology of Esophageal Cancer in North China. 1975. The epidemiology of esophageal cancer in north China. A preliminary report. Chin. Med. J. (Peking, Engl. Ed.) 1:167-183.

Corneliussen, P. E. 1972. Pesticide residues in total diet samples. VI. Pestic. Monit. J. 5:313-330.

Davies, I. J. T., M. Musa, and T. L. Dormandy. 1968. Measurements of plasma zinc. Part II. In malignant disease. J. Clin. Pathol. 21:363-365.

DeWys, W., and W. Pories. 1972. Inhibition of a spectrum of animal tumors by dietary zinc deficiency. J. Natl. Cancer Inst. 48:375-381.

DeWys, W., W. J. Pories, M. C. Richter, and W. H. Strain. 1970. Inhibition of Walker 256 carcinosarcoma growth by dietary zinc deficiency. Proc. Soc. Exp. Biol. Med. 135:17-22.

Dingwall-Fordyce, I., and R. E. Lane. 1963. A follow-up study of lead workers. Br. J. Ind. Med. 20:313-315.

DiPaolo, J. A., R. L. Nelson, and B. C. Casto. 1978. *In vitro* neoplastic transformation of Syrian hamster cells by lead acetate and its relevance to environmental carcinogenesis. Br. J. Cancer 38:452-455.

Doniach, I. 1958. Experimental induction of tumours of the thyroid by radiation. Br. Med. Bull. 14:181-183.

Duncan, J. R., and I. E. Dreosti. 1975. Zinc intake, neoplastic DNA synthesis, and chemical carcinogenesis in rats and mice. J. Natl. Cancer Inst. 55:195-196.

Durum, W. H., J. D. Hem, and S. G. Heidel. 1971. Reconnaissance of Selected Minor Elements in Surface Waters of the United States, October 1970. Geological Survey Circular 643. U.S. Geological Survey and U.S. Bureau of Sport Fisheries and Wildlife, U.S. Department of the Interior, Washington, D.C. 49 pp.

Edington, G. M. 1976. Dietary iodine and risk of breast, endometrial and ovarian cancer. Lancet 1:1413-1414.

Endo, H., M. Ishizawa, T. Endo, K. Takahashi, T. Utsunomiya, N. Kinoshita, K. Hidaka, and T. Baba. 1977. A possible process of conversion of food components to gastric carcinogens. Pp. 1591-1607 in H. H. Hiatt, J. D. Watson, and J. A. Winsten, eds. Origins of Human Cancer, Book C. Human Risk Assessment. Cold Spring Harbor Laboratory, Cold Spring Harbor, N.Y.

Eskin, B. A. 1978. Iodine and mammary cancer. Adv. Exp. Med. Biol. 91:293-304.

Eskin, B. A., D. G. Bartuska, M. R. Dunn, G. Jacob, and M. B. Dratman. 1967. Mammary gland dysplasia in iodine deficiency. J. Am. Med. Assoc. 200:691-695.

Eskin, B. A., H. I. Jacobson, V. Bolmarcich, and J. A. Murray. 1976. Breast atypia in altered iodine states: Intracellular changes. Senologia 1:51. Abstract 72.

Fairhall, L. T., and J. W. Miller. 1941. A study of the relative toxicity of the molecular components of lead arsenate. Public Health Rep. 56:1610-1625.

Fenton, M. R., J. P. Burke, F. D. Tursi, and F. P. Arena. 1980. Effect of a zinc-deficient diet on the growth of an IgM-secreting plasmacytoma (TEPC-183). J. Natl. Cancer Inst. 65:1271-1272.

Fisher, K. D., and C. J. Carr. 1974. Iodine in foods: Chemical methodology and sources of iodine in the human diet. Life Sciences Research Office, Federation of American Societies for Experimental Biology, Bethesda, Md. 105 pp.

Fong, L. Y. Y., A. Sivak, and P. M. Newberne. 1978. Zinc deficiency and methylbenzylnitrosamine-induced esophageal cancer in rats. J. Natl. Cancer Inst. 61:145-150.

Friberg, L., M. Piscator, G. F. Nordberg, and T. Kjellström. 1974. Cadmium in the Environment, 2nd edition. C.R.C. Press, Cleveland, Ohio. 248 pp.

Furst, A. 1977. Inorganic agents as carcinogens. Pp. 209-229 in H. F. Kraybill and M. A. Mehlman, eds. Advances in Modern Toxicology, Volume 3. Environmental Cancer. John Wiley and Sons, New York.

Furst, A. 1979. Problems in metal carcinogenesis. Pp. 83-92 in N. Kharasch, ed. Trace Metals in Health and Disease. Raven Press, New York.

Furst, A., M. Schlauder, and D. P. Sasmore. 1976. Tumorigenic activity of lead chromate. Cancer Res. 36:1779-1783.

Galy, P., R. Touraine, J. Brune, P. Gallois, P. Roudier, R. Loire, P. Lheureux, and T. Wiesendanger. 1963. [In French.] Les cancers broncho-pulmonaires de l'intoxication arsenicale chronique chez les viticulteurs du Beaujolais. Lyon Med. 210:735-744.

Golden, M. H. N., B. E. Golden, P. S. E. Harland, and A. A. Jackson. 1978. Zinc and immunocompetence in protein-energy malnutrition. Lancet 1:1226-1227.

Greeder, G. A., and J. A. Milner. 1980. Factors influencing the inhibitory effect of selenium on mice inoculated with Ehrlich ascites tumor cells. Science 209:825-827.

Griffin, A. C. 1979. Role of selenium in the chemoprevention of cancer. Adv. Cancer Res. 29:419-442.

Gunn, S. A., T. C. Gould, and W. A. D. Anderson. 1963. Cadmium-induced interstitial cell tumors in rats and mice and their prevention by zinc. J. Natl. Cancer Inst. 31:745-759.

Gunn, S. A., T. C. Gould, and W. A. D. Anderson. 1964. Effect of zinc on cancerogenesis by cadmium. Proc. Soc. Exp. Biol. Med. 115:653-657.

Gunn, S. A., T. C. Gould, and W. A. D. Anderson. 1967. Specific response of mesenchymal tissue in cancerigenesis by cadmium. Arch. Pathol. 83:493-499.

Guthrie, J. 1964. Histological effects of intra-testicular injections of cadmium chloride in domestic fowl. Br. J. Cancer 18:255-260.

Györkey, F., K. W. Min, J. A. Huff, and P. Györkey. 1967. Zinc and magnesium in human prostate gland: Normal, hyperplastic and neoplastic. Cancer Res. 27:1348-1353.

Haddow, A., F. J. C. Roe, C. E. Dukes, and B. C. V. Mitchley. 1964. Cadmium neoplasia: Sarcomata at the site of injection of cadmium sulphate in rats and mice. Br. J. Cancer 18:667-673.

Harr, J. R., J. F. Bone, I. J. Tinsley, P. H. Weswig, and R. S. Yamamoto. 1967. Selenium toxicity in rats. II. Histopathology. Pp. 153-178 in O. H. Muth, ed. Symposium: Selenium in Biomedicine. First International Symposium. AVI Publishing Co., Westport, Conn.

Harr, J. R., J. H. Exon, P. D. Whanger, and P. H. Weswig. 1972. Effect of dietary selenium on N-2-fluorenyl-acetamide(FAA)-induced cancer in vitamin E supplemented, selenium depleted rats. Clin. Toxicol. 5:187-194.

Hass, G. M., J. H. McDonald, R. Oyasu, H. A. Battifora, and J. T. Paloucek. 1967. Renal neoplasia induced by combinations of dietary lead subacetate and N-2-fluorenylacetamide. Pp. 377-412 in J. S. King, Jr., ed. Renal Neoplasia. Little, Brown Co., Boston.

Heath, J. C., M. R. Daniel, J. T. Dingle, and M. Webb. 1962. Cadmium as a carcinogen. Nature 193:592-593.

Holden, J. M., W. R. Wolf, and W. Mertz. 1979. Zinc and copper in self-selected diets. J. Am. Diet. Assoc. 75:23-28.

Hueper, W. C., and W. W. Payne. 1962. Experimental studies in metal carcinogenesis: Chromium, nickel, iron, arsenic. Arch. Environ. Health 5:445-462.

International Agency for Research on Cancer. 1973. Pp. 65-68 in IARC Monographs on the Evaluation of the Carcinogenic Risk of Chemicals to Man: Volume 2. Some Inorganic and Organometallic Compounds. International Agency for Research on Cancer, Lyon, France.

International Agency for Research on Cancer. 1980a. Case reports and epidemiological studies. Pp. 101-112 in IARC Monographs on the Evaluation of the Carcinogenic Risk of Chemicals to Humans. Volume 23: Some Metals and Metallic Compounds. International Agency for Research on Cancer, Lyon, France.

International Agency for Research on Cancer. 1980b. Lead and lead compounds. Pp. 325-415 in IARC Monographs on the Evaluation of the Carcinogenic Risk of Chemicals to Humans. Volume 23: Some Metals and Metallic Compounds, International Agency for Research on Cancer, Lyon, France.

Ip, C., and D. K. Sinha. 1981. Enhancement of mammary tumorigenesis by dietary selenium deficiency in rats with a high polyunsaturated fat intake. Cancer Res. 41:31-34.

Ito, N. 1973. Experimental studies on tumors of the urinary system of rats induced by chemical carcinogens. Acta Pathol. Jpn. 23:87-109.

Ito, N., Y. Hiasa, Y. Kamamoto, S. Makiura, S. Sugihara, M. Marugami, and E. Okajima. 1971. Histopathological analysis of kidney tumors in rats induced by chemical carcinogens. Gann 62:435-444.

Jacobs, M. M., T. S. Matney, and A. C. Griffin. 1977. Inhibitory effects of selenium on the mutagenicity of 2-acetyl-aminofluorene (AAF) and AAF derivatives. Cancer Lett. 2:319-322.

Jansson, B., G. B. Seibert, and J. F. Speer. 1975. Gastrointestinal cancer: Its geographic distribution and correlation to breast cancer. Cancer 36:2373-2384.

Jansson, B., M. M. Jacobs, and A. C. Griffin. 1978. Gastrointestinal cancer: Epidemiology and experimental studies. Adv. Exp. Med. Biol. 91:305-322.

Jensen, L. S. 1975. Modification of a selenium toxicity in chicks by dietary silver and copper. J. Nutr. 105:769-775.

Kada, T., K. Hirano, and Y. Shirasu. 1980. Screening of environmental chemical mutagens by the rec-assay system with Bacillus subtilis. Chem. Mutagens 6:149-173.

Kang, H. K., P. F. Infante, and J. S. Carra. 1980. Occupational lead exposure and cancer. Science 207:935-936.

Kanisawa, M., and H. A. Schroeder. 1967. Life term studies on the effects of arsenic, germanium, tin and vanadium on spontaneous tumors in mice. Cancer Res. 27:1192-1195.

Kazantzis, G., and W. J. Hanbury. 1966. The induction of sarcoma in the rat by cadmium sulphide and by cadmium oxide. Br. J. Cancer 20:190-199.

Kipling, M. D., and J. A. H. Waterhouse. 1967. Letter to the Editor: Cadmium and prostatic carcinoma. Lancet 1:730-731.

Klevay, L. M., S. J. Reck, and D. F. Barcome. 1979. Evidence of dietary copper and zinc deficiencies. J. Am. Med. Assoc. 241:1916-1918.

Kolonel, L. N. 1976. Association of cadmium with renal cancer. Cancer 37:1782-1787.

Kolonel, L. N., and W. Winkelstein, Jr. 1977. Letter to the Editor: Cadmium and prostatic carcinoma. Lancet 2:566-567.

Larsson, L.-G., A. Sandström, and P. Westling. 1975. Relationship of Plummer-Vinson disease to cancer of the upper alimentary tract in Sweden. Cancer Res. 35:3308-3316.

Latarjet, M., P. Galy, G. Maret, and P. Gallois. 1964. [In French.] Cancers broncho-pulmonaires et intoxication arsenicale chez des vignerons du Beaujolais. Mem. Acad. Chir. 90:384-390.

Lemen, R. A., J. S. Lee, J. K. Wagoner, and H. P. Blejer. 1976. Cancer mortality among cadmium production workers. Ann. N. Y. Acad. Sci. 271:273-279.

Lin, H. J., W. C. Chan, Y. Y. Fong, and P. M. Newberne. 1977. Zinc levels in serum, hair and tumors from patients with esophageal cancer. Nutr. Rep. Int. 15:635-643.

Lo, L. W., J. Koropatrick, and H. T. Stich. 1978. The mutagenicity and cytotoxicity of selenite and selenate for normal and DNA repair-deficient human fibroblasts. Mutat. Res. 49:305-312.

Luo, X. M., H. J. Wei, G. G. Hu, A. L. Shang, Y. Y. Liu, S. M. Lu, and S. P. Yang. 1981. Molybdenum and esophageal cancer in China. Fed. Proc. Fed. Am. Soc. Exp. Biol. 40:928. Abstract 3962.

MacKinnon, A. E., and J. Bancewicz. 1973. Sarcoma after injection of intramuscular iron. Br. Med. J. 2:277-279.

Mahaffey, K. R., P. E. Corneliussen, C. F. Jelinek, and T. A. Fiorino. 1975. Heavy metal exposure from foods. Environ. Health Perspect. 12:63-69.

Mao, P., and J. J. Molnar. 1967. The fine structure and histochemistry of lead-induced renal tumors in rats. Am. J. Pathol. 50:571-603.

Medina, D., and F. Shepherd. 1980. Selenium-mediated inhibition of mouse mammary tumorigenesis. Cancer Lett. 8:241-245.

Minkel, D. T., P. J. Dolhun, B. L. Calhoun, L. A. Saryan, and D. H. Petering. 1979. Zinc deficiency and growth of Ehrlich ascites tumor. Cancer Res. 39:2451-2456.

Nakamuro, K., K. Yoshikawa, Y. Sayato, H. Kurata, M. Tonomura, and A. Tonomura. 1976. Studies on selenium-related compounds. V. Cytogenetic effect and reactivity with DNA. Mutat. Res. 40:177-183.

National Academy of Sciences. 1971. Selenium in Nutrition. A report of the Subcommittee on Selenium, Committee on Animal Nutrition. National Academy of Sciences, Washington, D.C. 79 pp.

National Academy of Sciences. 1977a. Arsenic. A report of the Committee on Medical and Biologic Effects of Environmental Pollutants. National Academy of Sciences, Washington, D.C. 332 pp.

National Academy of Sciences. 1977b. Drinking Water and Health. A report of the Safe Drinking Water Committee, National Academy of Sciences, Washington, D.C. 939 pp.

National Academy of Sciences. 1980a. Drinking Water and Health, Volume 2. A report of the Safe Drinking Water Committee. National Academy Press, Washington, D.C. 393 pp.

National Academy of Sciences. 1980b. Pp. 162-163 in Recommended Dietary Allowances, 9th edition. A report of the Food and Nutrition Board. National Academy of Sciences, Washington, D.C.

Nelson, A. A., O. G. Fitzhugh, and H. O. Calvery. 1943. Liver tumors following cirrhosis caused by selenium in rats. Cancer Res. 3:230-236.

Nelson, W. C., M. H. Lykins, J. Mackey, V. A. Newill, J. F. Finklea, and D. I. Hammer. 1973. Mortality among orchard workers exposed to lead arsenate spray: A cohort study. J. Chronic Dis. 26:105-118.

Newman, J. A., V. E. Archer, G. Saccomanno, M. Kuschner, O. Auerbach, R. D. Grondahl, and J. C. Wilson. 1976. Histologic types of bronchogenic carcinoma among members of copper-mining and smelting communities. Ann. N. Y. Acad. Sci. 271:260-268.

Nishioka, H. 1975. Mutagenic activities of metal compounds in bacteria. Mutat. Res. 31:185-189.

Nordenson, I., G. Beckman, L. Beckman, and S. Nordström. 1978. Occupational and environmental risks in and around a smelter in northern Sweden. II. Chromosomal aberrations in workers exposed to arsenic. Hereditas 88:47-50.

Paton, G. R., and A. C. Allison. 1972. Chromosome damage in human cell cultures induced by metal salts. Mutat. Res. 16:332-336.

Pendergrast, W. J., B. K. Milmore, and S. C. Marcus. 1961. Thyroid cancer and thyrotoxicosis in the United States: Their relation to endemic goiter. J. Chronic Dis. 13:22-38.

Petering, H. G., H. H. Buskirk, and J. A. Crim. 1967. The effect of dietary mineral supplements of the rat on the antitumor activity of 3-ethoxy-2-oxobutyraldehyde bis(thiosemicarbazone). Cancer Res. 27:1115-1121.

Petres, J., and A. Berger. 1972. [In German; English Summary.] The effect of inorganic arsenic on DNA-synthesis of human lymphocytes in vitro. Arch. Dermatol. Forsch. 242:343-352.

Petres, J., and M. Hundeiker. 1968. [In German; English Summary.] "Chromosome pulverization" induced in vitro in cell cultures by sodium diarsenate. Arch. Klin. Exp. Dermatol. 231:366-370.

Petres, J., K. Schmid-Ullrich, and U. Wolf. 1970. [In German.] Chromosomenaberrationen an menschlichen Lymphozyten bei chronischen Arsenschäden. Dtsch. Med. Wochenschr. 95:79-80.

Petres, J., D. Baron, and M. Hagedorn. 1977. Effects of arsenic cell metabolism and cell proliferation: Cytogenetic and biochemical studies. Environ. Health Perspect. 19:223-227.

Pimentel, J. C., and A. P. Menezes. 1977. Liver disease in vineyard sprayers. Gastroenterology 72:275-283.

Poswillo, D. E., and B. Cohen. 1971. Inhibition of carcinogenesis by dietary zinc. Nature 231:447-448.

Potts, C. L. 1965. Cadmium proteinuria--the health of battery workers exposed to cadmium oxide dust. Ann. Occup. Hyg. 8:55-61.

Prasad, A. S. 1978. Trace Elements and Iron in Human Metabolism. Plenum Publishing Corp., New York and London. 392 pp.

Reichlmayr-Lais, A. M., and M. Kirchgessner. 1981. [In German; English Summary.] Essentiality of lead for growth and metabolism. Z. Tierphysiol. Tierernaehr. Futtermittelkd. 46:1-8.

Robinson, C. E. G., D. N. Bell, and J. H. Sturdy. 1960. Possible association of malignant neoplasm with iron-dextran injection. Br. Med. J. 2:648-650.

Robinson, T. R. 1976. The health of long service tetraethyl lead workers. J. Occup. Med. 18:31-40.

Roe, F. J. C., C. E Dukes, K. M. Cameron, R. C. B. Pugh, and B. C. V. Mitchley. 1964. Cadmium neoplasia: Testicular atrophy and Leydig cell hyperplasia and neoplasia in rats and mice following the subcutaneous injection of cadmium salts. Br. J. Cancer 18:674-681.

Rosenkranz, H. S., and L. A. Poirier. 1979. Evaluation of the mutagenicity and DNA-modifying activity of carcinogens and noncarcinogens in microbial systems. J. Natl. Cancer Inst. 62:873-892.

Rossman, T. G., M. S. Meyn, and W. Troll. 1977. Effects of arsenite on DNA repair in Escherichia coli. Environ. Health Perspect. 19:229-233.

Roth, F. 1957a. [In German.] Über die Spätfolgen des chronischen Arsenismus der Moselwinzer. Dtsch. Med. Wochenschr. 82:211-217.

Roth, F. 1957b. [In German; English Summary.] Arsen-Leber-Tumoren (Hämangioendotheliom). Z. Krebsforsch. 61:468-503.

Ruddell, W. S. J., E. S. Bone, M. J. Hill, and C. L. Walters. 1978. Pathogenesis of gastric cancer in pernicious anaemia. Lancet 1:521-523.

Schrauzer, G. N. 1976. Selenium and cancer: A review. Bioinorg. Chem. 5:275-281.

Schrauzer, G. N. 1979. Trace elements in carcinogenesis. Pp. 219-244 in H. H. Draper, ed. Advances in Nutritional Research, Volume 2. Plenum Publishing Corp., New York and London.

Schrauzer, G. N., D. A. White, and C. J. Schneider. 1977a. Cancer mortality correlation studies--III. Statistical associations with dietary selenium intakes. Bioinorg. Chem. 7:23-34.

Schrauzer, G. N., D. A. White, and C. J. Schneider. 1977b. Cancer mortality correlation studies--IV. Associations with dietary intakes and blood levels of certain trace elements, notably Se-antagonists. Bioinorg. Chem. 7:35-56.

Schrauzer, G. N., D. A. White, and C. J. Schneider. 1978. Selenium and cancer: Effects of selenium and of the diet on the genesis of spontaneous mammary tumors in virgin inbred female C3H/St mice. Bioinorg. Chem. 8:387-396.

Schroeder, H. A., and M. Mitchener. 1971a. Scandium, chromium (VI), gallium, yttrium, rhodium, palladium, indium in mice: Effects on growth and life span. J. Nutr. 101:1431-1438.

Schroeder, H. A., and M. Mitchener. 1971b. Selenium and tellurium in rats: Effects on growth, survival, and tumors. J. Nutr. 101:1531-1540.

Schroeder, H. A., and M. Mitchener. 1972. Selenium and tellurium in mice: Effects on growth, survival and tumors. Arch. Environ. Health 24:66-71.

Schroeder, H. A., J. J. Balassa, and W. H. Vinton, Jr. 1964. Chromium, lead, cadmium, nickel and titanium in mice: Effect on mortality, tumors and tissue levels. J. Nutr. 83:239-250.

Schroeder, H. A., J. J. Balassa, and W. H. Vinton, Jr. 1965. Chromium, cadmium and lead in rats: Effects on life span, tumors and tissue levels. J. Nutr. 86:51-66.

Schroeder, H. A., M. Mitchener, J. J. Balassa, M. Kanisawa, and A. P. Nason. 1968. Zirconium, niobium, antimony and fluorine in mice: Effect on growth, survival and tissue levels. J. Nutr. 95:95-101.

Schroeder, H. A., M. Mitchener, and A. P. Nason. 1970. Zirconium, niobium, antimony, vanadium and lead in rats: Life term studies. J. Nutr. 100:59-68.

Schwartz, M. K. 1975. Role of trace elements in cancer. Cancer Res. 35:3481-3487.

Schwarz, K. 1977. Essentiality versus toxicity of metals. Pp. 3-22 in S. S. Brown, ed. Clinical Chemistry and Chemical Toxicology of Metals. Elsevier/North-Holland Biomedical Press, Amsterdam, New York, and Oxford.

Scott, D., and A. Theologides. 1974. Hepatoma, erythrocytosis and increased serum erythropoietin developing in long-standing hemochromatosis. Am. J. Gastroenterol. 61:206-211.

Shakerin, M., and J. Paloucek. 1965. Intranuclear inclusions and renal tumors in rats fed lead subacetate. Lab. Invest. 14:592. Abstract.

Shamberger, R. J. 1970. Relation of selenium to cancer. I. Inhibitory effect of selenium on carcinogenesis. J. Natl. Cancer Inst. 44:931-936.

Shamberger, R. J., and D. V. Frost. 1969. Letter to the Editor: Possible protective effect of selenium against human cancer. Can. Med. Assoc. J. 100:682.

Shamberger, R. J., and C. E. Willis. 1971. Selenium distribution and human cancer mortality. CRC Crit. Rev. Clin. Lab. Sci. 2:211-221.

Shamberger, R. J., E. Rukovena, A. K. Longfield, S. A. Tytko, S. Deodhar, and C. E. Willis. 1973. Antioxidants and cancer. I. Selenium in the blood of normals and cancer patients. J. Natl. Cancer Inst. 50:863-870.

Shamberger, R. J., S. A. Tytko, and C. E. Willis. 1976. Antioxidants and cancer. Part VI. Selenium and age-adjusted human cancer mortality. Arch. Environ. Health 31:231-235.

Shamberger, R. J., K. D. Beaman, C. L. Corlett, and B. L. Kasten. 1978. Effect of selenium and other antioxidants on the mutagenicity of malonaldehyde. Fed. Proc. Fed. Am. Soc. Exp. Biol. 37:261. Abstract 265.

Shiraishi, Y., H. Kurahashi, and T. H. Yosida. 1972. Chromosomal aberrations in cultured human leukocytes induced by cadmium sulfide. Proc. Jpn. Acad. 48:133-137.

Simmon, V. F. 1979. In vitro assays for recombinogenic activity of chemical carcinogens and related compounds with Saccharomyces cerevisiae D3. J. Natl. Cancer Inst. 62:901-909.

Simmon, V. F., H. S. Rosenkranz, E. Zeiger, and L. A. Poirier. 1979. Mutagenic activity of chemical carcinogens and related compounds in the intraperitoneal host-mediated assay. J. Natl. Cancer Inst. 62:911-918.

Sirover, M. A., and L. A. Loeb. 1976. Infidelity of DNA synthesis <u>in</u> <u>vitro</u>: Screening for potential metal mutagens or carcinogens. Science 194:1434-1436.

Sissoëff, I., J. Grisvard, and E. Guille. 1976. Studies on metal ions-DNA interactions: Specific behaviour of reiterative DNA sequences. Prog. Biophys. Mol. Biol. 31:165-199.

Stadel, B. V. 1976. Dietary iodine and risk of breast, endometrial, and ovarian cancer. Lancet 1:890-891.

Steinherz, P. G., V. C. Canale, and D. R. Miller. 1976. Hepatocellular carcinoma, transfusion-induced hemochromatosis and congenital hypoplastic anemia (Blackfan-Diamond Syndrome). Am. J. Med. 60:1032-1035.

Stocks, P., and R. I. Davies. 1964. Zinc and copper content of soils associated with the incidence of cancer of the stomach and other organs. Br. J. Cancer 18:14-24.

Stoner, G. D., M. B. Shimkin, M. C. Troxell, T. L. Thompson, and L. S. Terry. 1976. Test for carcinogenicity of metallic compounds by the pulmonary tumor response in strain A mice. Cancer Res. 36:1744-1747.

Strain, W. H., E. G. Mansour, A. Flynn, W. J. Pories, A. J. Tomaro, and O. A. Hill, Jr. 1972. Letter to the Editor: Plasma-zinc concentration in patients with bronchogenic cancer. Lancet 1:1021-1022.

Sunderman, F. W., Jr. 1977. Metal carcinogenesis. Pp. 257-295 in R. A. Goyer and M. A. Mehlman, eds. Toxicology of Trace Elements. Hemisphere Publishing Corporation, Washington and London.

Sussman, E. B., I. Nydick, and G. F. Gray. 1974. Hemangioendothelial sarcoma of the liver and hemochromatosis. Arch. Pathol. 97:39-42.

Sweeney, G. D., K. G. Jones, F. M. Cole, D. Basford, and F. Krestynski. 1979. Iron deficiency prevents liver toxicity of 2,3,7,8-tetrachlorodibenzo-<u>p</u>-dioxin. Science 204:332-335.

Teodorescu, F., and A. Čalugăru. 1972. [In Romanian; French Summary.] Modificări cromozomiale produse în celulele măduvei osoase la şoblanul alb în urma intoxicaţiel cu acetat de plumb. Stud. Cercet. Biol. Seria Zool. 24:451-457.

Thompson, H. J., and P. J. Becci. 1980. Selenium inhibition of N-methyl-N-nitrosourea-induced mammary carcinogenesis in the rat. J. Natl. Cancer Inst. 65:1299-1301.

Thomson, C. D., and M. F. Robinson. 1980. Selenium in human health and disease with emphasis on those aspects peculiar to New Zealand. Am. J. Clin. Nutr. 33:303-323.

Tseng, W. P. 1977. Effects and dose-response relationships of skin cancer and blackfoot disease with arsenic. Environ. Health Perspect. 19:109-119.

Tseng, W. P., H. M. Chu, S. W. How, J. M. Fong, C. S. Lin, and S. Yeh. 1968. Prevalence of skin cancer in an endemic area of chronic arsenicism in Taiwan. J. Natl. Cancer Inst. 40:453-463.

Tsuchiya, K. 1977. Various effects of arsenic in Japan depending on the type of exposure. Environ. Health Perspect. 19:35-42.

U.S. Food and Drug Administration. 1980. Compliance Program Report of Findings, FY 1977. Total Diet Studies (Adult, 7320.73). Bureau of Foods, Food and Drug Administration, Washington, D.C. [33] pp.

Van Esch, G. J., and R. Kroes. 1969. The induction of renal tumours by feeding basic lead acetate to mice and hamsters. Br. J. Cancer 23:765-771.

Van Esch, G. J., H. Van Genderen, and H. H. Vink. 1962. The incidence of renal tumours by feeding of basic lead acetate to rats. Br. J. Cancer 16:289-297.

van Rensburg, S. J. 1981. Epidemiologic and dietary evidence for a specific nutritional predisposition to esophageal cancer. J. Natl. Cancer Inst. 67:243-251.

Venugopal, B., and T. D. Luckey. 1978. Lead. Pp. 185-195 in Metal Toxicity in Mammals--2. Chemical Toxicity of Metals and Metalloids. Plenum Press, New York and London.

Vitale, J. J., S. A. Broitman, E. Vavrousek-Jakuba, P. W. Rodday, and L. S. Gottlieb. 1978. The effects of iron deficiency and the quality and quantity of fat on chemically induced cancer. Adv. Exp. Med. Biol. 91:229-242.

Volgarev, M. N., and L. A. Tscherkes. 1967. Further studies in tissue changes associated with sodium selenate. Pp. 179-184 in O. H. Muth, ed. Symposium: Selenium in Biomedicine. First International Symposium. AVI Publishing Co., Westport, Conn.

Wahner, H. W., C. Cuello, P. Correa, L. F. Uribe, and E. Gaitan. 1966. Thyroid carcinoma in an endemic goiter area, Cali, Colombia. Am. J. Med. 40:58-66.

Waterhouse, J., C. Muir, P. Correa, and J. Powell, eds. 1976. Cancer Incidence in Five Continents, Volume 3. IARC Scientific Publications No. 15. International Agency for Research on Cancer, Lyon, France.

Williams, E. D., I. Doniach, O. Bjarnason, and W. Michie. 1977. Thyroid cancer in an iodide rich area. A histopathological study. Cancer 39:215-222.

World Health Organization. 1972. Evaluation of certain food additives and the contaminants mercury, lead, and cadmium. Sixteenth Report of the Joint FAO/WHO Expert Committee on Food Additives. W.H.O. Tech. Rep. Ser. 505:1-32.

Wynder, E. L., S. Hultberg, F. Jacobsson, and I. J. Bross. 1957. Environmental factors in cancer of the upper alimentary tract: A Swedish study with special reference to Plummer-Vinson (Paterson-Kelly) syndrome. Cancer 10:470-487.

Yagi, T., and H. Nishioka. 1977. DNA damage and its degradation by metal compounds. Sci. Eng. Rev. Doshisha Univ. 18:63-70.

Yamane, Y., and K. Sakai. 1973. Suppressive effect of concurrent administration of metal salts on carcinogenesis by 3'-methyl-4-(dimethylamino)azobenzene, and the effect of these metals on aminoazo dye metabolism during carcinogenesis. Gann 64:563-573.

Yang, C. S. 1980. Research on esophageal cancer in China: A review. Cancer Res. 40:2633-2644.

Zawirska, B., and K. Medraś. 1968. [In German.] Tumoren und Störungen des Porphyrinstoffweschels bei Ratten mit chronischer experimenteller Bleiintoxikation. Zentralbl. Allg. Pathol. Pathol. Anat. 111:1-12.

11 Alcohol

Estimates of per capita alcoholic beverage intake based on taxes paid on alcohol purchases in various countries may be moderately or extremely low. This is partly because alcoholic beverages purchased either illegally or by special sanctions from U.S. government agencies escape taxation, and thus, inclusion in the tax records from which the estimates are drawn. Studies based on surveys are also prone to error because consumers tend to underestimate their alcohol intake (DeLuca, 1981).

EPIDEMIOLOGICAL EVIDENCE

Specific Alcoholic Beverages

A number of reports implicate specific alcoholic beverages as risk factors for cancers at certain sites. Using data on per capita intake of various types of alcoholic beverages and standard mortality ratios in the 46 prefectures of Japan, Kono and Ikeda (1979) found only suggestive correlations for males between cancer of the esophagus and intake of both whiskey and shochu; cancer of the rectum and wine intake; and cancer of the prostate and shochu intake. There were no correlations for females. Cook (1971) and Collis et al. (1972) ascribed the high frequency of esophageal cancer in an African population to the consumption of an alcoholic beverage prepared from maize. In the Normandy region of France, people who consumed home-distilled apple brandy had an increased risk of esophageal cancer, compared to nondrinkers (Tuyns et al., 1979). Smoking enhanced this risk (Tuyns and Massé, 1973; Tuyns et el., 1977). In a very early study, Lamy (1910) reported an association between esophageal cancer and the consumption of absinthe by chronic alcoholics in France. In China, where earlier records indicated that esophageal cancer comprised approximately one-half of the gastrointestinal tract cancers, pai-kan, a strong alcoholic beverage, was cited as an etiological agent (Kwan, 1937; Wu and Loucks, 1951).

Recently, Hoey et al. (1981) reported that the consumption of alcohol (primarily red wine) increased the risk of adenocarcinoma of the stomach. In this study, which was conducted in Lyon, France, patients with gastric cancer consumed approximately 800 calories per day as alcohol compared to 400 calories per day for patients with other digestive diseases.

In a multi-ethnic population living in Hawaii, a direct association was observed for beer consumption and eight cancer sites (including tongue/mouth, pharynx, larynx, esophagus, stomach, pancreas, lung, and kidney) (Hinds et al., 1980). In the mainland United States, Breslow and Enstrom (1974) and Enstrom (1977) demonstrated a statistically significant association between per capita beer intake and colorectal cancer,

202

especially rectal cancer. Wynder and Shigematsu (1967) reported that a group of 314 male colorectal cancer patients contained a significantly higher proportion of beer drinkers than did one control group, but there were no differences between the cases and a second control group. In a study of 166 male bowel cancer patients in Great Britain, Stocks (1957) demonstrated a significant association with beer drinking. Bjelke (1973) reported a dose-response relationship for the risk of colorectal cancer and the frequency of beer and liquor consumption in a prospective study of 12,000 middle-aged Norwegian men. Dean et al. (1979) also reported a direct association based on a cohort study in Dublin. Conversely, case-control studies of bowel cancer in Finland, Kansas, and Norway by Pernu (1960), Higginson (1966), and Bjelke (1971, 1973) showed no significant relationship with beer drinking. Similarly, no associations were observed in a correlational analysis by Hinds et al. (1980) or in a cohort study by Jensen (1979).

Using international data and estimates of ethanol intake from beer, wine, and distilled spirits, Vitale et al. (1981) demonstrated a correlation coefficient of 0.78 for beer drinking and colorectal cancer in 20 countries. Poor correlations were obtained for colon cancer and intake of total ethanol, distilled spirits, or wine.

Thus, in certain populations throughout the world there appears to be an association between consumption of strong, locally prepared alcoholic beverages and esophageal cancer. There also appears to be a statistically significant association between beer drinking and colorectal cancers in certain countries but not in others. These associations with specific beverage types suggest that the effects may be due to intake of other contaminants in the beverages, rather than to consumption of ethanol per se.

As noted above, epidemiological studies have linked the consumption of alcoholic beverages to the development of cancers at various sites. In an ideal study to examine this relationship, alcohol abusers and "moderate" drinkers should be studied separately. In the abusers, alcohol may play a modifying or contributing role in carcinogenesis by inducing nutritional deficiency diseases that, in turn, may interact in the process of carcinogenesis in the host. This effect of alcohol may be different in moderate drinkers. However, because it is difficult to determine alcohol intake with accuracy, the distinction between alcohol abuse and moderate drinking in the studies described below is to some extent arbitrary.

Total Alcoholic Beverages

An association between cancer at various sites and alcohol abuse has been recognized for some time. In France, Piquet and Tison (1937) observed that 95% of their patients with esophageal cancer were alcohol abusers. In a study of 4,000 French patients, Schwartz and colleagues showed a significant correlation between mean daily alcohol consumption and frequency of cancers of the tongue, hypopharynx, and larynx (Schwartz, 1966; Schwartz et al., 1962, 1966). A large majority of the individuals with cancers at these sites were heavy drinkers. In a Finnish male cohort study, chronic alcoholics were found to have excess morbidity from cancers of the pharynx, esophagus, and lung (Hakulinen et al., 1974). On the basis of a literature survey, the World Health Organization (1964) concluded that excessive consumption of alcoholic beverages was associated with cancer of the mouth, larynx, and esophagus. Case-control studies conducted in the United States have established that excessive consumption of alcoholic beverages increases the risk of incurring cancer of the oral cavity, excluding the lip, glottis and supraglottic region, larynx, and esophagus (Bross and Coombs, 1976; Burch et al., 1981; Graham et al., 1977; Kaminonkowski and Fleshler, 1965; Keller and Terris, 1965; Keller et al., 1977; Moore, 1965; Rothman and Keller, 1972; Schottenfeld, 1979; Schottenfeld et al., 1974; Vincent and Marchetta, 1963; Wynder and Bross, 1961; Wynder et al., 1957a). Salient features of the earlier studies have been summarized by Keller et al. (1977) in a report prepared for the U.S. Congress.

Excessive alcohol consumption has also been linked with the development of hepatomas (MacDonald, 1956). Purtilo and Gottlieb (1973) noted that by far the greatest number of hepatomas were hepatocellular carcinomas, which were found in 72% of the hepatoma patients studied. Approximately one-half of the 98 patients in this series were alcohol abusers. The investigators suggested that chronic alcoholism contributed to the development of hepatomas by inducing cirrhosis. Keen and Martin (1971) suggested that aflatoxin consumed by African patients induced hepatomas indirectly by first inducing cirrhosis. Vogel and his associates (1970) found hepatitis-associated antigen (HAA) in African patients with hepatomas. Hepatitis B antigenemia has been frequently associated with hepatocellular carcinomas (Sherlock et al., 1970; Vogel et al., 1970; Wu and Lam, 1979). In general, hepatomas are found in individuals with cirrhosis. Thus, agents such as alcohol, hepatitis antigen, and aflatoxin, which result in hepatic injury leading to cirrhosis, may contribute to the development of hepatomas through this pathway. A number of etiologies have been proposed for the development of carcinomas through the hepatocellular regeneration that accompanies cirrhosis (Lieber et al., 1979).

There is a substantial amount of experimental evidence indicating that aflatoxin is a carcinogen as well as a hepatotoxin (Rogers and Newberne, 1971), but there is no direct evidence that hepatitis B virus is oncogenic. (See Chapter 12 for a discussion of primary liver cancer associated with exposure to hepatitis B viral infection.) No adequate studies have been conducted to determine whether alcohol per se is carcinogenic or cocarcinogenic in the develoment of hepatomas in the absence of cirrhosis.

Lieber et al. (1979) reported that a small number of alcohol abusers developed hepatocellular carcinomas in the absence of cirrhosis.

Although other investigators (e.g., Keller, 1978) reported similar findings, Lieber and colleagues suggested that the numbers were too small to ascertain if the tumor incidence was significantly greater in alcohol abusers than in moderate drinkers or nondrinkers. Additional studies are required to evaluate fully the role of ethanol in hepatocarcinogenesis.

Other sites in the digestive tract where cancer has also been associated with alcohol abuse include the gastric cardia (MacDonald, 1972) and the pancreas (Burch and Ansari, 1968).

Synergism Between Alcohol and Smoking

Alcohol consumers (especially abusers) are, more often than not, smokers. Flamant et al. (1964), assessing both variables, stressed the interaction between alcohol consumption and smoking for cancers of the oral cavity and the esophagus. Studies completed since then have confirmed these findings supporting an interactive role between tobacco and alcohol in tumorigenesis of the oral cavity, the larynx, and esophagus (Burch et al., 1981; Keller and Terris, 1965; Martínez, 1970; Pottern et al., 1981, Rothman and Keller, 1972; Wapnick et al., 1972). Avoidance of tobacco and alcohol by males could effect a marked reduction of these cancers (Rothman, 1980; Rothman and Keller, 1972). Flamant et al. (1964) suggested that alcohol abuse may be more important than smoking in the development of esophageal cancer, but smoking is more closely allied to cancers of the mouth and pharynx.

It is difficult to ascertain if moderate or heavy consumption of alcohol (other than the beverages specified above) enhances the risk of oral and upper respiratory tract cancer in nonsmokers. Synergistic effects of alcohol and smoking have been observed in smokers consuming 45 ml or more of ethanol per day (Schottenfeld, 1979). Cancer sites correlating with past ethanol consumption more strongly than with exposure to tobacco include the floor of the mouth, supraglottic region, hypopharynx, and esophagus (Omerović, 1976; Spalajkovic, 1976; Stevens, 1979). Since alcohol consumption involves direct exposure of the sites, Kissin (1975) suggested that ethanol exerts a direct local effect rather than a systemic one. Geographic, ethnic, and dietary factors may also be of some consequence in esophageal cancer (Pothe and Voigtsberger, 1976; Sadeghi et al., 1977; Schwartz et al., 1966; Steiner, 1956). A case-control study conducted by Graham et al. (1977) introduced still another variable. These investigators reported that the interaction of tobacco and alcohol in cancers of the oral cavity was apparent only in individuals with clinical evidence of inadequate dentition.

McCoy et al. (1979) noted that excessive ethanol consumption and exposure to tobacco may act synergistically to affect the risk of cancer of the upper alimentary and respiratory tracts. The much lower incidence of cancer at these sites in nondrinkers and nonsmokers suggested to these

researchers that excessive alcohol consumption may augment other processes such as impaired nutritional status, which may be associated with the
development of cancer at these sites.

Estimated ethanol intake, independent of smoking, was associated with
a modest, but increased risk for cancers of the upper respiratory tract
(McCoy and Wynder, 1979; Rothman and Keller, 1972). Williams and Horm
(1977) also observed that ethanol increased the risk for cancers at this
site when they controlled for smoking. A number of other reports have
indicated that there is a dose response between consumption of ethanol
(independent of the type of alcoholic beverage) and the risk of upper
respiratory tract cancer (Williams and Horm, 1977; Wynder and Stellman,
1977; Wynder et al., 1957b). In general, these studies focused on moderate to heavy consumers of ethanol.

Reports by Rothman (1980) and by Burch et al. (1981) indicate that
the risk for cancers of the oral cavity is slightly increased in smokers
reporting low to moderate consumption of ethanol (i.e., >12 to 45 ml, or
approximately 70 to 270 calories daily). However, because consumers tend
to underreport their ethanol intake (DeLuca, 1981), it is difficult to
interpret these findings.

Effect of Nutritional Status

Malnutrition may play a key role in the development of cancers of the
head and neck in alcohol abusers (Kissin and Kaley, 1974). These individuals frequently suffer from malnutrition because they often consume
from 25% to 50% (or more) of their daily calories as alcohol. In the
absence of chronic alcoholism and smoking, malnutrition or nutritional
imbalance have been found frequently in individuals with cancer of the
oral cavity and respiratory tract (Kissin and Kaley, 1974). For example, an association between Plummer-Vinson (also called Paterson-Kelly)
syndrome and iron deficiency with esophageal cancer has been observed in
Swedish women (Wynder and Fryer, 1958; Wynder and Klein, 1965). Since
the early 1950's, dietary supplementation with iron and vitamins has
markedly reduced the incidence of Plummer-Vinson syndrome as well as
esophageal cancer (Larsson et al., 1975). Esophageal cancer in Iran
(Kmet and Mahboubi, 1972), Sweden (Jacobsson, 1961), and Puerto Rico
(Martinez, 1970) is more frequent among the malnourished. Experimentally induced deficiency of lipotropes, riboflavin, vitamin A, or
zinc have been shown to enhance carcinogen-induced tumors in laboratory animals (Newberne and McConnell, 1980).

EXPERIMENTAL EVIDENCE

Postulated Mechanisms of Action in Carcinogenesis

Possible mechanisms through which alcohol might contribute to the
risk of cancer of the head and neck are: alcohol acting as a carcinogen,

cocarcinogen, or promoter; alcohol acting as a solvent facilitating transport of carcinogens across membranes; induction of microsomal enzymes by alcohol leading to activation and/or metabolism of carcinogens; alcohol as a source of putative carcinogenic contaminants in alcoholic beverages; alcohol-related nutritional deficiencies; and alcohol abuse associated with immunosuppression. These have been discussed by Kissin and Kaley (1974), Vitale and Gottlieb (1975), McCoy and Wynder (1979), Lieber et al. (1979), Schottenfeld (1979), and Vitale et al. (1981).

There are only a few experimental data to indicate that alcohol can act either as a carcinogen or cocarcinogen or that its solvent properties facilitate the transport of carcinogens across cell membranes. The relationship of alcohol-induced immunosuppression to tumorigenesis in animals has not been explored, and the role of alcohol-related nutritional deficiencies to carcinogenesis in animals is only in the preliminary stages of investigation.

Alcohol and Induction of Microsomal Enzymes

The chronic feeding of ethanol to laboratory animals can increase the activity of the hepatic microsomal enzymes responsible for bioactivation of procarcinogens (Rubin et al., 1970). Polycyclic hydrocarbons, e.g., benzo[a]pyrene, were activated to a greater extent when rats were fed ethanol than when they were fed a control diet (Seitz et al., 1978). In contrast, Capel et al. (1978) reported a decrease in benzo[a]pyrene-hydroxylase activity following chronic administration of ethanol. McCoy et al. (1979) demonstrated that ethanol fed to hamsters for 28 days increased the hydroxylation rates of two cyclic nitrosamines, N-nitrosopyrrolidine and N-nitrosonornicotine, which are found in mainstream and sidestream tobacco smoke. Enhanced mutagenicity of these hydroxylated compounds was assessed with the Ames test. The enhanced activation of both nitrosamines by ethanol provides some experimental evidence for the synergistic effect of chronic alcohol abuse and smoking in the induction of head and neck cancers. Microsomal activation of tobacco pyrolysate has been observed in the rat lung, and activation of benzo[a]pyrene occurs in cultures of small bowel tissue. The metabolic activation of these procarcinogens was increased in tissues chronically exposed to ethanol by injection (McCoy et al., 1979).

Occurrence of Putative Carcinogens in Alcoholic Beverages

Certain congeners of alcoholic beverages, e.g., nitrosamines (Lijinsky and Epstein, 1970) and fusel oil (Gibel et al., 1968), have been demonstrated to produce tumors of the stomach and esophagus in laboratory animals. Other putative carcinogens found in alcoholic beverages include polycyclic hydrocarbons, such as phenanthrene, fluoranthrene, benzanthracene, benzo[a]pyrene, and chrysene (Goff and

Fine, 1979; Masuda et al., 1966), and asbestos fibers, which often leach from filters into wines (Bignon et al., 1977; Gaudichet et al., 1978), beer (Biles and Emerson, 1968), and gin (Wehman and Plantholt, 1974).

SUMMARY AND CONCLUSIONS

The effects of alcohol consumption on cancer incidence have been studied in human populations. In some countries, including the United States, excessive beer drinking has been associated with an increased risk of colorectal cancer, especially rectal cancer. This observation has not been confirmed in most case-control or cohort studies. There is limited evidence that excessive alcohol consumption contributes to hepatic injury and cirrhosis, which in turn may lead to the formation of hepatomas. Excessive consumption of alcoholic beverages by smokers appears to act synergistically in increasing the risk for cancer of the mouth, larynx, esophagus, and the respiratory tract.

REFERENCES

Bignon, J., M. Bientz, G. Bonnaud, and P. Sebastien. 1977. [In French.] Letter to the Editor: Evaluation numérique des fibres d'amiante dans des échantillons de vins. Nouv. Presse Med. 6:1148-1149.

Biles, B., and T. R. Emerson. 1968. Examination of fibres in beer. Nature 219:93-94.

Bjelke, E. 1971. Case-control study of cancer of the stomach, colon, and rectum. Pp. 320-334 in R. L. Clark, R. C. Cumley, J. E. McCay, and M. M. Copeland, eds. Oncology 1970. Volume 5: A. Environmental Causes. B. Epidemiology and Demography. C. Cancer Education. Yearbook Medical Publishers, Chicago.

Bjelke, E. 1973. Epidemiologic Studies of Cancer of the Stomach, Colon, and Rectum; With Special Emphasis on the Role of Diet, Volumes I-IV. Ph.D. Thesis, University of Minnesota. 1,746 pp.

Breslow, N. E., and J. E. Enstrom. 1974. Geographic correlations between cancer mortality rates and alcohol-tobacco consumption in the United States. J. Natl. Cancer Inst. 53:631-639.

Bross, I. D. J., and J. Coombs. 1976. Early onset of oral cancer among women who drink and smoke. Oncology 33:136-139.

Burch, G. E., and A. Ansari. 1968. Chronic alcoholism and carcinoma of the pancreas: A correlative hypothesis. Arch. Intern. Med. 122:273-275.

Burch, J. D., G. R. Howe, A. B. Miller, and R. Semenciw. 1981. Tobacco, alcohol, asbestos, and nickel in the etiology of cancer of the larynx: A case-control study. J. Natl. Cancer Inst. 67:1219-1224.

Capel, I. D., M. Jenner, M. H. Pinnock, H. M. Dorrell, and D. C. Williams. 1978. The effect of chronic ethanol intake on the growth and spread of some murine tumors. Oncology 35:224-226.

Collis, C. H., P. J. Cook, J. K. Foreman, and J. F. Palframan. 1972. Letter to the Editor: Cancer of the oesophagus and alcoholic drinks in East Africa. Lancet 1:441.

Cook, P. 1971. Cancer of the oesophagus in Africa: A summary and evaluation of the evidence for the frequency of occurrence, and a preliminary indication of the possible association with the consumption of alcoholic drinks made from maize. Br. J. Cancer 25:853-880.

Dean, G., R. MacLennan, H. McLoughlin, and E. Shelly. 1979. Causes of death of blue-collar workers at a Dublin brewery, 1954-1973. Br. J. Cancer 40:581-589.

DeLuca, J. R., ed. 1981. Fourth Special Report to the U.S. Congress on Alcohol and Health. National Institute on Alcohol Abuse and Alcoholism, Public Health Service, U.S. Department of Health and Human Services, Rockville, Md. 206 pp.

Enstrom, J. E. 1977. Colorectal cancer and beer drinking. Br. J. Cancer 35:674-683.

Flamant, R., O. Lasserre, P. Lazar, J. Leguerinais, P. Denoix, and D. Schwartz. 1964. Differences in sex ratio according to cancer site and possible relationship with use of tobacco and alcohol: Review of 65,000 cases. J. Natl. Cancer Inst. 32:1309-1316.

Gaudichet, A., P. Sebastien, G. Dufour, G. Bonnaud, M. Bientz, J. Bignon, and J. Puisais. 1978. Asbestos fibers in wines: Relation to filtration process. J. Environ. Pathol. Toxicol. 2:417-425.

Gibel, W., G. P. Wildner, and K. Lohs. 1968. [In German; English Summary.] Cancerogenic and hepatotoxic effects of fusel oil. Arch. Geschwulstforsch. 32:115-125.

Goff, E. U., and D. H. Fine. 1979. Analysis of volatile N-nitrosamines in alcoholic beverages. Food Cosmet. Toxicol. 17:569-573.

Graham, S., H. Dayal, T. Rohrer, M. Swanson, H. Sultz, D. Shedd, and S. Fischman. 1977. Dentition, diet, tobacco, and alcohol in the epidemiology of oral cancer. J. Natl. Cancer Inst. 59:1611-1618.

Hakulinen, F., L. Lehtimäki, M. Lehtonen, and L. Teppo. 1974. Cancer morbidity among two male cohorts with increased alcohol consumption in Finland. J. Natl. Cancer Inst. 52:1711-1714.

Higginson, J. 1966. Etiological factors in gastrointestinal cancer in man. J. Natl. Cancer Inst. 37:527-545.

Hinds, M. W., L. N. Kolonel, J. Lee, and T. Hirohata. 1980. Associations between cancer incidence and alcohol/cigarette consumption among five ethnic groups in Hawaii. Br. J. Cancer 41:929-940.

Hoey, J., C. Montvernay, and R. Lambert. 1981. Wine and tobacco: Risk factors for gastric cancer in France. Am. J. Epidemiol. 113:668-674.

Jacobsson, F. 1961. The Paterson-Kelly (Plummer-Vinson) syndrome and carcinoma of the cervical oesophagus. Pp. 53-60 in N. C. Tanner and D. W. Smithers, eds. Neoplastic Disease at Various Sites, Volume 4. Tumors of the Esophagus. E. and S. Livingstone, Ltd., Edinburgh and London.

Jensen, O. M. 1979. Cancer morbidity and causes of death among Danish brewery workers. Int. J. Cancer 23:454-463.

Kamionkowski, M. D., and B. Fleshler. 1965. The role of alcoholic intake in esophageal carcinoma. Am. J. Med. Sci. 249:696-700.

Keen, P., and P. Martin. 1971. Is aflatoxin carcinogenic in man? The evidence in Swaziland. Trop. Geogr. Med. 23:44-53.

Keller, A. Z. 1978. Liver cirrhosis, tobacco, alcohol and cancer among blacks. J. Natl. Med. Assoc. 70:575-579.

Keller, A. Z., and M. Terris. 1965. The association of alcohol and tobacco with cancer of the mouth and pharynx. Am. J. Public Health 55:1578-1585.

Keller, M., D. M. Promisel, D. Spiegler, L. Light, and M. N. Davies, eds. 1977. Alcohol and cancer. Pp. 53-67 in Second Special Report to the U.S. Congress on Alcohol and Health. Public Health Service, Department of Health, Education, and Welfare, Rockville, Md.

Kissin, B. 1975. Epidemiologic investigations of possible biological interactions of alcohol and cancer of the head and neck. Ann. N.Y. Acad. Sci. 252:374-377.

Kissin, B., and M. M. Kaley. 1974. Alcohol and cancer. Pp. 481-511 in B. Kissin and H. Begleiter, eds. The Biology of Alcoholism. Volume 3. Clinical Pathology. Plenum Press, New York and London.

Kmet, J., and E. Mahboubi. 1972. Esophageal cancer in the Caspian littoral of Iran: Initial studies. Science 175:846-853.

Kono, S., and M. Ikeda. 1979. Correlation between cancer mortality and alcoholic beverage in Japan. Br. J. Cancer 40:449-455.

Kwan, K. W. 1937. Carcinoma of the esophagus. A statistical study. Chin. Med. J. (Peking) 52:237-254.

Lamy, L. 1910. [In French.] Étude de statistique clinique de 134 cas de cancer de l'oesophage et du cardia. Arch. Mal. Appar. Dig. Mal. Nutr. 4:451-475.

Larsson, L.-G., A. Sandström, and P. Westling. 1975. Relationship of Plummer-Vinson disease to cancer of the upper alimentary tract in Sweden. Cancer Res. 35:3308-3316.

Lieber, C. S., H. K. Seitz, A. J. Garro, and T. M. Worner. 1979. Alcohol-related diseases and carcinogenesis. Cancer Res. 39:2863-2886.

Lijinsky, W., and S. S. Epstein. 1970. Nitrosamines as environmental carcinogens. Nature 225:21-23.

MacDonald, R. A. 1956. Cirrhosis and primary carcinoma of the liver: Changes in their occurrence at the Boston City Hospital, 1897-1954. N. Engl. J. Med. 255:1179-1183.

MacDonald, W. C. 1972. Clinical and pathological features of adeno-carcinoma of the gastric cardia. Cancer 29:724-732.

Martínez, I. 1970. Retrospective and prospective study of carcinoma of the esophagus, mouth, and pharynx in Puerto Rico. Bol. Asoc. Med. P. R. 62:170-178.

Masuda, Y., K. Mori, T. Hirohata, and M. Kuratsune. 1966. Carcino-genesis in the esophagus. III. Polycyclic aromatic hydrocarbons and phenols in whisky. Gann 57:549-557.

McCoy, G. D., and E. L. Wynder. 1979. Etiological and preventive implications in alcohol carcinogenesis. Cancer Res. 39:2844-2850.

McCoy, G. D., C. B. Chen, S. S. Hecht, and E. C. McCoy. 1979. Enhanced metabolism and mutagenesis of nitrosopyrrolidine in liver fractions isolated from chronic ethanol-consuming hamsters. Cancer Res. 39:793-796.

Moore, C. 1965. Smoking and cancer of the mouth, pharynx, and larynx. J. Am. Med. Assoc. 191:283-286.

Newberne, P. M., and R. G. McConnell. 1980. Nutrient deficiencies in cancer causation. J. Environ. Pathol. Toxicol. 3(4):323-356.

Ómerović, V. H. 1976. [In Serbo-Croatian; English Summary.] Kronicni alkololizam: Njegova korelacija sa karcinomom oro-farinska. Med. Arh. 30:19-21.

Pernu, J. 1960. An epidemiological study on cancer of the digestive organs and respiratory system. Ann. Med. Intern. Fenn. Suppl. 33:1–117.

Piquet, J., and Tison. 1937. [In French.] Alcool et cancer de l'oesophage. Bull. Acad. Med. (Paris) 117:236–239.

Pothe, H., and P. Voigtsberger. 1976. [In German.] Zur Epidemiologie und Diagnostik des Ösophaguskarzinoms. Dtsch. Gesundheitswes. 31:2148–2152.

Pottern, L. M., L. E. Morris, W. J. Blot, R. G. Zeigler, and J. F. Fraumeni, Jr. 1981. Esophageal cancer among black men in Washington, D.C. I. Alcohol, tobacco, and other risk factors. J. Natl. Cancer Inst. 67:777–783.

Purtilo, D. T., and L. S. Gottlieb. 1973. Cirrhosis and hepatoma occurring at Boston City Hospital (1917–1968). Cancer 32:458–462.

Rogers, A. E., and P. M. Newberne. 1971. Nutrition and aflatoxin carcinogenesis. Nature 229:62–63.

Rothman, K. J. 1980. The proportion of cancer attributable to alcohol consumption. Prev. Med. 9:174–179.

Rothman, K., and A. Keller. 1972. The effect of joint exposure to alcohol and tobacco on risk of cancer of the mouth and pharynx. J. Chronic Dis. 25:711–716.

Rubin, E., P. Bacchin, H. Cang, and C. S. Lieber. 1970. Induction and inhibition of hepatic microsomal and mitochondrial enzymes by ethanol. Lab. Invest. 22:569–580.

Sadeghi, A., S. Behmard, H. Shafiepoor, and E. Zeighmani. 1977. Cancer of the esophagus in southern Iran. Cancer 40:841–845.

Schottenfeld, D. 1979. Alcohol as a co-factor in the etiology of cancer. Cancer 43:1962–1966.

Schottenfeld, D., R. C. Gantt, and E. L. Wynder. 1974. The role of alcohol and tobacco in multiple primary cancers of the upper digestive system, larynx and lung: A prospective study. Prev. Med. 3:277–293.

Schwartz, D. 1966. [In French; English Summary.] Alcool et cancer. Étude de géographie pathologique. Cancro 19:200–209.

Schwartz, D., J. Lellouch, R. Flamant, and P. F. Denoix. 1962. [In French; English Summary.] Alcool et cancer. Resultats d'une equête retrospective. Rev. Fr. Etud. Clin. Biol. 7:590-604.

Schwartz, D., O. Lasserre, R. Flamant, and J. Lellouch. 1966. [In French; English Summary.] Alcool et cancer: Étude de pathologie géographique portant sur 19 pays. Eur. J. Cancer 2:367-372.

Seitz, H. K., A. J. Garro, and C. S. Lieber. 1978. Effect of chronic ethanol ingestion on intestinal metabolism and mutagenicity of benzo(α)pyrene. Biochem. Biophys. Res. Commun. 85:1061-1066.

Sherlock, S., R. A. Fox, S. P. Niazi, and P. J. Scheuer. 1970. Chronic liver disease and primary liver-cell cancer with hepatitis-associated (Australia) antigen in serum. Lancet 1:1243-1247.

Spalajkovic, M. 1976. [In French.] Alcoolisme et cancer du larynx et de l'hypopharynx. J. Fr. Oto-Rhino-Laryngol. Audio-Phonol. Chiur. Maxillo-Fac. 25:49-50.

Steiner, P. E. 1956. The etiology and histogenesis of carcinoma of the esophagus. Cancer 9:436-452.

Stevens, M. H. 1979. Synergistic effect of alcohol on epidermoid carcinogenesis in the larynx. Otolaryngol. Head Neck Surg. 87:751-756.

Stocks, P. 1957. Cancer Incidence in North Wales and Liverpool Region in Relation to Habits and Environment. British Empire Cancer Campaign Thirtyfifth Annual Report, Supplement to Part II. Cancer Research Campaign, London. 156 pp.

Tuyns, A. J., and L. M. F. Massé. 1973. Mortality from cancer of the oesophagus in Brittany. Int. J. Epidemiol. 2:241-245.

Tuyns, A. J., G. Péquignot, and O. M. Jensen. 1977. [In French; English Summary.] Oesophageal cancer in Ille-et-Vilaine in relation to levels of alcohol and tobacco consumption: Multiplicative risks. Bull. Cancer 64:45-60.

Tuyns, A. J., G. Péquignot, and J. S. Abbatucci. 1979. Oesophageal cancer and alcohol consumption; importance of type of beverage. Int. J. Cancer 23:443-447.

Vincent, R. G., and F. Marchetta. 1963. The relationship of the use of tobacco and alcohol to cancer of the oral cavity, pharynx or larynx. Am. J. Surg. 106:501-505.

Vitale, J. J., and L. S. Gottlieb. 1975. Alcohol and alcohol-related deficiencies as carcinogens. Cancer Res. 35:3336-3338.

Vitale, J. J., S. A. Broitman, and L. S. Gottlieb. 1981. Alcohol and carcinogenesis. Pp. 291-301 in G. R. Newell and N. M. Ellison, eds. Nutrition and Cancer: Etiology and Treatment. Raven Press, New York.

Vogel, C. L., P. P. Anthony, N. Mody, and L. F. Barker. 1970. Hepatitis associated antigen in Ugandan patients with hepatocellular carcinoma. Lancet 2:621-624.

Wapnick, S., W. Castle, D. Nicholle, L. N. D. Zanamwe, and M. Gelfand. 1972. Cigarette smoking, alcohol and cancer of the oesophagus. S. Afr. Med. J. 46:2023-2026.

Wehman, H. J., and B. A. Plantholt. 1974. Asbestos fibrils in beverages. 1. Gin. Bull. Environ. Contam. Toxicol. 11:267-272.

Williams, R. R., and J. W. Horm. 1977. Association of cancer sites with tobacco and alcohol consumption and socioeconomic status of patients: Interview study from the Third National Cancer Survey. J. Natl. Cancer Inst. 58:525-547.

World Health Organization. 1964. Cancer agents that surround us. World Health 1964 (Sep.):16-17.

Wu, P. C., and K. C. Lam. 1979. Cytoplasmic hepatitis B surface antigen and the ground-glass appearance in hepatocellular carcinoma. Am. J. Clin. Pathol. 71:229-234.

Wu, Y. K., and H. H. Loucks. 1951. Carcinoma of the esophagus or cardia of the stomach: An analysis of 172 cases with 81 resections. Ann. Surg. 134:946-956.

Wynder, E. L., and I. J. Bross. 1961. A study of etiological factors in cancer of the esophagus. Cancer 14:389-413.

Wynder, E. L., and J. H. Fryer. 1958. Etiologic considerations of Plummer-Vinson (Paterson-Kelly) syndrome. Ann. Int. Med. 49:1106-1128.

Wynder, E. L., and U. E. Klein. 1965. The possible role of riboflavin deficiency in epithelial neoplasia. I. Epithelial changes of mice in simple deficiency. Cancer 18:167-180.

Wynder, E. L., and T. Shigematsu. 1967. Environmental factors of cancer of the colon and rectum. Cancer 20:1520-1561.

Wynder, E. L., and S. D. Stellman. 1977. Comparative epidemiology of tobacco-related cancers. Cancer Res. 37:4608-4622.

Wynder, E. L., I. J. Bross, and R. M. Feldman. 1957a. A study of the etiological factors in cancer of the mouth. Cancer 10:1300-1323.

Wynder, E. L., S. Hultberg, F. Jacobsson, and I. J. Bross. 1957b. Environmental factors in cancer of the upper alimentary tract: A Swedish study with special reference to Plummer-Vinson (Paterson-Kelly) syndrome. Cancer 10:470-487.

Section B The Role of Nonnutritive
Dietary Constituents

Section A presented the evidence linking nutrients to carcinogenesis. In this section, which contains Chapters 12 through 15, the committee has attempted to provide a perspective on the contribution of nonnutritive dietary components (food additives, contaminants, naturally occurring carcinogens, and mutagens) to the risk of cancer in humans. The factors that determined the selection of compounds included in Chapters 12 and 14 and the inherent difficulties in assessing the health effects of food additives and contaminants are discussed below. Chapter 12 focuses on naturally occurring substances that are suspected or known carcinogens, whereas the discussion in Chapter 13 concentrates on mutagens in food, some of which are also carcinogenic. The evidence for carcinogenicity of food additives and contaminants is reviewed in Chapter 14. The inhibitory properties of certain nonnutritive synthetic compounds, or some that are present naturally in foods, are presented in Chapter 15.

Technological advances in recent years have led to changes in the methods of food processing, a greater assortment of food products, and, as a result, changes in the consumption patterns of the U.S. population. The impact of these modifications on human health, especially the potential adverse effects of food additives and contaminants, has drawn considerable attention from the news media and the public. Advances in technology have resulted in an increased use of industrial chemicals, thereby increasing the potential for chemical contamination of drinking water and food supplies. The use of processed foods and, consequently, of additives has also increased substantially during the past four decades. Roberts (1981) estimates that more than 55% of the food consumed in the United States today has been processed to some degree before distribution to the consumer.

Clearly, the degree of concern about the health risks from food additives varies. For example, in ranking the probable sources of health hazard in the U.S. diet, the Food and Drug Administration (FDA) has consistently listed food additives in fifth or sixth place, well below microbiological contaminants and nutrient deficiencies. In contrast, consumers surveyed in five cities recommended that the FDA give high priority to assessing the safety of food additives (U.S. Food and Drug Administration, 1981).

FOOD ADDITIVES

In this report, the term "food additives" is often used generically to refer to <u>all</u> substances that may be added to foods. However, in the 1958 Food Additives Amendment to the Federal Food, Drug, and Cosmetic Act, the term has a more restricted legal definition:

"Food additive" means any substance the intended use of which results or may reasonably be expected to result, directly or indirectly, in its becoming a component or otherwise affecting the character of a food.... (U.S. Department of Health and Human Services, 1980, p. 4)

The 1958 amendment changed the rules under which food additives were regulated. Until then, a substance added to food was presumed safe until someone (usually the government through the FDA) could prove it otherwise; after 1958, FDA approval of safety was required prior to use. Because this change in the law would have placed an unmanageable burden on the manufacturers to conduct the tests required to prove the safety of the many hundreds of substances then added to foods, the definition of "food additive" was modified for regulatory purposes to exclude many classes of substances. The term now covers approximately 400 of the 2,600 to 2,700 substances intentionally added to foods (Code of Federal Regulations, 1981). Not included are approximately 500 food ingredients termed GRAS (Generally Recognized as Safe) substances; about 100 other "unpublished GRAS substances;" approximately 1,650 flavoring agents, most of which are classified as GRAS; prior-sanctioned food ingredients, consisting of about 100 substances approved by the U.S. Department of Agriculture (USDA) or the FDA prior to 1958; and approximately 30 color additives (U.S. Department of Health and Human Services, 1980). It would be difficult to prepare a list of all the compounds in these categories.

Table B-1 summarizes the classes of food ingredients covered in the Federal Food, Drug, and Cosmetic Act and provides examples of each. For each category, it also presents information concerning the applicability of the Delaney Clause--an amendment to the Act concerning the regulation of carcinogens. (This amendment and other regulatory actions are discussed below.)

CONTAMINANTS

Two other, much larger groups of added food constituents are also included in Table B-1. It is estimated that approximately 12,000 substances are introduced unintentionally during processing, and an unknown number of other contaminants are inadvertently added to the food supply. The first group (also called indirect additives) includes by-products of processing (e.g., caustics used in potato peeling, machinery cleaners, packaging components), as well as residues of permitted pesticides and of drugs given to animals. There are regulations restricting the concentrations and types of these compounds in food and the purposes for which they can be used. Contaminants in the second group, classified as unavoidable "added" constituents, are regulated when found. For example, after an accidental contamination by a hazardous chemical, the concentration of the chemical is compared to established "action levels" to determine if the foods are fit for human consumption.

THE DELANEY CLAUSE AND OTHER REGULATORY ACTIONS

The regulation of carcinogens has been a matter of special concern because it is covered by the Delaney Clause[1] of the Federal Food, Drug, and Cosmetic Act. The amendment prohibits the FDA from approving the use of any food additive found to cause cancer in animals or humans. It has been criticized as being too restrictive by setting a zero level of risk. In fact, it applies only to approximately 400 of the 2,700 substances intentionally added to foods, many of which are GRAS. If any GRAS substance is found to be carcinogenic, it would no longer be considered GRAS and would fall under the legal definition of a food additive, thereby becoming subject to the Delaney Clause.

In addition to the Delaney Clause, numerous amendments to the Federal Food, Drug, and Cosmetic Act have been made since the early 1960's (U.S. Department of Health and Human Services, 1980). It appears that the statutory provisions governing food safety are a patchwork of divergent, sometimes carefully considered, but sometimes offhand, legislative policies that invite uneven monitoring of different substances in foods and inconsistent treatment of comparable risks from different categories of food additives.

Recognizing the need to acquire better data and to standardize testing procedures and the criteria for acceptability, the FDA has recently initiated a review of direct food additives (U.S. Department of Health and Human Services, 1981). Similarly, the FAO/WHO Joint Expert Committee on Food Additives acknowledged that the safety of a large number of food additives remains to be examined or needs to be reevaluated (World Health Organization, 1980).

Many factors complicate the assessment of nonnutritive dietary constituents.

- Some food constituents are discrete chemical entities that are easy to test, whereas others are complex, poorly defined mixtures of natural origin.

- Although the Federal Food, Drug, and Cosmetic Act defines various categories of food ingredients, it is frequently difficult to determine how to classify certain substances that meet the definitions of more than one category (Code of Federal Regulations, 1981). Information about contaminants is even less precise.

- Although most additives and the known contaminants are present in minute quantities in the diet, little is known about the chronic effects of low levels of chemicals on human health, and even less is known about the potential for synergistic and/or antagonistic interactions among most of these substances in foods or in the body.

---

[1]Sec. 409(c)(1)(A).

TABLE B-1

The Federal Food, Drug, and Cosmetic Act[a]: Categories of Food Constituents

Category	Number of Compounds in Each Category[b]	Example(s)	Applicability of Delaney Clause
Natural Food Constituents			
Vitamins and minerals in foods	~70	Ascorbic acid in oranges; calcium in milk	NA[c]
Other chemical components of foods	?	Caffeine in coffee; nitrate in spinach	
Intentionally Added Substances	~2,700		
Direct additives, e.g., stabilizers, leavening agents, emulsifiers, antioxidants, sweeteners	~400	Yeasts, sodium bicarbonate, sodium hydroxide, lecithin, butylated hydroxyanisole (BHA), saccharin	Yes
Previously sanctioned additives, e.g., preservatives	~100	Sodium nitrite	NA
GRAS substances, e.g., spices, seasonings, multipurpose substances	~600	Cumin, carrageenin, BHA, butylated hydroxytoluene (BHT), acetic acid, lecithin, sulfuric acid, hydrochloric acid, vanilla, caffeine, sodium chloride, sucrose	NA
Flavoring ingredients (many are GRAS)	~1,700	Monosodium glutamate, vanilla, licorice	NA

Category	Number[b]	Examples	Premarket testing required?[a]
Color additives	~30	Food, Drug, and Cosmetic (FD&C) Blue #1, Orange B, Citrus Red #2, FD&C Yellow #5	Yes
Indirect Additives	~12,000		
Indirect additives, e.g., processing aids, packaging components	~10,000	Acetone, methyl alcohol, methylene chloride, polystyrene	Yes, except for GRAS substances[d]
Drugs given to animals, e.g., synthetic hormones, antibiotics	~200	Dinestrol diacetate, tylosin	To residues only
Pesticide residues, e.g., organochlorine compounds, carbamates	~1,400	Hexachlorobenzene, lindane, carbaryl	NA
Unavoidable "Added" Constituents (Contaminants)	?		
Fungi, microbial toxins, metal residues, industrial chemicals	?	Aflatoxin, patulin, poly-chlorinated biphenyls, mercury, beryllium	NA

[a] Code of Federal Regulations, 1981.
[b] Information on the numbers of substances is derived partially from lists of additives published by the Food and Drug Administration in the Code of Federal Regulations and partly from estimates based on the opinion of experts in the field (Merrill, 1978; Roberts, 1981).
[c] NA = Not applicable.
[d] Examples of indirect additives that are also GRAS substances are coconut oil, pulps, and sulfonic acid.

EXPOSURE OF HUMANS

To determine the risk of carcinogenesis from food additives and contaminants, it is necessary to know the extent to which humans are "typically" exposed, the degree of exposure in subgroups of the population, the carcinogenic potency of the compound, and the quantity and quality of the data concerning its toxicity and carcinogenicity.

Although humans are exposed to various additives and contaminants at levels ranging over several orders of magnitude, some generalizations can be made about exposure to different classes of substances. The National Science Foundation (1973) estimated that 0.5% (by weight) of the U.S. food supply consists of intentional food additives, and the per capita intake of food additives has increased approximately fourfold in the past decade. Currently, their use amounts to approximately 5 kg per capita annually, although as a measure of the average intake of food additives this may be misleading because approximately one-half of these additives are used in amounts of 0.5 mg or less (Roberts, 1981). Many intentional additives are nutritive substances, e.g., sugar, corn syrup, salt, and dextrose, which are used in large amounts (many kilograms per capita annually for sugar and corn syrup), whereas many others, e.g., lecithin, fumaric acid, and sodium bisulfite, are used in quantities that provide an intake of 10 to 50 g per capita annually. Table B-2 lists the annual usage of some major classes of food additives (Jorgenson, 1980).

Information about the use of indirect additives by the food industry is much less precise. Consequently, exposure of humans is difficult to estimate. It would depend to a large extent on the physical and chemical characteristics of the additive. For example, packaging materials can migrate into food. A concentration of 50 µg/kg in a product consumed at the rate of 50 g per day would lead to an intake of 2.5 µg of the additive daily, or <1 mg annually (Roberts, 1981). If the migratory substances are present in a concentration of 10 mg/kg in a food consumed at this rate, ∿200 mg of additive would be ingested annually (Roberts, 1981). Most pesticides and industrial chemicals are ingested in trace amounts, resulting in a daily intake of only a few milligrams or less of each compound per capita. The daily per capita intake of heavy metals ranges from 2.4 µg for mercury to 90.2 µg for lead.

The FDA's Market Basket Surveys conducted since the mid-1960's have monitored only a few substances and have excluded convenience foods. However, they have provided information on the levels of some pesticides, industrial chemicals, and heavy metals that are ingested as contaminants in the diet (U.S. Food and Drug Administration, 1980). With a few exceptions, information about the exposure to other classes of additives is estimated indirectly from the amount produced or used in the processing of foods rather than by direct measurement of actual consumption (National Academy of Sciences, 1972, 1973, 1978, 1979).

TABLE B-2

Use of Some Food Additives (Nutritive and Nonnutritive)
in the United States[a]

Category	Approximate Quantity (million kg/year)
Thickeners/stabilizers (hydrocolloids)	195 – 215
Flavors and enhancers	132 – 145
Emulsifiers (surfactants)	123 – 136
Acidulants	82 – 91
Chemical leavening agents	80 – 91
Colors	36 – 39
Humectants	27 – 32
Nutritional supplements (vitamins)	25 – 30
Preservatives	23 – 27
Enzymes	> 12
Dietary sweeteners (nonnutritive)	> 2.3
Antioxidants	2.3 – 3.6
Sugar[b]	9,000
Other	> 91

[a]Adapted from Jorgenson, 1980.
[b]Data from U.S. Department of Agriculture, 1980.

THE CARCINOGENICITY OF FOOD ADDITIVES AND CONTAMINANTS

Both additives and contaminants have been studied within the United States and abroad. During the past two decades, these studies have produced an immense body of literature on the health effects of food additives. For example, the Select Committee on GRAS Substances (SCOGS) has published 118 reports on 415 GRAS substances (Fisher and Allison, 1981), and the Flavor and Extracts Manufacturing Association (FEMA) has compiled approximately 70 reports (Oser and Ford, 1979), which contain the opinions of an FEMA expert committee on about 1,650 flavoring ingredients used in foods. Since 1958 the FAO/WHO Joint Expert Committee on Food Additives has prepared annual reports concerning the toxicity of several hundred additives (World Health Organization, 1958-1980). The International Agency for Research on Cancer (1972-1981) has published 24 monographs, many of which evaluate the carcinogenic risk of selected additives to humans. Before the 1970's, most reports concerned with the safety of additives were based on data from tests of acute or subchronic toxicity. These reports documented the general health effects of food ingredients, but did not necessarily contain comments on carcinogenicity, although they did identify substances found to be carcinogenic. More chronic feeding studies have been conducted during the past decade. However, the majority of food additives approved for use have not been tested specifically for carcinogenicity or mutagenicity. Table B-3 summarizes the classes of chemicals tested from 1953 to 1973 in the National Cancer Institute Carcinogenesis Bioassay Program (National Cancer Institute, 1975). Very few epidemiological studies have been conducted to study the effect of food additives. This is probably because of the difficulty of identifying populations with significantly different exposures to specific additives, and because of lack of sensitivity of epidemiological techniques to measure the effects of exposure to low levels of chemicals.

Eighty-three of the 415 GRAS substances reviewed by SCOGS have been tested by long-term feeding studies, but very few of these studies were designed to test for carcinogenicity. A total of 513 GRAS substances have been tested for mutagenicity and/or by long-term feeding studies. Because SCOGS was restricted to evaluating each substance only for its use as a GRAS substance, the determination of safety for many of the compounds is based on one specific use of the compound. For example, caffeine was evaluated for its use as an additive in cola beverages only, not for total exposure from all dietary sources, such as from coffee and tea (Fisher and Allison, 1981).

Flavoring ingredients have been assessed by FEMA to determine their safety for specific uses (Oser and Ford, 1979); however, not all ingredients have been tested for mutagenicity and carcinogenicity. Because several food-coloring agents are suspected or known carcinogens, the 30 or more compounds currently approved for this use in the United States have been studied extensively for carcinogenicity. Many pesticides, heavy metals, and industrial chemicals have also been examined

TABLE B-3

Categories of Compounds Bioassayed for Carcinogenicity
Between 1953 and 1973[a]

Category	Percent of Total Bioassayed
Pharmaceuticals	20.8
Pesticides	17.4
Industrial chemicals (organic)	15.2
Metallic compounds	6.7
Natural food products	5.7
Food chemicals	1.6
Tobacco ingredients	0.8
Environmental agents (general)	0.2
Miscellaneous (structural analogues, multiple uses)	31.6
	100.0

[a]Data from National Cancer Institute, 1975.

specifically for carcinogenicity and/or mutagenicity. Although many naturally occurring contaminants have also been tested for mutagenicity and a few for carcinogenicity, much less emphasis has generally been placed on this class of substances.

Table B-4 lists examples of suspected or proven carcinogens in each category of food ingredients. With the exception of saccharin, any direct food additive known to cause cancer in animals or humans has been banned from use in foods. For known carcinogens in some classes of additives, especially contaminants of natural origin, the FDA establishes tolerable levels. However, for residues of pesticides, the Environmental Protection Agency establishes limits (Acceptable Daily Intakes) (U.S. Department of Health and Human Services, 1980).

TABLE B-4

Some Food Additives and Contaminants Suspected or Proven
to be Carcinogenic in Laboratory Animals

Agent	Use/Source in Diet	Tumor Site	Species	Reference
Intentional Food Additives				
Cyclamates[a]	Nonnutritive sweetener	Bladder	Rats	International Agency for Research on Cancer, 1980
Saccharin[a]	Nonnutritive sweetener	Bladder	Several species	International Agency for Research on Cancer, 1980
Dulcin (p-phenethylurea)	Nonnutritive sweetener	Bladder, liver	Rats	International Agency for Research on Cancer, 1976b
Xylitol[b]	Sweetener	Bladder	Female mice	Hunter et al., 1978b
Sucrose[b]	Sweetener	Liver	Female mice	Hunter et al., 1978a
Amaranth (FD&C Red #2)	Food color	Nonspecific	Female rats	International Agency for Research on Cancer, 1975
FD&C Red #32	Food color	Lung, mammary tissue	Mice	International Agency for Research on Cancer, 1975
FD&C Orange #2	Food color	Intestinal, local	Mice	International Agency for Research on Cancer, 1975
Butter yellow (N,N-dimethyl-4-aminoazobenzene)	Food color	Liver	Rats and mice	International Agency for Research on Cancer, 1975
Safrole[a]	Flavoring agent	Liver	Rats and mice	International Agency for Research on Cancer, 1976a
Oil of calamus	Flavoring agent	Small intestine	Rats	Gross et al., 1967
Cinnamyl anthranilate	Flavoring agent	Liver, kidney, and pancreas	Mice and rats	International Agency for Research on Cancer, 1978a
Diethylpyrocarbonate	Preservative	Lung	Mice	Kraybill, 1977
8-Hydroxyquinoline	Preservative	Multiple sites	Rats and mice	International Agency for Research on Cancer, 1977
Thioacetamide	Seed grain mordant	Liver	Rats	International Agency for Research on Cancer, 1974b
Butylated hydroxytoluene[a]	Antioxidant	Lung (promotor)	Mice	Witschi et al., 1981
Trichloroethylene	Extractant	Liver	Mice	International Agency for Research on Cancer, 1979a
Carrageenin	Emulsifier	Sarcomas	Rats	Cater, 1961
Myrj 45 (polyoxyethylene monostearate)	Antistaling agent	Bladder	Rats	Kraybill, 1977
Tannic acid[a]	Wine, fruits	Liver	Rats	International Agency for Research on Cancer, 1976a

Compound	Source/Use	Site	Species	Reference
Tween-60 (sorbitan monostearate)	Antibloom agent in chocolates	Skin, also a promoting agent	Rats and hamsters	Kraybill, 1977
Carboxymethylcellulose	Ice cream stabilizer	Subcutaneous tissue	Rats	Kraybill, 1977
Unintentional Additives				
Polyvinyl chloride (vinyl chloride monomer)[a]	Packaging material	Several sites	Several species	Feron et al., 1981
Acrylonitrile[a]	Packaging material	Forestomach, central nervous system, Zymbal's gland	Rats	Norris, 1977
DES (diethylstilbestrol)[a]	Animal drug residue	Multiple sites	Several species	International Agency for Research on Cancer, 1979b
Various organochlorine pesticides[a]	Residues in diet	Liver	Mice	International Agency for Research on Cancer, 1974a
Parathion[a]	Residues in diet	Adrenals	Rats	National Cancer Institute, 1979
PAH's (polycyclic aromatic hydrocarbons), e.g., benzo[a]pyrene[a]	Air pollution; charcoal broiling	Several sites	Several species	International Agency for Research on Cancer, 1973
PCB's (polychlorinated biphenyls)[a]	Freshwater fish, packaging materials	Liver	Rats	International Agency for Research on Cancer, 1978b
Cycads and cycasin[a]	Cycad nuts	Liver, kidney, intestine	Rats	International Agency for Research on Cancer, 1976a
Aflatoxin[a]	Milk, mold in cereals, peanuts, corn	Liver, stomach, kidneys	Several species	International Agency for Research on Cancer, 1976a
Nitrosamines[a]	Nitrite and amines in foods	Several sites	Rat	National Academy of Sciences, 1981
Tannins[a]	Tea, wine	Liver, sarcomas	Mice	International Agency for Research on Cancer, 1976a
Bracken fern[a]	Fern species	Bladder	Several species	Hirono et al., 1979
Thiourea[a]	Laburnum shrubs	Several sites	Rats	International Agency for Research on Cancer, 1974b
Pyrrolizidine alkaloids[a]	Herbal medicine, teas, and food plants	Liver	Rats	International Agency for Research on Cancer, 1976b
Patulin[a]	Mold in apple juice	Local sarcomas	Rats	Dickens and Jones, 1961

[a]Compounds considered in Chapters 12, 13, 14, or 15.
[b]Compounds considered in Chapter 7.

B-11

ASSESSMENT OF EFFECTS ON HUMAN HEALTH

Lack of adequate data on a large number of substances precludes a comprehensive assessment of the risk to humans exposed to food additives and contaminants. Therefore, Chapters 12, 13, 14, and 15 contain examples of nonnutritive substances selected from Table B-4 to illustrate the carcinogenic potential of this vast group of substances. The selection of these examples was determined by the extent to which humans are exposed through the general diet and the reliability of the data pertaining to these exposures.

Any assessment of the health effects of food additives and contaminants must take into consideration not only the extent to which humans are exposed through the average diet, but also the wide range of exposure for subgroups of the population, the wide range in the carcinogenic potency of these compounds, and the potential for synergistic and/or antagonistic effects of the numerous compounds that are present in the average diet.

REFERENCES

Cater, D. B. 1961. The carcinogenic action of carrageenin in rats. Br. J. Cancer 15:607-614.

Code of Federal Regulations. 1981. Title 21, Parts 1-99, 100-169, and 170-199. Office of the Federal Register, National Archives and Records Service, General Services Administration, Washington, D. C.

Dickens, F., and H. E. H. Jones. 1961. Carcinogenic activity of a series of reactive lactones and related substances. Br. J. Cancer 15:85-100.

Feron, V. J., C. F. M. Hendriksen, A. J. Speek, H. P. Til, and B. J. Spit. 1981. Lifespan oral toxicity study of vinyl chloride in rats. Food Cosmet. Toxicol. 19:317-333.

Fisher, K. D., and R. G. Allison. 1981. Food Additives as Candidates for Carcinogenicity Testing. Paper prepared for the Committee on Diet, Nutrition, and Cancer for its meeting of February 17-18, 1981. National Academy of Sciences, Washington, D. C. 36 pp. [unpublished].

Gross, M. A., W. I. Jones, E. L. Cook, and C. C. Boone. 1967. Carcinogenicity of oil of calamus. Proc. Am. Assoc. Cancer Res. 8:24. Abstract 93.

Hirono, I., H. Mori, M. Haga, M. Fujii, K. Yamada, Y. Hirata, H. Takanashi, E. Uchida, S. Hosaka, I. Ueno, T. Matsushima, K. Umezawa, and A. Shirai. 1979. Edible plants containing carcinogenic pyrrolizidine alkaloids in Japan. Pp. 79-87 in E. C. Miller, J. A. Miller, I. Hirono, T. Sugimura, and S. Takayama, eds. Naturally Occurring Carcinogens-Mutagens and Modulators of Carcinogenesis. Japan Scientific Societies Press, Tokyo; University Park Press, Baltimore, Md.

Hunter, B., J. Colley, A. E. Street, R. Heywood, D. E. Prentice, and G. Magnusson. 1978a. Xylitol Tumorigenicity and Toxicity Study in Long-Term Dietary Administration To Rats (Final Report). Huntingdon Research Centre, Huntingdon, Cambridgeshire, England. Volumes 11-14 of Xylitol. F. Hoffman La Roche Company, Ltd., Basel, Switzerland. 2250 pp.

Hunter, B., C. Graham, R. Heywood, D. E. Prentice, F. J. C. Roe, and D. N. Noakes. 1978b. Tumorigenicity and Carcinogenicity Study with Xylitol in Long-Term Dietary Administration to Mice (Final Report). Huntingdon Research Centre, Huntingdon, Cambridgeshire, England. Volumes 20-23 of Xylitol. F. Hoffman La Roche Company, Ltd., Basel, Switzerland. 1500 pp.

International Agency for Research on Cancer. 1973. IARC Monographs
    on the Evaluation of the Carcinogenic Risk of Chemicals to Man.
    Volume 3. Certain Polycyclic Aromatic Hydrocarbons and Heterocyclic
    Compounds. International Agency for Research on Cancer, Lyon,
    France. 271 pp.

International Agency for Research on Cancer. 1974a. IARC Monographs on
    the Evaluation of the Carcinogenic Risk of Chemicals to Man. Volume
    5. Some Organochlorine Pesticides. International Agency for Re-
    search on Cancer, Lyon, France. 241 pp.

International Agency for Research on Cancer. 1974b. IARC Monographs
    on the Evaluation of the Carcinogenic Risk of Chemicals to Man.
    Volume 7. Some Anti-Thyroid and Related Substances, Nitrofurans and
    Industrial Chemicals. International Agency for Research on Cancer,
    Lyon, France. 326 pp.

International Agency for Research on Cancer. 1975. IARC Monographs
    on the Evaluation of the Carcinogenic Risk of Chemicals to Man.
    Volume 8. Some Aromatic Azo Compounds. International Agency for
    Research on Cancer, Lyon, France. 357 pp.

International Agency for Research on Cancer. 1976a. IARC Monographs
    on the Evaluation of the Carcinogenic Risk of Chemicals to Man.
    Volume 10. Some Naturally Occurring Substances. International
    Agency for Research on Cancer, Lyon, France. 353 pp.

International Agency for Research on Cancer. 1976b. IARC Monographs
    on the Evaluation of the Carcinogenic Risk of Chemicals to Man.
    Volume 12. Some Carbamates, Thiocarbamates and Carbazides.
    International Agency for Research on Cancer, Lyon, France. 282 pp.

International Agency for Research on Cancer. 1977. IARC Monographs
    on the Evaluation of the Carcinogenic Risk of Chemicals to Man.
    Volume 13. Some Miscellaneous Pharmaceutical Substances.
    International Agency for Research on Cancer, Lyon, France. 255 pp.

International Agency for Research on Cancer. 1978a. IARC Monographs
    on the Evaluation of the Carcinogenic Risk of Chemicals to Man.
    Volume 16. Some Aromatic Amines and Related Nitro Compounds--Hair
    Dyes, Colouring Agents and Miscellaneous Industrial Chemicals.
    International Agency for Research on Cancer, Lyon, France. 400 pp.

International Agency for Research on Cancer. 1978b. IARC Monographs on
    the Evaluation of the Carcinogenic Risk of Chemicals to Humans.
    Volume 18. Polychlorinated Biphenyls and Polybrominated Biphenyls.
    International Agency for Research on Cancer, Lyon, France. 140 pp.

International Agency for Research on Cancer. 1979a. IARC Monographs
    on the Evaluation of Carcinogenic Risk of Chemicals to Humans.
    Volume 20. Some Halogenated Hydrocarbons. International Agency for
    Research on Cancer, Lyon, France. 609 pp.

International Agency For Research on Cancer. 1979b. IARC Monographs on the Evaluation of the Carcinogenic Risk of Chemicals to Humans. Volume 21, Sex Hormones (II). International Agency for Research on Cancer, Lyon, France. 583 pp.

International Agency for Research on Cancer. 1980. IARC Monographs on the Evaluation of the Carcinogenic Risk of Chemicals to Humans. Volume 22, Some Non-Nutritive Sweetening Agents. International Agency for Research on Cancer, Lyon, France. 208 pp.

Jorgensen, D. J. 1980. The need of additives in industry. Pp. 652–677 in H. D. Graham, ed. The Safety of Foods. Second edition. AVI Publishing Company, Westport, Conn.

Kraybill, H. F. 1976. Food chemicals and food additives. Pp. 245–318 in P. M. Newberne, ed. Trace Substances and Health: A Handbook. Part 1. Marcel Dekker, New York and Basel.

Merrill, R. A. 1978. Regulating carcinogens in food: A legislator's guide to the food safety provisions of the Federal Food, Drug, and Cosmetic Act. Mich. Law Rev. 77:171–250.

National Academy of Sciences. 1972. A Comprehensive Survey of Industry on the Use of Food Chemicals Generally Recognized as Safe (GRAS) (Comprehensive GRAS Survey). A report prepared by the Subcommittee on Review of GRAS List--Phase II. National Academy of Sciences, Washington, D.C. 41 pp.

National Academy of Sciences. 1973. The Use of Chemicals in Food Production, Processing, Storage, and Distribution. A report prepared by the Committee on Food Protection, Food and Nutrition Board. National Academy of Sciences, Washington, D.C. 34 pp.

National Academy of Sciences. 1978. 1975 Resurvey of the Annual Poundage of Food Chemicals Generally Recognized as Safe (GRAS). Committee on GRAS List Survey--Phase III. National Academy of Sciences, Washington, D.C. 23 pp.

National Academy of Sciences. 1979. The 1977 Survey of Industry on the Use of Food Additives. Volume 1, Description of the Survey; Volume 2, Summarized Data; Volume 3, Estimates of Daily Intake. Food and Nutrition Board, National Academy of Sciences, Washington, D.C. 2,135 pp. Available from the National Technical Information Service, Springfield, Va. as Publication No. PB 80-113418.

National Academy of Sciences. 1981. The Health Effects of Nitrate, Nitrite, and N-Nitroso Compounds. Part 1 of a 2-Part Study by the Committee on Nitrite and Alternative Curing Agents in Food. National Academy Press, Washington, D.C. 544 pp.

National Cancer Institute. 1975. Survey of Compounds Which Have Been Tested for Carcinogenic Activity. 1972–1973 Volume. National Institutes of Health, U.S. Department of Health, Education, and Welfare, Bethesda, Md. 1638 pp.

National Cancer Institute. 1979. Bioassay of Methyl Parathion for Possible Carcinogenicity. NCI Carcinogenesis Technical Report Series No. 157. DHEW Publication No. (NIH) 79-1713. Carcinogenesis Testing Program, National Cancer Institute, Bethesda, Md. 112 pp.

National Science Foundation. 1973. Chemicals and Health. Report of the Panel on Chemicals and Health of the President's Science Advisory Committee, September 1973. Science and Technology Policy Office, National Science Foundation, Washington, D.C. 211 pp.

Norris, J. M. 1977. Status Report on the 2 Year Study Incorporating Acrylonitrile in the Drinking Water of Rats. Health and Environmental Research, The Dow Chemical Company, Midland, Mich. [14] pp. (unpublished).

Oser, B. L., and R. A. Ford. 1979. Recent progress in the consideration of flavoring ingredients under the food additives amendment. 12. GRAS substances. Food Technol. 33(7):65-73.

Roberts, H. R. 1981. Food safety in perspective. Pp. 1-13 in H. R. Roberts, ed. Food Safety. John Wiley & Sons, New York.

U.S. Department of Agriculture. 1980. Sugar and Sweetener Report 5(8): 1-54.

U.S. Department of Health and Human Services. 1980. Food and Drug Administration Acts. Federal Food, Drug, and Cosmetic Act, as Amended January 1980; Public Health Service Act, Biological Products; Radiation Control for Health and Safety Act; Fair Packaging and Labeling Act. HHS Publication No. (FDA) 80-1051. Food and Drug Administration, U.S. Department of Health and Human Services, Rockville, Md. 169 pp.

U.S. Department of Health, Education, and Welfare. 1981. Toxicological Principles and Procedures for Direct Food Additive Cyclic Review U.S. Department of Health, Education, and Welfare, Washington, D.C. (unpublished)

U.S. Food and Drug Administration. 1980. Compliance Program Report of Findings. FY 77 Total Diet Studies--Adult (7320.73). Bureau of Foods, Food and Drug Administration, Washington, D.C. [33] pp.

U.S. Food and Drug Administration. 1981. Consumers participate in FDA's priority setting process. FDA Consumer Update 18:1-3.

Witschi, H. P., P. J. Hakkinen, and J. P. Kehrer. 1981. Modification of lung tumor development in A/J mice. Toxicology 21:37-45.

World Health Organization. 1958-1980. Reports of the Joint FAO/WHO Expert Committee on Food Additives. World Health Organization Technical Report Series (Twenty-four reports to date). World Health Organization, Geneva, Switzerland.

World Health Organization. 1980. Evaluation of Certain Food Additives. Twenty-Third Report of the Joint FAO/WHO Expert Committee on Food Additives. WHO Tech. Rep. Ser. 648:1-45.

12 Naturally Occurring Carcinogens

The production of toxic compounds by living cells has long been recognized. Some of these chemicals, especially those produced by microbes and plant cells, have carcinogenic activity. Although some of these compounds are integral components of foods that are relatively common in the diet of humans, many of them have been found either in unusual food sources or in foods contaminated by microorganisms or unwanted plant materials. The potential hazards to human health posed by these components or contaminants of foods range from slight to very great. For example, very low levels of exposure to chemicals with relatively weak carcinogenic activity in laboratory animals may pose little risk to human populations. On the other hand, the presence of aflatoxin B_1 in foods is a matter of great concern, since aflatoxin B_1 is a potent carcinogen for a number of species and epidemiological data suggest that this carcinogen may play a role in the development of cancer in humans living in some parts of Africa and in the Far East (Peers et al., 1976; van Rensburg et al., 1974).

Much of the literature on the carcinogenic products of living cells has been collected and evaluated by working groups of the International Agency for Research on Cancer (1976) and by the National Research Council (National Academy of Sciences, 1973). Accordingly, these comprehensive reviews are often cited in this chapter instead of the primary literature. In addition, several recent reviews on naturally occurring carcinogens include exhaustive lists of primary references pertaining to these carcinogens. The overviews also cite literature on certain aspects of these carcinogens not covered in this chapter, such as their metabolic activation and deactivation, the reactions of electrophilic derivatives with cellular macromolecules, and the biochemical and biological consequences of the latter reactions (Hirono, 1981; Miller and Miller, 1979; Miller et al., 1979; Schoental, 1976).

MYCOTOXINS

By definition, mycotoxins are toxic secondary products resulting from the metabolism of molds. In this chapter, the committee has reviewed only those toxic metabolites of mold that occur as natural contaminants of food or feed or that demonstrate some evidence of carcinogenicity in mammals when administered orally. Although at least 45 mycotoxins have been identified as eliciting some type of carcinogenic or mutagenic response, only 17 of them have been reported to occur naturally in food or feed (Stoloff, in press) (or only 13, if the aflatoxin group is considered as a single compound).

The selection of the mycotoxins discussed in this section was based on the extent of their occurrence in food and/or the data demonstrating their carcinogenicity. These compounds include: aflatoxins, sterigmatocystin, ochratoxin A, zearalenone, T-2 toxin, patulin, penicillic acid, griseofulvin, luteoskyrin, cyclochlorotine, and ergot.

Aflatoxins

A very extensive effort has gone into the study of this group of mycotoxins, especially to examine its most potent member, aflatoxin B_1. Much more is known about the occurrence and toxicity of the aflatoxins than about any other mycotoxin and, probably, most other natural contaminants.

The scattered data pertaining to worldwide occurrence of aflatoxins in food were compiled for a conference on mycotoxins, which was sponsored by the Food and Agriculture Organization, the United Nations Environment Program, and the World Health Organization (1977). More recently, Stoloff (in press) compiled data on the occurrence of aflatoxins in the United States.

The aflatoxin-producing molds <u>Aspergillus flavus</u> and <u>A</u>. <u>parasiticus</u> are ubiquitous. They are frequently encountered as outgrowths on stored commodities under conditions prevailing in many tropical areas. In the United States, aflatoxin contamination is generally restricted to those crops invaded by the aflatoxin-producing molds before harvest: most frequently peanuts, corn, and cottonseed, and to a much lesser extent tree nuts, including almonds, walnuts, pecans, and pistachios. The extent of contamination is greater in the southeastern United States.

In the United States, humans are exposed to aflatoxin mostly from corn and peanuts (U.S. Food and Drug Administration, 1979). Other direct dietary sources, such as tree nuts, are of minor significance, either because contamination is infrequent or because only small quantities are consumed.

It is unlikely that secondary exposures result from the ingestion of aflatoxin residues in tissues of animals fed aflatoxin-contaminated feed (Stoloff, 1979), except for aflatoxin M_1, a metabolite that appears in the milk of lactating mammals exposed to aflatoxins. But, although large amounts of milk are consumed, this exposure is negligible compared to the direct exposure from peanuts and corn.

Aflatoxins are classified as unavoidable contaminants. In the United States, the maximum allowable limit of total aflatoxins in consumer peanut products is currently 20 μg/kg (U.S. Food and Drug Administration, 1980b).

Epidemiological Evidence. Oettlé (1965) was the first investigator to draw serious attention to the hypothesis that aflatoxin ingestion might cause liver cancer. He suggested that the geographic distribution of liver cancer in Africa could be explained by differing levels of exposure to aflatoxin in the diet. Keen and Martin (1971) reported an apparent association between the consumption of groundnuts contaminated with aflatoxin and the occurrence of liver cancer in different areas of Swaziland. Alpert et al. (1971) made a similar correlation of contaminated foodstuffs and incidence of hepatoma by tribe and by province or district in Uganda. In a later study in Swaziland, Peers et al. (1976) analyzed aflatoxin levels in foods consumed by a representative sample of the population in 11 geographic areas. He reported a significant correlation between aflatoxin contamination and incidence of primary liver cancer among adult males. A similar study in the Murang'a district of Kenya (Peers and Linsell, 1973) indicated that there was a correlation between aflatoxin levels in dietary staples of three district subdivisions and the incidence of liver cancer. Mozambique has particularly high rates of liver cancer, perhaps the highest in the world, and studies of aflatoxin contamination of foods indicated that the estimated daily intake of aflatoxin in that country was higher than that reported for any other country (van Rensburg et al., 1974). One problem recognized by the researchers in all of these studies is the inadequacy of the data on liver cancer incidence, since cancer registration is not well established in these areas.

Detailed studies of aflatoxin contamination of ingested foodstuffs have also been conducted in Thailand, where there was an overall correlation between estimated aflatoxin intakes in two regions and liver cancer incidence (Shank et al., 1972a,b; Wogan, 1975). The frequency with which aflatoxin was detected in foods has also been correlated with liver cancer mortality in Guangxi province in China (Armstrong, 1980). In Taiwan, where liver cancer mortality rates are high, Tung and Ling (1968) reported that dietary staples (e.g., peanuts and peanut oil, which is widely used in cooking) are frequently contaminated with aflatoxin.

Linsell and Peers (1977) observed a strong correlation between estimated levels of aflatoxin ingested and liver cancer incidence from various studies conducted in Africa and Asia. They further noted that there were no areas where high levels of aflatoxin ingestion have been associated with low rates of liver cancer.

Although the studies described above suggest that aflatoxin causes primary hepatocellular carcinoma (PHC), numerous other reports have also documented a high correlation between PHC and exposure to hepatitis B virus (Chien et al., 1981; Prince et al., 1975; Simons et al., 1972; Tong et al., 1971; Vogel et al., 1970). These studies do not indicate whether present or past exposure to this virus is more closely associated with the development of PHC. However, Kew et al. (1979)

reported that active hepatitis B viral infection is present in approximately 80% to 90% of the patients with PHC. Approximately 5% to 10% of the victims of hepatitis B infection actually develop chronic active hepatitis with persistent liver damage. The liver cells of these individuals are believed to regenerate more rapidly, thereby increasing the likelihood that a biochemical lesion that initiates neoplasia will become fixed in the genes of the subsequent cell population.

The worldwide occurrence of hepatitis B viral infection is similar to that of primary hepatocellular carcinoma. However, it is possible that the influences of aflatoxin and hepatitis B virus on the risk for PHC are not completely independent. Van Rensburg (1977) reviewed the evidence for both risk factors and concluded that preexisting viral infection is probably a prerequisite for malignant transformation by aflatoxin.

The possibility that aflatoxin may also be involved in the etiology of esophageal cancer is suggested by the correlation between mortality from esophageal cancer and the consumption of large amounts of pickled vegetables and other fermented or moldy food in Linxian county of Henan province in northern China (Yang, 1980). Although Aspergillus flavus has been isolated from some products, it is difficult to determine the role of aflatoxin in the etiology of this disease because these foods also contain other fungal species, mutagens, and carcinogens, including N-nitroso compounds.

Epidemiological studies have not been undertaken in Western countries, but there have been reports indicating the presence of aflatoxin B_1 in autopsy samples from liver cancer patients in Czechoslovakia (Dvořačková et al., 1977), New Zealand (Becroft and Webster, 1972), and the United States (Siraj et al., 1981). Siraj et al. (1981) detected aflatoxin B_1 in four of the six liver samples obtained from patients with PHC in the United States. The significance of these findings is not yet known.

Experimental Evidence: Carcinogenicity. Aflatoxin B_1 is the most potent hepatocarcinogen known, being about 1,000 times more powerful than butter yellow (p-dimethylaminoazobenzene) in rats. The carcinogenicity of aflatoxins has been examined in several studies in a variety of species and strains of laboratory animals, including mice, marmosets, tree shrews, trout, ducks, rhesus monkeys, hamsters, and several strains of rats (Wogan, 1973). Of the various species tested, the male Fischer 344 rat was the most sensitive to aflatoxin-induced carcinogenesis (Wogan, 1973).

Aflatoxin B_1 induced mainly hepatocellular carcinomas in rats. However, other studies in rats have indicated that it may also induce a very low incidence of carcinomas of the glandular stomach (Butler and Barnes, 1966), cancers of the colon (Newberne and Rogers, 1973; Wogan and Newberne, 1967), renal epithelial neoplasia (Epstein et al., 1969),

and lung adenomas (Newberne et al., 1967). Within a susceptible
species and strain, males are much more susceptible than females to
challenge with aflatoxin (Wogan and Newberne, 1967).

Mice are resistant to aflatoxin-induced carcinogenesis under conditions that result in 100% tumor incidence in Fischer rats. However,
hepatomas were induced in 82 of 105 inbred (C57BL X C3H)F_1 mice injected intraperitoneally during the first 7 days after birth with doses
of aflatoxin B_1 as low as 1.25 μg/g body weight (bw) and killed 82
weeks later (Vesselinovitch et al., 1972).

In comparison to Fischer rats, nonhuman primates (170 animals in 12
different investigations) were relatively resistant to aflatoxin-induced
carcinogenesis (Stoloff and Friedman, 1976). Liver tumors do not occur
spontaneously in monkeys (O'Gara and Adamson, 1972), but a female rhesus
monkey developed a primary liver carcinoma after ingesting approximately
500 mg of aflatoxin B_1 over a 6-year period (Adamson et al., 1973). In
another study, one of nine marmosets developed liver tumors after 50 weeks
on a diet (5 days a week) containing aflatoxin B_1 at 2 μg/g (Lin et al.,
1974). However, the authors also observed liver cirrhosis,which is not a
symptom of aflatoxicosis in rats. Reddy et al. (1976) reported that 9 of
18 tree shrews intermittently fed aflatoxin B_1 at 2 μg/g diet developed
liver cancers after 74 to 172 weeks of treatment.

Experimental Evidence: Mutagenicity. Aflatoxin B_1 was shown to be
mutagenic to Salmonella typhimurium strains TA98 and TA100 with and without S9 fraction (Ueno et al., 1978). It was positive in the Bacillus
subtilis rec assay (Ueno and Kubota, 1976). In FM3A mouse cells, aflatoxin induced 8-azaguanine-resistant mutants as well as chromosome aberrations (Umeda et al., 1977). Aflatoxin M_1, the metabolite of aflatoxin
B_1, was mutagenic in the Ames test (Wong and Hsieh, 1976), but inactive
in B. subtilis rec assay (Ueno and Kubota, 1976).

Other Mycotoxins

Table 12-1 summarizes the data on the occurrence, carcinogenicity,
and mutagenicity of mycotoxins other than aflatoxins that may be found
in food. Although most of these mycotoxins are mutagenic in bacterial
systems and other short-term tests and/or are carcinogenic in laboratory
animals, there are no epidemiological studies pertaining to their role
in neoplasia in humans.

Summary and Conclusions: Aflatoxins and Other Mycotoxins

A consistent body of evidence, all based on correlational data,
associates the contamination of foods by aflatoxin with a high incidence
of liver cancer in parts of Africa and Asia, but there is no epidemiological evidence that aflatoxin contamination of foodstuffs is related to

TABLE 12-1

Occurrence, Carcinogenicity, and Mutagenicity of Mycotoxins Other than Aflatoxins

Mycotoxin and Occurrence	Epidemiological Evidence	Carcinogenicity	Mutagenicity
Sterigmatocystin: Occasionally found in obviously moldy feed and moldy cheese rind, and less often in green coffee beans (Stoloff, in press).	No data available.	Oral administration induced liver tumors in rats (Purchase and van Der Watt, 1970).	Positive in Ames test (Ueno et al., 1978) and in B. subtilis rec assay (Ueno and Kubota, 1976). Mutagenic and clastogenic in mouse cells (Umeda et al., 1977).
Ochratoxin A: Frequent in grains and related foods; less often in white beans and green coffee beans (Stoloff, in press).	Circumstantial evidence that it may play a role in kidney tumors in the Balkans, but no epidemiological studies have been conducted.	Oral administration to mice induced liver and kidney tumors (Kanisawa and Suzuki, 1978).	Not mutagenic in Ames test (Wehner et al., 1978).
Zearalenone: Frequent in feed grains, maize, and soybeans; related to periodic Fusarium roseum infection of the grains (Stoloff, in press).	Might be involved in cervical cancer in South Africa (Martin and Keen, 1978; however, no epidemiological studies have been conducted.	Oral administration not carcinogenic to rats (Becci et al., in press), but carcinogenic to B6C3F$_1$ mice (National Cancer Institute, in press).	Negative in Ames test (Ueno et al., 1978), but positive in B. subtilis rec assay (Ueno and Kubota, 1976).
T-2 Toxin: Limited survey information due to inadequate analytical methods. Has been found in maize, barley, safflower seeds, and sorghum invaded by Fusarium tricinctum (Stoloff, in press).	Circumstantial evidence that it may be involved in esophageal cancer in China and South Africa; however, no epidemiological studies have been conducted.	Intragastric administration of LD$_{50}$ dose to rats induced cancer of digestive tract and brain (Schoental et al., 1979).	Negative in Ames test (Ueno et al., 1978), and in B. subtilis rec assay (Ueno and Kubota, 1976).
Patulin: Ubiquitous in apple juice and some other fruits subject to soft rot by Penicillium expansum (Stoloff, in press).	No data available.	Subcutaneous injection produced sarcomas in rats (Dickens and Jones, 1965). Chronic administration per os to rats was not carcinogenic (Becci et al., 1981).	Negative in Ames test (Wehner et al., 1978); positive in B. subtilis rec assay (Ueno and Kubota, 1976). Induced mutations in mouse cells (Umeda et al., 1977).
Penicillic Acid: Limited data indicate occurrence in dried beans and in corn with mold damage known as "blue eye" (Stoloff, in press).	No data available.	Produced local sarcomas when injected under the skin of rats (Dickens and Jones, 1965).	Negative in Ames test (Wehner et al., 1978) and in B. subtilis rec assay (Ueno and Kubota, 1976); induced DNA breaks in HeLa cells (Umeda et al., 1972).
Griseofulvin: Used as systematic fungicide in treatment of mycoses. No information on natural occurrence.	No data available.	Dietary administration induced liver tumors in mice (International Agency for Research on Cancer, 1976).	Negative in Ames test (Wehner et al., 1978) and in B. subtilis rec assay (Ueno and Kubota, 1976).
Luteoskyrin and Cyclochlorotine: Penicillium islandicum, which produces these toxins in laboratory cultures, is a common component of grain mycoflora. No evidence of natural occurrence of those toxins in the grains (International Agency for Research on Cancer, 1976).	No data available.	Dietary luteoskyrin induced hepatic tumors in mice (International Agency for Research on Cancer, 1976). Few liver tumors developed in mice fed cyclochlorotine (International Agency for Research on Cancer, 1976).	Luteoskyrin is negative in Ames test (Ueno et al., 1978), but positive in S. typhimurium TM677 (Stark et al., 1978).
Ergot: The dried sclerotium of the fungus Claviceps purpurea that grows on rye and certain other grasses. It contains many alkaloids and physiologically active substances (Miller, 1973).	No data available.	Ergot fed to rats at 5% of the diet for 2 years induced neurofibromas of the ears, which regressed when feeding of ergot was stopped and reappeared when ergot feeding resumed (Nelson et al., 1942).	No data available.

cancer risk in the United States. Epidemiological studies have also
indicated a high correlation between primary hepatocellular carcinoma
and exposure to hepatitis B viral infection. Aflatoxin is carcinogenic
in several species of animals, including rats, mice, trout, ducks,
monkeys, and marmosets, and there is evidence of dose response. It
induces mainly tumors of the liver and, to a lesser extent, tumors in
the kidney, lung, stomach, and colon, more readily in males and in the
young. The carcinogenicity of aflatoxin is paralleled by its
mutagenicity in various systems.

There is no reliable information about the role of other mycotoxins
in carcinogenesis in humans.

HYDRAZINES IN MUSHROOMS

Epidemiological Evidence. No epidemiological studies have been
conducted to determine the effects of hydrazines on carcinogenesis in
humans.

Agaricus bisporus

Agaricus bisporus is a commonly eaten cultivated mushroom in
Europe, North America, and other parts of the world. The exact
consumption figures for Agaricus bisporus are unknown, but the U.S.
Department of Agriculture (1981) has estimated that approximately 213
million kilograms of this mushroom were available for consumption
(production and imports) in the United States during 1980.

Agaricus bisporus contains agaritine -- β-N-[γ-L(+)-glutamyl]-4-
hydroxymethylphenylhydrazine (Toth et al., 1978) -- and 4-(hydroxy-
methyl)benzenediazonium ion (Levenberg, 1962). 4-Hydroxymethylphenyl-
hydrazine and 4-methylphenylhydrazine, which are breakdown products of
agaritine, have also been found in A. bisporus (Levenberg, 1964).

Experimental Evidence: Carcinogenicity. N'-Acetyl-4-(hydroxy-
methyl)phenylhydrazine as a 0.0625% solution in drinking water administered continuously to Swiss mice from 6 weeks of age to the end of
their lives induced lung and blood vessel tumors (Toth et al., 1978).

4-(Hydroxymethyl)benzenediazonium tetrafluoroborate administered
to Swiss mice in 26 weekly subcutaneous injections at 50 μg/g bw
resulted in an increased incidence of tumors of the subcutis and skin
(Toth et al., 1981).

4-Methylphenylhydrazine hydrochloride administered to Swiss mice in
7 weekly intragastric instillations of 250 μg/g bw induced lung and
blood vessel tumors (Toth et al., 1977).

Experimental Evidence: Mutagenicity. N'-Acetyl-4-(hydroxy-methyl)phenylhydrazine was most mutagenic in S. typhimurium TA1537 without metabolic activation, and it exhibited marginal DNA-modifying activity only when the S9 fraction was included (Rogan et al., in press).

4-(Hydroxymethyl)benzenediazonium tetrafluoroborate was weakly mutagenic in TA1535 and strongly mutagenic in TA1537, exhibiting toxicity in both strains (Rogan et al., in press).

Agaritine produced equivocal results in both in vitro assays. There was a slight enhancement of mutagenicity in S. typhimurium TA1537 without metabolic activation, and marginal DNA-modifying activity in the presence of S9 fraction (Rogan et al., in press).

4-Methylphenylhydrazine hydrochloride was also found to be mutagenic with and without S9 fraction in S. typhimurium TA98 and TA100 (Shimizu et al., 1978).

Gyromitra esculenta

Each year, approximately 1 million people throughout the world eat the mushroom Gyromitra esculenta (Simons, 1971); 100,000 of these people reside in the United States (S. Miller, personal communication). The literature contains more than 500 reports of poisonings resulting from the ingestion of this mushroom. Some of these incidents were fatal (Franke et al., 1967).

Experimental Evidence: Carcinogenicity. Eleven hydrazines and hydrazones have been identified in G. esculenta. Studies have been conducted to determine the carcinogenicity of many of these compounds.

Continuous administration of 0.0078% N-methyl-N-formylhydrazine (MFH) in drinking water to 6-week-old outbred Swiss mice for life produced tumors of the liver, lung, gallbladder, and bile duct. A higher dose (0.0156% MFH) given under identical conditions had no tumorigenic effect, since it proved too toxic for the animals (Toth and Nagel, 1978). Subsequently, the carcinogenicity of MFH was confirmed in mice (Toth and Patil, 1980, 1981) and in Syrian hamsters (Toth and Patil, 1979).

Acetaldehyde methylformylhydrazone, the main ingredient of G. esculenta, was administered to Swiss mice in propylene glycol in 52 weekly intragastric instillations at 100 µg/g bw (Toth et al., 1981). The treatment induced tumors of the lungs, preputial glands, forestomach, and clitoral glands.

Drinking water solutions of 0.001% hydrazine, 0.01% methylhydrazine, and 0.001% methylhydrazine sulfate were administered continuously to 5- and 6-week-old randomly bred Swiss mice for their lifetimes. Hydrazine and methylhydrazine sulfate significantly increased the incidence of lung tumors in Swiss mice, whereas methylhydrazine enhanced the development of this neoplasm by shortening its latent period (Toth, 1972).

A 0.01% solution of methylhydrazine was administered daily in the drinking water of 6-week-old randomly bred Syrian golden hamsters for the remainder of their lifetimes. The treatment produced malignant histiocytomas of the liver and tumors of the cecum (Toth and Shimizu 1973).

Experimental Evidence: Mutagenicity. N-Methyl-N-formylhydrazine, which is present in G. esculenta, was mutagenic only in S. typhimurium TA1537 without activation and had no DNA-modifying activity (Rogan et al., in press).

Methylhydrazine was mutagenic in S. typhimurium TA1535 and TA1537. The addition of S9 fraction activating system enhanced the mutagenicity in both strains (Rogan et al., in press). The DNA-modifying activity was observed earlier by von Wright et al. (1977).

Summary and Conclusions: Hydrazines

Studies have shown that some chemical constituents of the Agaricus bisporus mushroom are carcinogenic in mice and mutagenic in bacterial systems. One constituent has also been shown to be carcinogenic in hamsters. But the findings of these studies are not sufficient for conclusions to be drawn concerning the risk to humans.

Some derivatives of hydrazines in the fungus Gyromitra esculenta have proven carcinogenic in a number of organs and tissues of mice and hamsters. Two of them were mutagenic in bacterial systems. There are no epidemiological studies concerning the carcinogenicity of these mushrooms in humans.

PLANT CONSTITUENTS AND METABOLITES

Pyrrolizidine Alkaloids

Pyrrolizidine alkaloids occur in many nonedible plant species, including the genera Senecio (ragworts), Crotalaria (rattleboxes), and Heliotropium (heliotropes), in amounts ranging from trace amounts to as much as 5% of the dry weight. In general, members of this group that contain a nuclear double bond alpha to an esterified carbinol are very potent toxins in the liver and lung of rodents and certain farm livestock (Hirono, 1981; Hirono et al., 1979; International Agency for Research on Cancer, 1976).

Experimental Evidence: Carcinogenicity. Monocrotaline, retrorsine, lasiocarpine, heliotrine, senkirkine, symphytine, and petasitenine, all of which are α, β-unsaturated esters, are carcinogenic when administered to rats orally or parenterally under conditions that permit long-term survivals. Most frequently, tumor induction has involved multiple doses of the alkaloids at moderate levels (e.g., a 0.01% solution of petasitenine in drinking water for 480 days) (Hirono et al., 1979), but low incidences of tumors after long latent periods have apparently resulted from only one or a few doses. Tumors have also been induced in rats after the administration of plants, such as coltsfoot (Tussilago farfara) or comfrey (Symphytum sp.), which contain high levels of pyrrolizidine alkaloids. The tumors occur most frequently in the liver, but some have developed in other tissues, including the skin and lungs.

Plants containing the pyrrolizidine alkaloids may contaminate forages and food grains. Such contamination has resulted in acute and chronic poisoning of livestock in some parts of the world (Schoental, 1976). Humans may also be exposed by consuming such alkaloid-containing plants as drugs or foods. For example, one species of comfrey (Symphytum officinale) is consumed as a green vegetable in Japan (Hirono et al., 1979). The carcinogenic potency of some pyrrolizidine alkaloids and their widespread occurrence have led to the suggestion that these α,β-unsaturated esters may play a role in the induction of hepatic cancer in humans in some parts of the world; however, there are no reliable data to support this hypothesis.

Experimental Evidence: Mutagenicity. Retrorsine, lasiocarpine, heliotrine, senkirkine, symphytine, and petasitenine, but not monocrotaline, have been shown to be mutagenic in the Salmonella/microsome assay (Hirono et al., 1979; Wehner et al., 1979; Yamanaka et al., 1979).

Allylic and Propenylic Benzene Derivatives

Numerous allylic and propenylic benzene derivatives are present in the essential oils of a wide variety of plants (Guenther, 1948-1952; Guenther and Althausen, 1949), and some of these plants or their extracts are used as flavoring agents for human foods or as medicines consumed by humans. Of the known naturally occurring allylic benzene derivatives, safrole (1-allyl-3,4-methylenedioxybenzene), which is a major component of oil of sassafras, and estragole (1-allyl-4-methoxybenzene), which is present in tarragon and anise, have been the most comprehensively studied.

Experimental Evidence: Carcinogenicity. Safrole has induced low-to-moderate incidences of hepatic tumors in adult rats fed at levels of 0.5% or more of the diet for as long as 2 years (International Agency for Research on Cancer, 1976). Both safrole and estragole induced hepatic tumors and subcutaneous angiosarcomas within 18 months after they were fed to adult female CD-1 mice at levels of 0.25%-0.5% for approximately 1 year (Miller et al., 1979). Administration of less than

1 mg of either compound or of methyl eugenol to CD-1 or (C57BL/6 x C3H/He)F$_1$ male mice prior to weaning resulted in a high incidence of hepatomas by the age of 12 months (Miller et al., 1979).

Experimental Evidence: Mutagenicity. Safrole was mutagenic in vitro and in the host-mediated assay (Green and Savage, 1978). However, McCann et al. (1975), Swanson et al. (1979), and Wislocki et al. (1977) reported that it was not mutagenic in the Ames test. It was positive in Bacillus subtilis rec assay (Rosenkranz and Poirier, 1979) and in Saccharomyces cerevisiae D3 (Simmon, 1979).

Estragole was mutagenic to S. typhimurium TA100 (Swanson et al., 1979). Eugenol was not mutagenic to Ames Salmonella strains in vitro and in the host-mediated assay (Green and Savage, 1978; Swanson et al., 1979).

Bracken Fern Toxin(s)

Bracken fern (Pteridium aquilinum) occurs widely in nature and is consumed by humans in several parts of the world, especially in Japan (Hirono, 1981). For at least 30 years, it has been known that consumption of this plant causes damage to the bone marrow and intestinal mucosa of cattle, but the precise compound(s) responsible for these toxic effects have not been identified.

Epidemiological Evidence: Carcinogenicity. In a prospective cohort study in Japan, Hirayama (1979) found a significantly higher risk of esophageal carcinoma associated with the daily intake of hot gruel or bracken fern every day, especially in people who ate both foods daily. However, Howe et al. (1980) found no association between bladder cancer and consumption of fiddlehead greens (related to bracken fern) in a case-control study in Canada.

Experimental Evidence: Carcinogenicity. The carcinogenicity of bracken fern was first suspected by Pamukcu in 1960, who found polyps in the urinary bladder mucosa of cattle fed large amounts of bracken fern for long periods (Pamukcu and Bryan, 1979). Since that time, ingestion of high levels of bracken fern (25% to 40% of the diet) has been found to result in the formation of urinary bladder carcinomas in cattle, urinary bladder carcinomas and intestinal adenocarcinomas in rats, urinary bladder tumors in guinea pigs, pulmonary adenomas in mice, and intestinal adenocarcinomas in Japanese quail (Evans, 1976).

Hirono (1981) reported that the greatest concentration of the toxin(s) is present in young plants before the fronds have uncurled, and the carcinogenic activity of the rhizome is greater than that of the stalk or fronds. The toxicity of the fern is reduced, but not eliminated, by cooking.

A number of studies have been conducted to identify the carcinogenic agent(s) in bracken fern (Evans, 1976; Hirono, 1981; Pamukcu and Bryan, 1979). Quercetin (3,3',4',5,7-pentahydroxyflavone) occurs as a conjugate in bracken fern and in numerous other plants. In culture, this compound has induced morphological transformation of cryopreserved golden hamster embryo cells (Umezawa et al., 1977) and mutations in S. typhimurium (Bartholomew and Ryan, 1980), but its carcinogenicity in rats continues to be disputed. In one study, administration of 0.1% quercetin in the diet of rats for as long as 1 year resulted in an 80% incidence of intestinal tumors and a 20% incidence of urinary bladder tumors (Pamukcu et al., 1980). However, in another laboratory, administration of quercetin as 1% or 5% of the diet for 540 days or as 10% of the diet for 850 days did not result in a significant incidence of tumors in ACI rats (Hirono et al., 1981).

Interest in the possibility that bracken fern might play a role in the induction of cancers stems from the knowledge that it is used by humans as food in several parts of the world (Hirono, 1981). Indirect evidence for its carcinogenicity is derived from observations that milk from cows fed high levels of bracken fern contained compounds that were shown to be carcinogenic in rats. Carcinomas of the intestine, urinary bladder, and kidney pelvis were observed in rats fed high levels of fresh or powdered milk from cows that had consumed 1 g of bracken fern per kilogram of body weight daily for approximately 2 years, but not in rats fed milk from control cows (Pamukcu et al., 1978).

Estrogenic Compounds

The plant estrogens include estrone (from palm kernels), genistein (from soybean and clover), coumestrol (from alfalfa and other forage crops), and mirestrol (from certain legumes) (Schoental, 1976; Stob, 1973). Zearalenone, a product of Fusarium molds that sometimes infect grains, also possesses estrogenic activity.

Plant estrogens are very weak estrogens compared to the hormones from animals; however, they can occur in relatively large amounts. For example, fat-free soybeans may contain as much as 0.1% of genistein (Verdeal et al., 1980).

Experimental Evidence: Carcinogenicity. Other than one report on zearalenone (discussed earlier in this chapter), there are no data pertaining to the carcinogenicity of plant estrogens. Some nonsteroidal phytoestrogens that are natural components of some foods compete for estrogen receptors in rat uterine cytosol in tissue sections from 7,12-dimethylbenz[a]anthracene-induced mammary tumors, and in mammary tumor tissue from humans (Verdeal et al., 1980). The significance of these findings in the etiology of neoplasia in humans is not known.

Experimental Evidence: Mutagenicity. Genistein and coumestrol were not mutagenic in the Salmonella microsome assay (Bartholomew and Ryan, 1980).

Coffee

Epidemiological Evidence: Carcinogenicity: Coffee drinking has been associated with elevated risk for bladder cancer in several case-control studies (Bross and Tidings, 1973; Cole, 1971; Fraumeni et al., 1971; Howe et al., 1980; Miller et al., 1978; Simon et al., 1975; Wynder and Goldsmith, 1977). However, with only two possible exceptions in males (Bross and Tidings, 1973; Wynder and Goldsmith, 1977), there has been no evidence of a dose-response relationship, and it appears that the association is not causal.

A direct association of coffee consumption with risk of pancreatic cancer based on case-control data was reported by MacMahon et al. (1981). They provided evidence for a dose-response relationship. In another report, Lin and Kessler (1981) noted an association between pancreatic cancer and the use of decaffeinated coffee specifically. In an earlier geographical correlation of per capita food intake and mortality from cancer, Stocks (1970) observed a significant association between coffee drinking and pancreatic cancer.

Other reported associations of coffee drinking with cancer have been scattered and inconsistent. Martínez (1969) found an association between oral and esophageal cancers combined and consumption of hot beverages, mostly coffee, whereas Stocks (1970) did not find a significant correlation between coffee consumption and esophageal cancer. Shennan (1973) reported a direct correlation between per capita coffee intake and mortality from renal carcinoma (r=0.8), and the association, though less strong, appeared also in the correlational data of Armstrong and Doll (1975). On the other hand, case-control studies of renal cancer (Armstrong et al., 1976; Wynder et al., 1974) have not confirmed this association. Stocks (1970) also found a direct correlation of prostate cancer mortality with per capita coffee intake. This finding did not appear in a similar analysis by Armstrong and Doll (1975), who reported an association with per capita fat intake and a high correlation between these two dietary factors.

Experimental Evidence: Carcinogenicity. Sprague-Dawley rats were fed a diet containing 5% instant coffee for 2 years. No bladder tumors were noted in rats fed diets containing the equivalent of up to 85 cups of coffee per day (Zeitlin, 1972).

Maximum tolerated doses of regular and decaffeinated instant coffees (6% of the diet) fed to Sprague-Dawley rats for 2 years produced no evidence of carcinogenesis (Würzner et al., 1977). The authors also reported that high levels of caffeine led to a lower incidence of tumors. However, Challis and Bartlett (1975) reported that readily oxidized phenolic compounds--which are constituents of coffee--catalyze nitrosamine formation from nitrite and secondary amines at gastric pH. For example, these experiments showed that 4-methylcatechol and the phenolic component of chlorogenic acid (approximately 13% of the dry weight of the soluble constituents of coffee), exerted catalytic effects on nitrosamine formation. This finding implies that several foodstuffs and beverages, including coffee, may have cocarcinogenic properties.

Experimental Evidence: Mutagenicity. Coffee is mutagenic to Salmonella typhimurium strain TA100, whether it is brewed, instant, or decaffeinated (Aeschbacher and Würzner, 1980; Aeschbacher et al., 1980; Nagao et al., 1979). Although caffeine has been reported to be mutagenic to bacteria (Clarke and Wade, 1975; Demerec et al., 1948, 1951; Gezelius and Fries, 1952; Glass and Novick, 1959; Johnson and Bach, 1965; Kubitschek and Bendigkeit, 1958, 1964; Novick, 1956), it could not have been responsible for the mutagenicity of coffee observed in these reports, since decaffeinated coffee was as mutagenic as regular coffee and caffeine itself was not detected as a mutagen under the test conditions used (Aeschbacher et al., 1980; Nagao et al., 1979).

Methylxanthines

Experimental Evidence: Carcinogenicity. Another widely consumed class of compounds are the methylxanthines, which include caffeine. There appear to be no published studies on the carcinogenicity of caffeine in laboratory animals following chronic oral administration. In one as yet unpublished study (Takayama, personal communication), Wistar rats were divided into three dose groups each containing 50 males and 50 females. The first two groups were given 0.2% and 0.1% caffeine in their drinking water for 18 months beginning at the age of 8 weeks. Then, normal water without caffeine was given to the surviving animals for an additional 6 months. The third group, which served as the control group, was given normal water throughout the experiment. All remaining animals were sacrificed 24 months after the caffeine treatment had begun. The investigators concluded that there was no significant increase in the incidence of any type of tumors in caffeine-treated animals, as compared to control animals.

Experimental Evidence: Mutagenicity. The methylxanthines--a class of compounds that are present in tea and coffee--are mutagenic in at least some test systems. Three of the compounds--caffeine, theophylline, and theobromine--have been reported to be mutagenic to bacteria and to cause abnormalities in the chromosomes of plant cells (see reviews by Kihlman, 1977, and Timson, 1975). However, the mutagenic effects of these compounds in mammals have not been clearly demonstrated in vivo. Caffeine can enhance the genetic effects of other chemicals, even in vivo (Frei and Venitt, 1975; Jenssen and Ramel, 1978). This activity is presumably due to the ability of caffeine to inhibit repair of DNA damage caused by chemical mutagens.

Cycasin

Cycasin (methylazoxymethanol-β-glucoside) is one of the most potent carcinogens found in plants (International Agency for Research on Cancer, 1976; Magee et al., 1976). This compound and at least one related glucoside (macrozamin) are present in the palmlike cycad trees of the family Cycadaceae. These trees have provided food for natives and their livestock in tropical and subtropical regions. The sliced nuts are generally extracted with water prior to use, but acute poisonings have been reported.

In Guam and Okinawa, which have high rates of liver cancer, the ingestion of cycasin in cycad nuts has been proposed as an etiologic factor. However, in a descriptive study conducted in the Miyako Islands of Okinawa, investigators found no correlation between mortality from hepatoma and the ingestion of cycad nuts (Hirono et al., 1970). Therefore, there is no evidence for the carcinogenicity of cycasin in humans.

Experimental Evidence: Carcinogenicity. When administered orally, cycasin is highly carcinogenic in the liver, kidney, and colon of rats, and also induces tumors in other species (Laquer and Spatz, 1968). The tissues of rats contain low levels of β-glucosidase, which hydrolyzes cycasin. However, the hydrolysis generally depends on the action of intestinal bacteria (Matsumoto et al., 1972). The product, methylazoxymethanol (MAM), decomposes at neutral pH to an electrophilic intermediate that methylates nucleic acids and proteins both in vitro and in vivo (Matsumoto and Higa, 1966). These findings and the carcinogenic activity of MAM (Laquer and Spatz, 1968) have implicated MAM as a proximate carcinogenic metabolite of cycasin. The methylating species formed from MAM and cycasin appears to be similar or identical to that formed during the metabolic activation of the synthetic carcinogen nitrosodimethylamine, which has carcinogenic properties similar to those of cycasin (Magee et al., 1976).

Experimental Evidence: Mutagenicity. Cycasin was not mutagenic in the standard Ames test (Ames et al., 1975), but it became mutagenic when preincubated with almond β-glucosidase (Matsushima et al., 1979).

Thiourea

Thiourea occurs naturally in laburnum shrubs and in certain fungi (e.g., Verticillium albo-atrum and Bortrylio cinerea).

Experimental Evidence: Carcinogenicity. Thiourea has been shown to cause thyroid tumors, hepatic adenomas, and epidermoid carcinomas of Zymbal's gland when administered to rats as 0.2% of the drinking water or diet for as long as 2 years (International Agency for Research on Cancer, 1974).

Experimental Evidence: Mutagenicity. Thiourea was negative in the standard Ames Salmonella/microsome assay (Simmon, 1979), but positive in the host-mediated assay (Simmon et al., 1979). It also induced transformations in hamster embryo cells (Pienta, 1981).

Tannic Acid and Tannins

Tannins are contained in many plants. These compounds are divided into two groups--the nonhydrolyzable condensed tannins and the hydrolyzable tannins, which are subdivided into ellagitannins or gallotannins. Commercially, the term tannic acid generally applies to hydrolyzable gallotannins, including taratannic acid. Tannins are widely distributed in plants, and are present naturally in small amounts in coffee and tea. Tannic acid has also been used by U.S. food processors as a clarifying agent in the brewing and wine industries and as a flavoring agent in such products as butter, caramel, fruit, brandy, maple, syrup, and nuts (National Academy of Sciences, 1965).

Experimental Evidence: Carcinogenicity. The investigations of Korpássy showed that subcutaneous administration of tannic acid in doses of 150 to 200 mg/kg bw produced skin necrosis, ulcers, and hepatic tumors in rats (Korpássy, 1959, 1961; Korpássy and Mosonyi, 1950, 1951). No adequate studies have been conducted to test the carcinogenicity of orally administered tannins.

In mice, repeated subcutaneous injections of three condensed nonhydrolyzable tannins produced liver tumors and sarcomas (Kirby, 1960).

Experimental Evidence: Mutagenicity. Tannic acid was found not to be genotoxic or mutagenic to Saccharomyces cerevisiae D4 and Ames S. typhimurium strains with and without metabolic activation (Litton Bionetics, Inc., 1975). Tannins from various sources such as apple juice, grape juice, wine, and betel nuts were found to be strongly clastogenic for Chinese hamster ovary cells, but they lacked the capacity to induce mutations in the Ames test (Stich and Powrie, in press).

Coumarin

Coumarin is present in a number of plants, including tonka beans, cassia, and woodruff, and in their essential oils (International Agency for Research on Cancer, 1976).

Experimental Evidence: Carcinogenicity. Coumarin (o-hydroxycinnamic acid-δ-lactone) has induced bile duct carcinomas in rats fed 0.35% to 0.5% of the compound in the diet for approximately 18 months.

Experimental Evidence: Mutagenicity. Coumarin was negative in the E. coli pol A assay (Rosenkranz and Leifer, 1981). It interferes with excision repair processes in ultraviolet-damaged DNA and with host cell reactivation of ultraviolet-irradiated phage T1 in E. coli WP2 (Grigg, 1972).

Parasorbic Acid

Parasorbic acid occurs in concentrations ranging from 0.2 to 2 μg/g in the ripe berries of the Moravian mountain ash Sorbus aucuparia var. edulis. It has not been found in a number of common fruits (pears, apples, lemons, cranberries, grapes, oranges, or tomatoes) (International Agency for Research on Cancer, 1976).

Experimental Evidence: Carcinogenicity. Sarcomas resulted within 2 years in rats that had received repeated subcutaneous injections of parasorbic acid in total doses of either 13 or 128 mg per animal (International Agency for Research on Cancer, 1976).

Experimental Evidence: Mutagenicity. No studies concerning the mutagenicity of parasorbic acid could be identified.

METABOLITES OF ANIMAL ORIGIN

Tryptophan and Its Metabolites

Experimental Evidence: Carcinogenicity. Dogs fed high levels of tryptophan (7 g/day, i.e., 7 times the amount fed to controls) for long periods developed hyperplasia of the urinary bladder (Radomski et al., 1971). When tryptophan was given to rats as 2% of the diet after sub-carcinogenic doses of a nitrofuran, tryptophan exerted a promoting effect on the formation of tumors in the urinary bladder (Cohen et al., 1979). In other studies, four metabolites of tryptophan (3-hydroxyky-nurenine, 3-hydroxyanthranilic acid, 2-amino-3-hydroxyacetophenone, and xanthurenic acid-8-methyl ether) each induced bladder tumors when implanted as pellets in the urinary bladders of mice (Clayson and Garner, 1976). However, attempts to relate the development of tumors in the urinary bladder of humans to abnormalities in the metabolism of tryptophan have not been definitive (Clayson and Garner, 1976).

Experimental Evidence: Mutagenicity. Tryptophan and its metabolites were not mutagenic in the Salmonella/microsome assay (Bowden et al., 1976).

Hormones

Experimental Evidence: Carcinogenicity. A number of endogenous peptide and steroid hormones facilitate the development of tumors of the endocrine glands of laboratory animals (Clifton and Sridharan, 1975; Furth, 1975). However, because humans consume only very small amounts of hormones from the tissues of animals and because there is no indication that hormones from food sources are significant factors in the development of cancer in humans, they are not considered in this report. One exception is diethylstilbestrol (DES), which is discussed in Chapter 14.

FERMENTATION PRODUCT

Ethyl Carbamate (Urethan)

Ethyl carbamate, or urethan, is a fermentation product. The detection of low levels of ethyl carbamate in wines treated with the synthetic sterilant diethyl pyrocarbonate (Ehrenberg et al., 1976) led to investigations into the natural occurrence of ethyl carbamate. These studies have demonstrated that naturally fermented foods and beverages (e.g., wines, bread, beers, and yogurt) contain detectable, but very low levels of ethyl carbamate, usually less than 5 μg/kg. The ethyl carbamate probably results from the reaction of ethanol and carbamoyl phosphate--both normal metabolic products in the yeast (Ough, 1976).

Experimental Evidence: Carcinogenicity. For many years, ethyl carbamate has been studied as a synthetic carcinogen in the rat, mouse, and hamster. Its ability to induce tumors has been demonstrated by administering the compound during the prenatal and preweanling periods as well as to adult animals. Ethyl carbamate is active when administered orally, by inhalation, or by subcutaneous or intraperitoneal injection. The susceptible tissues include the lungs, lymphoid tissue, skin, liver, mammary gland, and Zymbal's gland. Most frequently, tumors are induced with doses ranging from 0.5 to 3 mg/g bw (International Agency for Research on Cancer, 1974; Mirvish, 1968). However, lung adenomas were induced in mice with a single dose of 0.01 mg/g bw (Nomura, 1975).

The significance of naturally occurring ethyl carbamate in foods in the development of human cancer is unknown, but the levels are very low in comparison to those used to induce tumors in laboratory animals (i.e., the consumption of 5 μg/day by a 70-kg person would provide an annual intake of approximately 0.05 μg/g bw).

Experimental Evidence: Mutagenicity. Urethan was not mutagenic to Ames Salmonella strains (Simmon, 1979) or in the host-mediated assay (Simmon et al., 1979). However, it did induce transformations in hamster embryo cells (Pienta, 1981).

NITRATE, NITRITE, AND N-NITROSO COMPOUNDS

Because many N-nitrosodialkylamines, N-nitrosoalkylamides, and N-nitrosoalkylimides are strong carcinogens under a variety of conditions and in many species (Magee and Barnes, 1967; Magee et al., 1976) and because certain N-nitroso compounds have been detected in foods, in gastrointestinal contents, and in blood or urine (Fine et al., 1977; Hicks et al., 1977; Sen et al., 1980; Spiegelhalder et al., 1980; Stephany and Schuller, 1980), there has been much concern during the past 10 to 15 years about the role of N-nitroso compounds in the etiology of human cancer.

In recent years, a number of observations have also led to concern about potential risks to human health resulting from the use of nitrate and nitrite as preservatives in meats and other cured products. Nitrate can be reduced to nitrite, which can interact with dietary substrates such as amines or amides to produce N-nitroso compounds. Because the health effects of nitrate, nitrite, and N-nitroso compounds have been reviewed in depth by the Committee on Nitrite and Alternative Curing Agents in Food (National Academy of Sciences, 1981), only a brief summary is presented in this section.

Nitrate and nitrite are widely distributed in foods in varying concentrations, depending on a number of factors such as agricultural practices and storage conditions. It is difficult to estimate with any precision the exposure of humans to these ions because of differing lifestyles and dietary habits and the limitations in analytical techniques for measuring them and in the methods for determining food consumption. The Committee on Nitrite and Alternative Curing Agents in Food estimated that the average U.S. diet provides approximately 75 mg of nitrate and 0.8 mg of nitrite daily (National Academy of Sciences, 1981). Vegetables contribute most of the nitrate ingested. Other dietary sources include nitrate-rich drinking water and fruit juices. More than one-third of the average daily intake of nitrite is contributed by the ingestion of cured meats, approximately one-third by baked goods and cereals, and less than one-fifth by vegetables.

Two additional factors must be considered when determining exposure to nitrate and nitrite: Vegetables contain both inhibitors (e.g., ascorbic acid) and catalysts (e.g., phenols) of nitrosation reactions. These modifiers tend to affect the extent of in vivo nitrosation and, thus, the synthesis of N-nitroso compounds. Evidence indicates that in vivo nitrosation occurs when amines and/or amides and nitrate and/or nitrite are ingested simultaneously (National Academy of Sciences, 1981). The key factors that determine the extent of these reactions in the stomach are the gastric pH; the concentrations of the nitrate and/or nitrite and the nitrosatable amines and/or amides; the rates of nitrosation of the substrate; and types and amounts of nitrosation modifiers in the stomach.

Humans may also be exposed to preformed nitrosamines that occur as contaminants in some foods, chiefly in nitrate- or nitrite-treated products (Gough et al., 1978; Spiegelhalder et al., 1980; Stephany and Schuller, 1980). The largest single dietary source of nitrosamines was beer until recently, when maltsters reduced the concentrations by modifying the malting processes. The most important sources of nitrosamines in the diet are now cured meat products, especially bacon, which contributes approximately 0.17 µg of nitrosopyrrolidine per person daily. In the United States, the intake of nitrosamines from all dietary sources, including beer, is estimated to be approximately 1.1 µg/day.

Nitrate can be converted to nitrite by bacterial reduction in the saliva. Roughly 25% of ingested nitrate is recirculated into saliva, and approximately 20% of salivary nitrate is reduced to nitrite (National Academy of Sciences, 1981).

The formation of nitrate by bacteria in the large intestine (heterotrophic nitrification) has been postulated as one mechanism to account for differences in ingestion and urinary excretion of nitrate by humans (Tannenbaum et al., 1978). However, these conclusions appear to be erroneous since studies in germfree rodents indicate that such reactions are not important (Green et al., 1981). Moreover, the nitrate content of ingested food, water, and air may have been underestimated in the earlier studies. Recent studies suggest that mammalian tissues synthesize nitrate and that this may partially explain excess urinary nitrate excretion (Green et al., 1981; Parks et al., 1981). However, the amount of nitrate produced endogenously appears to be less than that suggested in earlier studies by Tannenbaum et al. (1978).

The formation of N-nitroso compounds in vivo has been well documented in laboratory animals (Mirvish et al., 1980). In humans, the evidence is sparse. However, one recent study provides direct evidence that nitrosamines are synthesized in humans following the ingestion of an amine (proline) and nitrate (Ohshima and Bartsch, 1981). In that experiment, the ingestion of a large excess of ascorbic acid or α-tocopherol effectively reduced the endogenous formation of nitrosamines.

Epidemiological Evidence

Studies conducted in Colombia, Chile, Japan, Iran, China, England, and the United States (Hawaii) have indicated that there is an association between increased incidence of cancers of the stomach and the esophagus and exposures to high levels of nitrate or nitrite in the diet or drinking water. (See, for example, Armijo and Coulson, 1975; Armijo et al., 1981; Correa et al., 1975; Cuello et al., 1976; Haenszel et al., 1972; Higginson, 1966; Meinsma, 1964).

Exposures to nitrate, nitrite, or N-nitroso compounds were not directly measured in these epidemiological studies. The associations with cancer were based either on correlations of high risk population groups with corresponding exposures in food and water supplies, or on comparisons of the frequency of consumption of foods containing these substances (plus secondary amines) by gastric cancer patients and by controls.

Bladder cancer has been correlated with nitrate in the water supply or with urinary tract infections in some epidemiological studies (Howe et al., 1980; Wynder et al., 1963). However, Howe et al. (1980) reported that there was no difference between cases and controls in consumption of nitrite-preserved meats, such as hams and sausages. Nevertheless, it is of interest that nitrosamines, which are presumably formed from dietary precursors, have been found in the urine of patients with urinary tract infections and could presumably be carcinogenic in the bladder (Hicks et al., 1977; Radomski et al., 1978).

The Committee on Nitrite and Alternative Curing Agents in Food concluded that these reports do not provide conclusive evidence of a causal relationship, and that alternative explanations for the findings have not been ruled out (National Academy of Sciences, 1981).

Studies of occupational exposure have not contributed significant information on possible associations between N-nitroso compounds and cancer risk.

Experimental Evidence: Carcinogenicity

The data on the carcinogenicity of nitrate and nitrite in animals are not definitive. The few experiments conducted in animals have provided no evidence that nitrate is carcinogenic (Greenblatt and Mirvish, 1973; Lijinsky et al., 1973; Sugiyama et al., 1979).

There have been very few adequate studies to test the carcinogenicity of nitrite. Most of the information is derived from data on tumor incidence in experiments that were designed primarily to study nitrosation in animals given nitrite and amine simultaneously. These data were compared with data on control animals given nitrite alone (usually in drinking water). Because the control animals were usually sacrificed after a few months, there may not have been sufficient time for tumors to develop (Aoyagi et al., 1980; Inai et al., 1979; Mirvish et al., 1980; Shank and Newberne, 1976).

In a larger lifetime study conducted for the U.S. Food and Drug Administration, Newberne (1978, 1979) fed various doses of nitrite to groups of approximately 68 male and 68 female Sprague-Dawley rats under a variety of conditions. In comparison to the controls, the treated

rats had not only a higher incidence of malignant tumors of the lymphatic system, but also a higher incidence of alterations (immunoblastic
cell proliferation) in the spleen and, occasionally, in the lymph nodes
of the treated groups (Newberne, 1979). These results were interpreted
by the author to indicate that nitrite may be an enhancer or promoter
of carcinogenesis in rats. However, a Joint Committee of Experts, which
was established to review the study, diagnosed fewer lymphomas than
those reported by Newberne (U.S. Food and Drug Administration, 1980a).
The discrepancy between the two diagnoses involved the differentiation
of lymphomas from extramedullary hematopoiesis, plasmacytosis, or his-
tiocytic sarcoma. Furthermore, the Joint Committee was unable to confirm the diagnosis of immunoblastic hyperplasia.

In addition, the Committee on Nitrite and Alternative Curing Agents
in Food reviewed 21 reports in which the carcinogenicity of nitrite was
examined (National Academy of Sciences, 1981). The committee concluded
that three of the 21 reports were too brief to evaluate adequately. Of
the remaining 18 studies, 9 were conducted in rats, 8 in mice, and 1 in
guinea pigs. The experimental design was inadequate in many cases, and
varied greatly with regard to the end points for carcinogenicity. However, none of the remaining 18 studies provided sufficient evidence
that nitrite was carcinogenic (see, for example, Greenblatt et al.,
1973; Lijinsky et al., 1980).

The absence of evidence that nitrite is a direct carcinogen does
not diminish the possibility that it can interact with specific components of diets consumed by humans and animals or with endogenous metabolites to produce N-nitroso compounds that induce cancer.

N-Nitroso compounds have been studied extensively to determine
their carcinogenic effects. Druckrey and his colleagues (1967)
reported tests in rats exposed to 65 N-nitroso compounds, most of
which were potent carcinogens. Lijinsky and Reuber (1981) examined
many other N-nitroso compounds for their carcinogenic potential, mainly
in rats. Approximately 300 different N-nitroso compounds have been
tested, and a majority of them have been shown to induce cancer in
various tissues of one or more species of laboratory animals when
administered by any of several routes (Preussmann and Steward, personal
communication, 1981). In addition to both nitrosodimethylamine and
nitrosodiethylamine, a number of other N-nitroso compounds detected
in the environment are carcinogenic in animals (see, for example,
Druckrey et al., 1967; Preussmann et al., 1981).

The carcinogenic action of several N-nitroso compounds can be
inhibited in systems where the formation of N-nitroso compounds has
been prevented (Mirvish, 1981). Nitrosation is inhibited when ascorbic
acid and a variety of other agents compete with the nitrosatable agent
for the available nitrite in the acidic conditions of the stomach. A
number of other agents that interact readily with nitrite can inhibit
nitrosation. Among these are other isomers of ascorbic acid, sorbic

acid, some phenols, and α-tocopherol. Most of these interactions have been observed at the chemical rather than at the biological level.

Formation of N-nitroso compounds can also be enhanced since a variety of ions, especially thiocyanate and iodide, may catalyze the nitrosation reaction in the stomach (Mirvish et al., 1975). Since these ions are present in foodstuffs, these catalysts could be important in determining the outcome.

The additive or synergistic effects of N-nitroso compounds on other carcinogens with similar organotropy has been emphasized by Schmähl (1980).

Experimental Evidence: Mutagenicity

Nitrate does not appear to be directly mutagenic (Konetzka, 1974). In microbial systems, nitrite may be mutagenic by three different mechanisms (Zimmerman, 1977): deamination of DNA bases in single-stranded DNA; formation of 2-nitroinosine, intrastrand, or interstrand lesions leading to helix distortions in double-stranded DNA; and formation of mutagenic N-nitroso compounds by combination with nitrosatable substrates. Except for the results of one study in which a high dose of nitrite was used, there is no evidence that nitrite is mutagenic in mammalian systems.

Many N-nitroso compounds have been found to be mutagenic in a variety of test systems, including bacterial tests and Drosophila, and under a variety of conditions (Montesano and Bartsch, 1976).

Summary and Conclusions: Nitrate, Nitrite, and N-Nitroso Compounds

Epidemiological evidence suggesting that nitrate, nitrite, and N-nitroso compounds play a role in the development of cancer in humans is largely circumstantial. However, the findings from several epidemiological studies of certain geographical/nationality groups are consistent with the hypothesis that exposure of humans to high levels of nitrate and/or nitrite may be associated with an increased incidence of cancers of the stomach and esophagus. In these studies, the level, duration, and time of exposure were not studied in relation to cancer incidence, and exposure to other known or suspected carcinogens was not excluded.

In animals, nitrate has not been shown to be carcinogenic or mutagenic per se. The data on nitrite, which has been tested more extensively than nitrate, indicate that nitrite is probably not carcinogenic but that it is mutagenic, at least in microbial systems.

As a group, the N-nitroso compounds are clearly carcinogenic in numerous species of animals in which they have been tested. Positive results have been obtained for nearly all of the approximately 300 N-nitroso compounds tested for carcinogenicity in one or more species. Many of these compounds are also mutagenic.

The Committee on Nitrite and Alternative Curing Agents in Food recommended that exposure to nitrate, nitrite, and N-nitroso compounds should be reduced (National Academy of Sciences, 1981).

SUMMARY AND CONCLUSIONS

This chapter contains an assessment of the carcinogenicity and mutagenicity of some naturally occurring substances, mainly mycotoxins and compounds of plant origin.

Aflatoxin, a mycotoxin that occurs in grains and other food commodities, is carcinogenic in several species of animals, including mice, rats, trout, ducks, and monkeys, and there is evidence of a dose response. In addition, it has been shown to be mutagenic in bacterial and mammalian systems. Several other mycotoxins that are found in food are carcinogenic and/or mutagenic in laboratory tests. However, with the exception of aflatoxin, which has been implicated in liver cancer in some parts of the world, there is no epidemiological evidence concerning other mycotoxins and neoplasia in humans.

Hydrazine derivatives of two mushrooms—Agaricus bisporus and Gyromitra esculenta—both of which are consumed throughout the world, appear to be carcinogenic in mice and, under certain conditions, in hamsters, and are mutagenic in bacteria. However, the significance of these findings for risk to humans cannot be determined since there are no epidemiological data.

Several pyrrolizidine alkaloids, e.g., monocrotaline, are carcinogenic in animals and/or mutagenic in several test systems. Tumors develop in rats fed plants such as coltsfoot, which contain these alkaloids. Cycad nuts, which are eaten in some parts of the world, contain cycasin (methylazoxymethanol-β-glucoside), a compound known to be carcinogenic in animals. It is also mutagenic in the Ames test after addition of β-glucosidase. However, no evidence has been presented for the carcinogenicity of pyrrolizidine alkaloids and cycasin in humans, although there is unsubstantiated speculation that they may be involved in the development of neoplasia in humans.

Other plant constituents, such as methylxanthines, thiourea, tannins, coumarin, parasorbic acid, safrole, estragole, and eugenol, and plant estrogens, such as zearalenone, are carcinogenic in laboratory animals and/or mutagenic in bacterial or mammalian cell systems. However, the significance of these findings for human health is not known since there are no data from studies in humans.

Nitrosamines--compounds derived from the reaction of nitrite with amines--are carcinogenic in numerous species of laboratory animals and mutagenic in several experimental systems. Nitrate appears to be neither carcinogenic nor mutagenic, whereas nitrite is probably not directly carcinogenic, but it is mutagenic in microbial systems. There is some inconclusive epidemiological evidence that nitrate, nitrite, and N-nitroso compounds play a role in the development of gastric and esophageal cancer.

Many of the naturally occurring substances discussed in this chapter have been found to be carcinogenic in laboratory animals and/ or mutagenic in bacterial and other systems, thereby posing a potential risk of cancer in humans. However, there have been no pertinent epidemiological studies concerning their impact on humans except for those on aflatoxins and those on nitrate, nitrite, and N-nitroso compounds. The compounds thus far shown to be carcinogenic in animals have been reported to occur in the average U.S. diet in small amounts; however, there is no evidence that any of these substances individually makes a major contribution to the total risk of cancer in the United States. This lack of sufficient data should not be interpreted as an indication that these or other compounds subsequently found to be carcinogenic do not present a hazard. Further investigations are necessary. Efforts should be made to minimize or avoid the exposure of humans to compounds that are carcinogenic or mutagenic in experimental systems.

REFERENCES

Adamson, R. H., P. Correa, and D. W. Dalgard. 1973. Occurrence of a primary liver carcinoma in a rhesus monkey fed aflatoxin B_1. J. Natl. Cancer Inst. 50:549-553.

Aeschbacher, H. U., and H. P. Würzner. 1980. An evaluation of instant and regular coffee in the Ames mutagenicity test. Toxicol. Lett. 5: 139-145.

Aeschbacher, H. U., C. Chappuis, and H. P. Würzner. 1980. Mutagenicity testing of coffee: A study of problems encountered with the Ames Salmonella test system. Food Cosmet. Toxicol. 18:605-613.

Alpert, M. E., M. S. R. Hutt, G. N. Wogan, and C. S. Davidson. 1971. Association between aflatoxin content of food and hepatoma frequency in Uganda. Cancer 28:253-260.

Ames, B. N., J. McCann, and E. Yamasaki. 1975. Methods for detecting carcinogens and mutagens with the Salmonella/mammalian-microsome mutagenicity test. Mutat. Res. 31:347-363.

Aoyagi, M., N. Matsukura, E. Uchida, T. Kawachi, T. Sugimura, S. Takayama and M. Matsui. 1980. Induction of liver tumors in Wistar rats by sodium nitrite given in pellet diet. J. Natl. Cancer Inst. 65:411-413.

Armijo, R., and A. H. Coulson. 1975. Epidemiology of stomach cancer in Chile--The role of nitrogen fertilizers. Int. J. Epidemiol. 4:301-309.

Armijo, R., A. Gonzalez, M. Orellana, A. H. Coulson, J. W. Sayre, and R. Detels. 1981. Epidemiology of gastric cancer in Chile: II--Nitrate exposures and stomach cancer frequency. Int. J. Epidemiol. 10:57-62.

Armstrong, B. 1980. The epidemiology of cancer in the People's Republic of China. Int. J. Epidemiol. 9:305-315.

Armstrong, B., and R. Doll. 1975. Environmental factors and cancer incidence and mortality in different countries, with special reference to dietary practices. Int. J. Cancer 15:617-631.

Armstrong, B., A. Garrod, and R. Doll. 1976. A retrospective study of renal cancer with special reference to coffee and animal protein consumption. Br. J. Cancer 33:127-136.

Bartholomew, R. M., and D. S. Ryan. 1980. Lack of mutagenicity of some phytoestrogens in the Salmonella/mammalian microsome assay. Mutat. Res. 78:317-321.

Becci, P. J., F. G. Hess, W. D. Johnson, M. A. Gallo, J. G. Babish, G. E. Cox, R. E. Dailey, and R. A. Parent. 1981. Long-term carcinogenicity and toxicity studies of patulin in the rat. J. Appl. Toxicol. 1:256-261.

Becci, P. J., G. E. Cox, J. M. Taylor, and R. A. Parent. In press. Long term carcinogenicity and toxicity studies of zearalenone in the rat. J. Appl. Toxicol.

Becroft, D. M. O., and D. R. Webster. 1972. Letter to the Editor: Aflatoxins and Rey's disease. Br. Med. J. 4:117.

Bowden, J. P., K.-T. Chung, and A. W. Andrews. 1976. Mutagenic activity of tryptophan metabolites produced by rat intestinal microflora. J. Natl. Cancer Inst. 57:921-924.

Bross, I. D. J., and J. Tidings. 1973. Another look at coffee drinking and cancer of the urinary bladder. Prev. Med. 2:445-451.

Butler, W. H., and J. M. Barnes. 1966. Carcinoma of the glandular stomach in rats given diets containing aflatoxin. Nature 209:90.

Challis, B. C., and C. D. Bartlett. 1975. Possible cocarcinogenic effects of coffee constituents. Nature 254:532-533.

Chien, M.-C., M. J. Tong, K.-J. Lo, J.-K. Lee, D. R. Milich, G. N. Vyas, and B. L. Murphy. 1981. Hepatitis B viral markers in patients with primary hepatocellular carcinoma in Taiwan. J. Natl. Cancer Inst. 66:475-479.

Clarke, C. H., and M. J. Wade. 1975. Evidence that caffeine, 8-methoxypsoralen and steroidal diamines are frameshift mutagens for E. coli K-12. Mutat. Res. 28:123-125.

Clayson, D. B., and R. C. Garner. 1976. Carcinogenic aromatic amines and related compounds. Pp. 366-461 in C. E. Searle, ed. Chemical Carcinogens. ACS Monograph 173. American Chemical Society, Washington, D.C.

Clifton, K. H., and B. N. Sridharan. 1975. Endocrine factors and tumor growth. Pp. 249-285 in F. F. Becker, ed. Cancer: A Comprehensive Treatise. Biology of Tumors: Volume 3. Cellular Biology and Growth. Plenum Press, New York and London.

Cohen, S. M., M. Arai, J. B. Jacobs, and G. H. Friedell. 1979. Promoting effect of saccharin and DL-tryptophan in urinary bladder carcinogenesis. Cancer Res. 39:1207-1217.

Cole, P. 1971. Coffee-drinking and cancer of the lower urinary tract. Lancet 1:1335-1337.

Correa, P., W. Haenszel, C. Cuello, S. Tannenbaum, and M. Archer. 1975. A model for gastric cancer epidemiology. Lancet 2:58-60.

Cuello, C., P. Correa, W. Haenszel, G. Gordillo, C. Brown, M. Archer, and S. Tannenbaum. 1976. Gastric cancer in Colombia. I. Cancer risk and suspect environmental agents. J. Natl. Cancer Inst. 57:1015-1020.

Demerec, M., B. Wallace, and E. M. Witkin. 1948. The gene. Carnegie Inst. Washington Yearb. 47:169-176.

Demerec, M., G. Bertani, and J. Flint. 1951. A survey of chemicals for mutagenic action on E. coli. Am. Nat. 85:119-136.

Dickens, F., and H. E. H. Jones. 1965. Further studies on the carcinogenic action of certain lactones and related substances in the rat and mouse. Br. J. Cancer 19:392-403.

Druckrey, H., R. Preussmann, S. Ivankovic, D. Schmähl, J. Afkham, G. Blum, H. D. Mennel, M. Müller, P. Petropoulos, and H. Scheider. 1967. [In German; English Summary.] Organotropic carcinogenic effects of 65 different N-nitroso-compounds on BD-rats. Z. Krebsforsch. 69:103-201.

Dvořačková, I., V. Kusák, D. Veselý, J. Veselá, and P. Nesnídal. 1977. Aflatoxin and encephalopathy with fatty degeneration of viscera (Reye). Ann. Nutr. Aliment. 31:977-989.

Ehrenberg, L., I. Fedorcsak, and F. Solymosy. 1976. Diethyl pyrocarbonate in nucleic acid research. Prog. Nucleic Acid Res. Mol. Biol. 16:189-262.

Epstein, S. M., B. Bartus, and E. Farber. 1969. Renal epithelial neoplasms induced in male Wistar rats by oral aflatoxin B_1. Cancer Res. 29:1045-1050.

Evans, I. A. 1976. The bracken carcinogen. Pp. 690-700 in C. E. Searle, ed. Chemical Carcinogens. ACS Monograph 173. American Chemical Society, Washington, D.C.

Fine, D. H., R. Ross, D. P. Rounbehler, A. Silvergleid, and L. Song. 1977. Formation in vivo of volatile N-nitrosamines in man after ingestion of cooked bacon and spinach. Nature 265:753-755.

Food and Agriculture Organization, United Nations Environment Program, and World Health Organization. 1977. Global perspective on myco-toxins, Document W/G5491, Agenda Item 4, Conference on Mycotoxins, Nairobi, Kenya. (unpublished)

Franke, S., U. Freimuth, and P. H. List. 1967. [In German.] Über die Giftigkeit der Frühjahrslorchel Gyromitra (Helvella) esculenta Fr. 14. Mitteilung: Pilzinhaltsstoffe. Arch. Toxicol. 22:293-332.

Fraumeni, J. F., Jr., J. Scotto, and L. J. Dunham. 1971. Letter to the Editor: Coffee-drinking and bladder cancer. Lancet 2:1204.

Frei, J. V., and S. Venitt. 1975. Chromosome damage in the bone marrow of mice treated with the methylating agents methyl methane-sulphonate and N-methyl-N-nitrosourea in the presence or absence of caffeine, and its relationship with thymoma induction. Mutat. Res. 30:89-95.

Furth, J. 1975. Hormones as etiological agents in neoplasia. Pp. 75-120 in F. F. Becker, ed. Cancer: A Comprehensive Treatise. Volume 1, Etiology: Chemical and Physical Carcinogenesis. Plenum Press, New York and London.

Gezelius, K., and N. Fries. 1952. Phage resistant mutants in Escheri-chia coli by caffeine. Hereditas 38:112-114.

Glass, E. A., and A. Novick. 1959. Induction of mutation in chloram-phenicol-inhibited bacteria. J. Bacteriol. 77:10-16.

Gough, T. A., K. S. Webb, and R. F. Coleman. 1978. Estimate of the volatile nitrosamine content of UK food. Nature 272:161-163.

Green, L. C., S. R. Tannenbaum, and P. Goldman. 1981. Nitrate synthe-sis in the germfree and conventional rat. Science 212:56-58.

Green, N. R., and J. R. Savage. 1978. Screening of safrole, eugenol, their ninhydrin positive metabolites and selected secondary amines for potential mutagenicity. Mutat. Res. 57:115-121.

Greenblatt, M., and S. S. Mirvish. 1973. Dose-response studies with with concurrent administration of piperazine and sodium nitrite to strain A mice. J. Natl. Cancer Inst. 50:119-124.

Greenblatt, M., V. R. C. Kommineni, and W. Lijinsky. 1973. Brief communication: Null effect of concurrent feeding of sodium nitrite and amino acids to MRC rats. J. Natl. Cancer Inst. 50:799-802.

Grigg, C. W. 1972. Effects of coumarin, pyronin Y, 6,9-dimethyl 2-methylthiopurine and caffeine on excision repair and recombination repair in Escherichia coli. J. Gen. Microbiol. 70:221-230.

Guenther, E. 1948-1952. The Essential Oils. Volume 1, 427 pp., 1949; Volume 3, 777 pp., 1949; Volume 4, 752 pp., 1950; Volume 5, 507 pp., 1952; Volume 6, 481 pp., 1952. D. Van Nostrand Co., New York, Toronto, and London.

Guenther, E., and D. Althausen. 1949. The Essential Oils. Volume 2, 852 pp. D. Van Nostrand Co., New York, Toronto, and London.

Haenszel, W., M. Kurihara, M. Segi, and R. K. C. Lee. 1972. Stomach cancer among Japanese in Hawaii. J. Natl. Cancer Inst. 49:969-988.

Hicks, R. M., T. A. Gough, and C. L. Walters. 1977. Demonstration of the presence of nitrosamines in human urine: Preliminary observations on a possible etiology for bladder cancer in association with chronic urinary tract infection. Pp. 465-475 in E. A. Walker, L. Griciute, M. Castegnaro, R. E. Lyle, and W. Davis, eds. Environmental Aspects of N-Nitroso Compounds. IARC Scientific Publications No. 19. International Agency for Research on Cancer, Lyon, France.

Higginson, J. 1966. Etiological factors in gastrointestinal cancer in man. J. Natl. Cancer Inst. 37:527-545.

Hirayama, T. 1979. Epidemiological evaluation of the role of naturally occurring carcinogens and modulators of carcinogenesis. Pp. 359-380 in E. C. Miller, J. A. Miller, I. Hirono, T. Sugimura, and S. Takayama, eds. Naturally Occurring Carcinogens-Mutagens and Modulators of Carcinogenesis. Japan Scientific Societies Press, Tokyo; University Park Press, Baltimore, Md.

Hirono, I. 1981. Natural carcinogenic products of plant origin. CRC Crit. Rev. Toxicol. 8:235-277.

Hirono, I., H. Kachi, and T. Kato. 1970. A survey of acute toxicity of cycads and mortality rate from cancer in the Miyako Islands, Okinawa. Acta Pathol. Jpn. 20:327-337.

Hirono, I., H. Mori, M. Haga, M. Fujii, K. Yamada, Y. Hirata, H. Takanashi, E. Uchida, S. Hosaka, I. Ueno, T. Matsushima, K. Umezawa, and A. Shirai. 1979. Edible plants containing carcinogenic pyrrolizidine alkaloids in Japan. Pp. 79-87 in E. C. Miller, J. A. Miller, I. Hirono, T. Sugimura, and S. Takayama, eds. Naturally Occurring Carcinogens-Mutagens and Modulators of Carcinogenesis. Japan Scientific Societies Press, Tokyo; University Park Press, Baltimore, Md.

Hirono, I., I. Ueno, S. Hosaka, H. Takanashi, T. Matsushima, T. Sugimura, and S. Natori. 1981. Carcinogenicity examination of quercetin and rutin in ACI rats. Cancer Lett. 13:15-21.

Howe, G. R., J. D. Burch, A. B. Miller, G. M. Cook, J. Esteve, B. Morrison, P. Gordon, L. W. Chambers, G. Fodor, and G. M. Winsor. 1980. Tobacco use, occupation, coffee, various nutrients, and bladder cancer. J. Natl. Cancer Inst. 64:701-713.

Inai, K., Y. Aoki, and S. Tokuoka. 1979. Chronic toxicity of sodium nitrite in mice, with reference to its tumorigenicity. Gann 70:203-208.

International Agency for Research on Cancer. 1974. Thiourea. Pp. 95-109 in IARC Monographs on the Evaluation of the Carcinogenic Risk of Chemicals to Man. Volume 7, Some Anti-Thyroid and Related Substances, Nitrofurans and Industrial Chemicals. International Agency for Research on Cancer, Lyon, France.

International Agency for Research on Cancer. 1976. IARC Monographs on the Evaluation of the Carcinogenic Risk of Chemicals to Man. Volume 10, Some Naturally Occurring Substances. International Agency for Research on Cancer, Lyon, France. 353 pp.

Jennssen, D., and C. Ramel. 1978. Factors affecting the induction of micronuclei at low doses of X-rays, MMS and dimethylnitrosamine in mouse erythroblasts. Mutat. Res. 58:51-65.

Johnson, H. G., and M. K. Bach. 1965. Apparent suppression of mutation rates in bacteria by spermine. Nature 208:408-409.

Kanisawa, M., and S. Suzuki. 1978. Induction of renal and hepatic tumors in mice by ochratoxin A, a mycotoxin. Gann 69:599-600.

Keen, P., and P. Martin. 1971. The toxicity and fungal infestation of foodstuffs in Swaziland in relation to harvesting and storage. Trop. Geogr. Med. 23:35-43.

Kew, M. C., J. Desmyter, A. F. Bradburne, and G. M. Macnab. 1979. Hepatitis B virus infection in southern African blacks with hepatocellular cancer. J. Natl. Cancer Inst. 62:517-520.

Kihlman, B. A. 1977. Caffeine and Chromosomes. Elsevier Scientific Publishing Company, Amsterdam, New York, and Oxford.

Kirby, K. S. 1960. Induction of tumours by tannin extracts. Br. J. Cancer 14:147-150.

Konetzka, W. A. 1974. Mutagenesis by nitrate reduction. P. 37 in Abstracts of the Annual Meeting of the American Society for Microbiology 1974, May 12-17, 1974, Chicago, Ill. American Society for Microbiology, Washington, D.C. Abstract G106.

Korpássy, B. 1959. The hepatocarcinogenicity of tannic acid. Cancer Res. 19:501-504.

Korpássy, B. 1961. Tannins as hepatic carcinogens. Prog. Exp. Tumor Res. 2:245-290.

Korpássy, B., and M. Mosonyi. 1950. The carcinogenic activity of tannic acid. Liver tumours induced in rats by prolonged subcutaneous administration of tannic acid solutions. Br. J. Cancer 4:411-420.

Korpássy, B., and M. Mosonyi. 1951. The carcinogenic action of tannic acid effect of casein on the development of liver tumours. Acta Morphol. Acad. Sci. Hung. 1:37-54.

Kubitschek, H. E., and H. E. Bendigkeit. 1958. Delay in the appearance of caffeine-induced T5 resistance in Escherichia coli. Genetics 43: 647-661.

Kubitschek, H. E., and H. E. Bendigkeit. 1964. Mutation in continuous cultures. I. Dependence of mutational response upon growth-limiting factors. Mutat. Res. 1:113-120.

Laqueur, G. L., and M. Spatz. 1968. Toxicology of cycasin. Cancer Res. 28:2262-2267.

Levenberg, B. 1962. An aromatic diazonium compound in the mushroom Agaricus bisporus. Biochim. Biophys. Acta 63:212-214.

Levenberg, B. 1964. Isolation and structure of agaritine, a - glutamyl-substituted arylhydrazine derivative from Agaricaceae. J. Biol. Chem. 239:2267-2273.

Lijinsky, W., and M. D. Reuber. 1981. Carcinogenic effect of nitrosopyrrolidine, nitrosopiperidine and nitrosohexamethyleneimine in Fischer rats. Cancer Lett. 12:99-103.

Lijinsky, W., M. Greenblatt, and C. Kommineni. 1973. Feeding studies of nitrilotriacetic acid and derivatives in rats. J. Natl. Cancer Inst. 50:1061-1063.

Lijinsky, W., M. D. Reuber, and W. B. Manning. 1980. Potent carcinogenicity of nitrosodiethanolamine in rats. Nature 288:589-590.

Lin, J. J., C. Liu, and D. J. Svoboda. 1974. Long-term effects of aflatoxin B_1 and viral hepatitis on marmoset liver. Lab. Invest. 30:267-278.

Lin, R. S., and I. I. Kessler. 1981. A multifactorial model for pancreatic cancer in man: Epidemiological evidence. J. Am. Med. Assoc. 245:147-152.

Linsell, C. A., and F. G. Peers. 1977. Aflatoxin and liver cell cancer. Trans. R. Soc. Trop. Med. Hyg. 71:471-473.

Litton Bionetics, Inc. 1975. Mutagenic evaluation of compound 001401554 tannic acid. Prepared for the Bureau of Foods, Food and Drug Administration under Contract No. 73-56. Litton Bionetics, Inc., Kensington, Md. 33 pp.

MacMahon, B., S. Yen, D. Trichopoulos, K. Warren, and G. Nardi. 1981. Coffee and cancer of the pancreas. N. Engl. J. Med. 304:630-633.

Magee, P. N., and J. M. Barnes. 1967. Carcinogenic nitroso compounds. Adv. Cancer Res. 10:163-246.

Magee, P. N., R. Montesano, and R. Preussmann. 1976. N-Nitroso compounds and related carcinogens. Pp. 491-625 in C. E. Searle, ed. Chemical Carcinogens. ACS Monograph 173. American Chemical Society, Washington, D.C.

Martin, P. M. D., and P. Keen. 1978. The occurrence of zearalanone in raw and fermented products from Swaziland and Lesotho. Sabouraudia 26:15-22.

Martínez, I. 1969. Factors associated with cancer of the esophagus, mouth and pharynx in Puerto Rico. J. Natl. Cancer Inst. 42:1069-1094.

Matsumoto, H., and H. H. Higa. 1966. Studies on methylazoxymethanol, the aglycone of cycasin: Methylation of nucleic acids in vitro. Biochem. J. 98:20C-22C.

Matsushima, T., H. Matsumoto, A. Shirai, M. Sawamura, and T. Sugimura. 1979. Mutagenicity of the naturally occurring carcinogen cycasin and synthetic methylazoxymethanol conjugates in Salmonella typhimurium. Cancer Res. 39:3780-3782.

McCann, J., E. Choi, E. Yamasaki, and B. N. Ames. 1975. Detection of carcinogens as mutagens in the Salmonella/microsome test: Assay of 300 chemicals. Proc. Natl. Acad. Sci. U.S.A. 72:5135-5139.

Meinsma, L. 1964. [In Dutch; English Summary.] Nutrition and cancer. Voeding 25:357-365.

Miller, C. T., C. I. Neutel, R. C. Nair, L. D. Marrett, J. M. Last, and W. E. Collins. 1978. Relative importance of risk factors in bladder carcinogenesis. J. Chronic Dis. 31:51-56.

Miller, E. C., and J. A. Miller. 1979. Naturally occurring chemical carcinogens that may be present in foods. Pp. 123-165 in A. Neuberger and T. H. Jukes, eds. International Review of Biochemistry, Volume 27. Biochemistry of Nutrition 1. University Park Press, Baltimore, Md.

Miller, E. C., J. A. Miller, I. Hirono, T. Sugimura, and S. Takayama, eds. 1979. Naturally Occurring Carcinogens-Mutagens and Modulators of Carcinogenesis. Japan Scientific Societies Press, Tokyo; University Park Press, Baltimore, Md. 399 pp.

Miller, J. A. 1973. Naturally occurring substances that can induce tumors. Pp. 508-549 in Toxicants Occurring Naturally in Foods, Second edition. Food and Nutrition Board, National Academy of Sciences, Washington, D.C.

Miller, J. A., E. C. Miller, and D. H. Phillips. In press. The metabolic activation and carcinogenicity of alkylbenzenes that occur naturally in many spices. In H. Stich, ed. Carcinogens and Mutagens in the Environment. Volume 1, Food Products. CRC Press, Boca Raton, Fla.

Mirvish, S. S. 1968. The carcinogenic action and metabolism of urethan and N-hydroxyurethan. Adv. Cancer Res. 11:1-42.

Mirvish, S. S. 1981. Inhibition of the formation of carcinogenic N-nitroso compounds by ascorbic acid and other compounds. Pp. 557-587 in J. H. Burchenal and H. F. Oettgen, eds. Cancer: Achievements, Challenges, and Prospects for the 1980s, Volume 1. Grune and Stratton, New York, London, Toronto, Sydney, and San Francisco.

Mirvish, S. S., A. Cardesa, L. Wallcave, and P. Shubik. 1975. Induction of mouse lung adenomas by amines or ureas plus nitrite and by N-nitroso compounds: Effect of ascorbate, gallic acid, thiocyanate, and caffeine. J. Natl. Cancer Inst. 55:633-636.

Mirvish, S. S., K. Karlowski, D. F. Birt, and J. P. Sams. 1980. Dietary and other factors affecting nitrosomethylurea (NMU) formation in the rat stomach. Pp. 271-277 in E. A. Walker, L. Griciute, M. Castegnaro, M. Börzsönyi, and W. Davis, eds. N-Nitroso Compounds: Analysis, Formation and Occurrence. IARC Scientific Publications No. 31. International Agency for Research on Cancer, Lyon, France.

Montesano, R., and H. Bartsch. 1976. Mutagenic and carcinogenic N-nitroso compounds: Possible environmental hazards. Mutat. Res. 32:179-227.

Nagao, M., Y. Takahashi, K. Wakabayashi, and T. Sugimura. 1979. Mutagens in coffee and tea. Mutat. Res. 68:101-106.

National Academy of Sciences. 1965. Chemicals Used in Food Processing. Food and Nutrition Board, National Academy of Sciences, Washington, D.C. 296 pp.

National Academy of Sciences. 1973. Toxicants Occurring Naturally in Foods. Second edition. Food and Nutrition Board, National Academy of Sciences, Washington, D.C. 624 pp.

National Academy of Sciences. 1981. The Health Effects of Nitrate, Nitrite, and N-Nitroso Compounds. Part 1 of a 2-Part Study by the Committee on Nitrite and Alternative Curing Agents in Food. National Academy Press, Washington, D.C. 544 pp.

National Cancer Institute. In press. Carcinogenesis bioassay of zearalenone. NTP-81-37. National Toxicology Program, National Cancer Institute, Bethesda, Md.

Nelson, A. A., O. G. Fitzhugh, H. J. Morris, and H. O. Calvery. 1942. Neurofibromas of rat ears produced by prolonged feeding of crude ergot. Cancer Res. 2:11-15.

Newberne, P. M. 1978. Final Report on Contract No. FDA 74-2181. Dietary Nitrite in the Rat. May 18, 1978. Food and Drug Administration, U.S. Department of Health, Education, and Welfare, Washington, D.C. 162 pp.

Newberne, P. M. 1979. Nitrite promotes lymphoma incidence in rats. Science 204:1079-1081.

Newberne, P. M., and A. E. Rogers. 1973. Rat colon carcinomas associated with aflatoxin and marginal vitamin A. J. Natl. Cancer Inst. 50:439-448.

Newberne, P. M., C. E. Hunt, and G. N. Wogan. 1967. Neoplasms in the rat associated with administration of urethan and aflatoxin. Exp. Mol. Pathol. 6:285-299.

Nomura, T. 1975. Letter to the Editor: Urethan (ethyl carbamate) as a cosolvent of drugs commonly used parenterally in humans. Cancer Res. 35:2895-2899.

Novick, A. 1956. Mutagens and antimutagens. Brookhaven Symp. Biol. 8:201-215.

Oettlé, A. G. 1965. The aetiology of primary carcinoma of the liver in Africa: A critical appraisal of previous ideas with an outline of the mycotoxin hypothesis. S. Afr. Med. J. 39:917-825.

O'Gara, R. W., and R. H. Adamson. 1972. Spontaneous and induced neoplasms in nonhuman primates. Pp. 190-238 in R. N. Fiennes, ed. Pathology of Simian Primates. Part I: General Pathology. S. Karger, Basel, Munich, Paris, London, New York, and Sydney.

Ohshima, H., and H. Bartsch. 1981. Quantitative estimation of endogenous nitrosation in humans by monitoring $\underline{N}$-nitrosoproline excreted in the urine. Cancer Res. 41:3658-366$\overline{2}$.

Ough, C. S. 1976. Ethylcarbamate in fermented beverages and foods. I. Naturally occurring ethylcarbamate. J. Agric. Food Chem. 24:323-328.

Pamukcu, A. M., and G. T. Bryan. 1979. Bracken fern, a natural urinary bladder and intestinal carcinogen. Pp. 89-99 in E. C. Miller, J. A. Miller, I. Hirono, T. Sugimura, and S. Takayama, eds. Naturally Occurring Carcinogens-Mutagens and Modulators of Carcinogenesis. Japan Scientific Societies Press, Tokyo; University Park Press, Baltimore, Md.

Pamukcu, A. M., E. Ertürk, S. Yalçiner, U. Milli, and G. T. Bryan. 1978. Carcinogenic and mutagenic activities of milk from cows fed bracken fern (Pteridium aquilinum). Cancer Res. 38:1556-1560.

Pamukcu, A. M., S. Yalçiner, J. F. Hatcher, and G. T. Bryan. 1980. Quercetin, a rat intestinal and bladder carcinogen present in bracken fern (Pteridium aquilinum). Cancer Res. 40:3468-3472.

Parks, N. J., K. A. Krohn, C. A. Mathis, J. H. Chasko, K. R. Geiger, M. E. Gregor, and N. F. Peek. 1981. Nitrogen-13-labeled nitrite and nitrate: Distribution and metabolism after intratracheal administration. Science 212:58-61.

Peers, F. G., and C. A. Linsell. 1973. Dietary aflatoxins and liver cancer--A population based study in Kenya. Br. J. Cancer 27:473-484.

Peers, F. G., G. A. Gilman, and C. A. Linsell. 1976. Dietary afla- toxins and human liver cancer. A study in Swaziland. Int. J. Cancer 17:167-176.

Pienta, R. J. 1981. Transformation of Syrian hamster embryo cells by diverse chemicals and correlation with their reported carcinogenic and mutagenic activities. Chem. Mutagens 6:175-202.

Preussmann, R., B. Spiegelhalder, G. Eisenbrand, G. Würtele, and I. Hofmann. 1981. Urinary excretion of $\underline{N}$-nitrosodiethanolamine in rats following its epicutaneous and intrathecal administration and its formation in vivo following skin application of diethanolamine. Cancer Lett. 13:227-231.

Prince, A. N., W. Szmuness, J. Michon, J. Demaille, G. Diebolt, J. Linhard, C. Quenum, and M. Sankale. 1975. A case/control study of the associa- tion between primary liver cancer and hepatitis B infection in Senegal. Int. J. Cancer 16:376-383.

Purchase, I. F. H., and J. J. van der Watt. 1970. Carcinogenicity of sterigmatocystin. Food Cosmet. Toxicol. 8:289-295.

Radomski, J. L., E. M. Glass, and W. B. Deichmann. 1971. Transitional cell hyperplasia in the bladders of dogs fed DL-tryptophan. Cancer Res. 31:1690-1694.

Radomski, J. L., D. Greenwald, W. L. Hearn, N. L. Block, and F. M. Woods. 1978. Nitrosamine formation in bladder infections and its role in the etiology of bladder cancer. J. Urol. 120:48-58.

Reddy, J. K., D. J. Svoboda, and M. S. Rao. 1976. Induction of liver tumors by aflatoxin B_1 in the tree shrew (Tupaia glis), a non- human primate. Cancer Res. 36:151-160.

Rogan, E. G., B. A. Walker, R. Gingell, D. Nagel, and B. Toth. In press. Microbial mutagenicity of selected hydrazines. Mutation Res.

Rosenkranz, H. S., and Z. Leifer. 1981. Determining the DNA-modifying activity of chemicals using DNA-polymerase deficient Escherichia coli. Chem. Mutagens 6:109-147

Rosenkranz, H. S., and L. A. Poirier. 1979. Evaluation of the mutagenicity and DNA-modifying activity of carcinogens and noncarcinogens in microbial systems. J. Natl. Cancer Inst. 62:873-891.

Schmähl, D. 1980. Combination effects in chemical carcinogenesis. Arch. Toxicol. Suppl. 4:29-40.

Schoental, R. 1976. Carcinogens in plants and microorganisms. Pp. 626-689 in C. E. Searle, ed. Chemical Carcinogens. ACS Monograph 173. American Chemical Society, Washington, D.C.

Schoental, R., A. Z. Joffe, and B. Yagen. 1979. Cardiovascular lesions and various tumors found in rats given T-2 toxin, a trichothecene metabolite of *Fusarium*. Cancer Res. 39:2179-2189.

Sen, N. P., S. Seaman, and M. McPherson. 1980. Further studies on the occurrence of volatile and non-volatile nitrosamines in foods. Pp. 457-463 in E. A. Walker, L. Griciute, M. Castegnaro, M. Börzsönyi, and W. Davis, eds. N-Nitroso Compounds: Analysis, Formation and Occurrence. IARC Scientific Publications No. 31. International Agency for Research on Cancer, Lyon, France.

Shank, R. C., and P. M. Newberne. 1976. Dose-response study of the carcinogenicity of dietary sodium nitrite and morpholine in rats and hamsters. Food Cosmet. Toxicol. 14:1-8.

Shank, R. C., N. Bhamarapravati, J. E. Gordon, and G. N. Wagan. 1972a. Dietary aflatoxins and human liver cancer. IV. Incidence of primary liver cancer in two municipal populations of Thailand. Food Cosmet. Toxicol. 10:171-179.

Shank, R. C., J. E. Gordon, G. N. Wogan, A. Nondasuta, and B. Subhamani. 1972b. Dietary aflatoxins and human liver cancer. III. Field survey of rural Thai families for ingested aflatoxins. Food Cosmet. Toxicol. 10:71-84.

Shennan, D. H. 1973. Letter to the Editor: Renal carcinoma and coffee consumption in 16 countries. Br. J. Cancer 28:473-474.

Shimizu, H., K. Hayashi, and N. Takemura. 1978. Relationships between the mutagenic and carcinogenic effects of hydrazine derivatives. Nippon Eiseigaku Zasshi 33:474-485.

Simmon, V. F. 1979. In vitro assays for recombinogenic activity of chemical carcinogens and related compounds with *Saccharomyces cerevisiae* D3. J. Natl. Cancer Inst. 62:901-909.

Simmon, V. F., H. S. Rosenkranz, E. Zeiger, and L. A. Poirer. 1979. Mutagenic activity of chemical carcinogens and related compounds in the intraperitoneal host-mediated assay. J. Natl. Cancer Inst. 62:911-918.

Simon, D., S. Yen, and P. Cole. 1975. Coffee drinking and cancer of the lower urinary tract. J. Natl. Cancer Inst. 54:587-591.

Simons, D. M. 1971. The mushroom toxins. Del. Med. J. 43:177-187.

Simons, M. J., E. H. Yap, and K. Shanmugaratnam. 1972. Australia antigen in Singapore Chinese patients with hepatocellular carcinoma and comparison groups: Influence of technique sensitivity on differential frequencies. Int. J. Cancer 10:320-325.

Siraj, M. Y., A. W. Hayes, P. D. Unger, G. R. Hogan, N. J. Ryan, and B. B. Wray. 1981. Analysis of aflatoxin B_1 in human tissues with high-pressure liquid chromatography. Toxicol. Appl. Pharmacol. 58:422-430.

Spiegelhalder, B., G. Eisenbrand, and R. Preussmann. 1980. Occurrence of volatile nitrosamines in foods: A survey of the West German market. Pp. 467-477 in E. A. Walker, L. Griciute, M. Castegnaro, M. Börzsönyi, and W. Davis, eds. N-Nitroso Compounds: Analysis, Formation and Occurrence. IARC Scientific Publications No. 31. International Agency for Research on Cancer, Lyon, France.

Stark, A. A., J. M. Townsend, G. N. Wogan, A. L. Demain, A. Manmade, and A. C. Ghosh. 1978. Mutagenicity and antibacterial activity of mycotoxins produced by Penicillium islandicum Sopp and Penicillium regulosum. J. Environ. Pathol. Toxicol. 2:313-324.

Stephany, R. W., and P. L. Schuller. 1980. Daily dietary intakes of nitrate, nitrite, and volatile N-nitrosamines in the Netherlands using the duplicate portion sampling technique. Oncology 37:203-210.

Stich, H. F., and W. D. Powrie. In press. Plant phenolics as genotoxic agents and as modulators for the mutagenicity of other food compounds. In H. Stich, ed. Carcinogens and Mutagens in the Environment. Volume 1, Food Products. CRC Press, Boca Raton, Fla.

Stob, M. 1973. Estrogens in foods. Pp. 550-557 in Toxicants Occurring Naturally in Foods, Second edition. Food and Nutrition Board, National Academy of Sciences, Washington, D.C.

Stocks, P. 1970. Cancer mortality in relation to national consumption of cigarettes, solid fuel, tea and coffee. Br. J. Cancer 24:215-225.

Stoloff, L. 1979. Mycotoxin residues in edible animal tissues. Pp. 157-166 in Interactions of Mycotoxins in Animal Production. Proceedings of a Symposium. National Academy of Sciences, Washington, D.C.

Stoloff, L. In press. Mycotoxins as potential environmental carcinogens. In H. Stich, ed. Carcinogens and Mutagens in the Environment. Volume 1, Food Products. CRC Press, Boca Raton, Fla.

Stoloff, L., and L. Friedman. 1976. Information bearing on the evaluation of the hazard to man from aflatoxin ingestion. PAG Bulletin 6:21-32.

Sugiyama, K., T. Tanaka, and H. Mori. 1979. [In Japanese; English Summary.] Carcinogenicity examination of sodium nitrate in mice. Gifu Daigaku Igakubu Kiyo 27:1-6.

Swanson, A. B., D. D. Chambliss, J. C. Blomquist, E. C. Miller, and J. A. Miller. 1979. The mutagenicities of safrole, estragole, eugenol, trans-anethole, and some of their known or possible metabolites for Salmonella typhimurium mutants. Mutat. Res. 60:143-153.

Tannenbaum, S. R., D. Fett, V. R. Young, P. D. Land, and W. R. Bruce. 1978. Nitrite and nitrate are formed by endogenous synthesis in the human intestine. Science 200:1487-1489.

Timson, J. 1975. Theobromine and theophylline. Mutat. Res. 32:169-177.

Tong, M. J., S.-C. Sun, B. T. Schaeffer, N.-K. Chang, K.-J. Lo, and R. L. Peters. 1971. Hepatitis-associated antigen and hepatocellular carcinoma in Taiwan. Ann. Intern. Med. 75:687-691.

Toth, B. 1972. Hydrazine, methylhydrazine and methylhydrazine sulfate carcinogenesis in Swiss mice. Failure of ammonium hydroxide to interfere in the development of tumors. Int. J. Cancer 9:109-118.

Toth, B., and D. Nagel. 1978. Tumors induced in mice by N-methyl-N-formylhydrazine of the false morel Gyromitra esculenta. J. Natl. Cancer Inst. 60:201-204.

Toth, B., and K. Patil. 1979. Carcinogenic effects in the Syrian golden hamster of N-methyl-N-formylhydrazine of the false morel mushroom Gyromitra esculenta. J. Cancer Res. Clin. Oncol. 93:109-121.

Toth, B., and K. Patil. 1980. The tumorigenic effect of low dose levels of N-methyl-N-formylhydrazine in mice. Neoplasma 27:25-31.

Toth, B., and K. Patil. 1981. Gyromitrin as a tumor inducer. Neo-
    plasma 28:559-564.

Toth, B., and H. Shimizu. 1973. Methylhydrazine tumorigenesis in
    Syrian golden hamsters and the morphology of malignant histiocy-
    tomas. Cancer Res. 33:2744-2753.

Toth, B., A. Tompa, and K. Patil. 1977. Tumorigenic effect of 4-methyl-
    phenylhydrazine hydrochloride in Swiss mice. Z. Krebsforsch. Klin.
    Onkol. 89:245-252.

Toth, B., D. Nagel, K. Patil, J. Erickson, and K. Antonson. 1978.
    Tumor induction with the N'-acetyl derivative of 4-hydroxymethyl-
    phenylhydrazine, a metabolite of agaritine of Agaricus bisporus.
    Cancer Res. 38:177-180.

Toth, B., J. Smith, and K. Patil. 1981. Cancer induction in mice
    with acetaldehyde methylformylhydrazone of the false morel mush-
    room. J. Natl. Cancer Inst. 67:881-887.

Tung, T. C., and K. H. Ling. 1968. Study on aflatoxin of food-
    stuffs in Taiwan. J. Vitaminol. 14(Supplement):48-52.

Ueno, Y., and K. Kubota. 1976. DNA-attacking ability of carcinogenic
    mycotoxins in recombination-deficient mutant cells of Bacillus .
    subtilis. Cancer Res. 36:445-451.

Ueno, Y., K. Kubota, T. Ito, and Y. Nakamura. 1978. Mutagenicity
    of carcinogenic mycotoxins in Salmonella typhimurium. Cancer Res.
    38:536-542.

Umeda, M., T. Yamamoto, and M. Saito. 1972. DNA-strand breakage of
    HeLa cells induced by several mycotoxins. Jpn. J. Exp. Med. 42:527-
    535.

Umeda, M., T. Tsutsui, and M. Saito. 1977. Mutagenicity and induci-
    bility of DNA single-strand breaks and chromosome aberrations by
    various mycotoxins. Gann 68:619-625.

Umezawa, K., T. Matsushima, T. Sugimura, T. Hirakawa, M. Tanaka, Y.
    Katoh, and S. Takayama. 1977. In vitro transformation of hamster
    embryo cells by quercetin. Toxicol. Lett. 1:175-178.

U. S. Department of Agriculture. 1981. Mushrooms. (Press Release.)
    Vg 2-1-2 (8-81). Crop Reporting Board, Statistical Reporting Ser-
    vice, U. S. Department of Agriculture, Washington, D.C. 4 pp.

U. S. Food and Drug Administration. 1979. Assessment of Estimated
    Risk Resulting from Aflatoxins in Consumer Peanut Products and Other

Food Commodities. Bureau of Foods, U.S. Food and Drug Administration, Washington, D.C. 29 pp.

U. S. Food and Drug Administration. 1980a. Re-evaluation of the Pathology Findings of Studies on Nitrite and Cancer: Histologic Lesions in Sprague-Dawley Rats. Final Report Submitted by Universities Associated for Research and Education in Pathology, Inc. Food and Drug Administration, Department of Health and Human Services, Washington, D.C. 231 pp.

U. S. Food and Drug Administration. 1980b. Nuts. Chapter 12 in Compliance Policy Guidelines. Division of Field Regulatory Guidance, Bureau of Foods, Food and Drug Administration, Washington, D.C.

van Rensburg, S. J. 1977. Role of epidemiology in the elucidation of mycotoxin health risks. Pp. 699-711 in J. V. Rodricks, C. W. Hesseltine, and M. S. Mehlman, eds. Mycotoxins in Human and Animal Health. Pathotox Publishers, Park Forest South, Ill.

van Rensburg, S. J., J. J. van der Watt, I. F. H. Purchase, L. P. Coutinho, and R. Markham. 1974. Primary liver cancer rate and aflatoxin intake in a high cancer area. S. Afr. Med. J. 48:2508a-2508d.

Verdeal, K., R. Brown, T. Richardson, and D. Ryan. 1980. Affinity of phytoestrogens for estradiol-binding proteins and effects of coumesterol on growth of 7,12-dimethylbenz[a]anthracene-induced rat mammary tumors. J. Natl. Cancer Inst. 64:285-290.

Vesselinovitch, S. D., N. Mihailovich, G. N. Wogan, L. S. Lombard, and K. V. N. Rao. 1972. Aflatoxin B_1, a hepatocarcinogen in the infant mouse. Cancer Res. 32:2289-2291.

Vogel, C. L., P. P. Anthony, N. Mody, and L. F. Barker. 1970. Hepatitis-associated antigen in Ugandan patients with hepatocellular carcinoma. Lancet 2:621-624.

von Wright, A., A. Niskanen, and H. Pyysalo. 1977. The toxicities and mutagenic properties of ethylidene gyromitrin and N-methylhydrazine with Escherichia coli as test organism. Mutat. Res. 56:105-110.

Wehner, F. C., P. G. Thiel, S. J. van Rensburg, and I. P. C. Demasius. 1978. Mutagenicity to Salmonella typhimurium of some Aspergillus and Penicillium mycotoxins. Mutat. Res. 58:193-203.

Wehner, F. C., P. G. Thiel, and M. du Rand. 1979. Mutagenicity of the mycotoxin emodin in the Salmonella/microsome system. Appl. Environ. Microbiol. 37:658-660.

Wislocki, P. G., E. C. Miller, J. A. Miller, E. C. McCoy, and H. S. Rosenkranz. 1977. Carcinogenic and mutagenic activities of safrole, 1'-hydroxysafrole, and some known or possible metabolites. Cancer Res. 37:1883-1891.

Wogan, G. N. 1973. Aflatoxin carcinogenesis. Pp. 309-344 in H. Busch, ed. Methods in Cancer Research, Volume 7. Academic Press, New York and London.

Wogan, G. N. 1975. Dietary factors and special epidemiological situations of liver cancer in Thailand and Africa. Cancer Res. 35:3499-3502.

Wogan, G. N., and P. M. Newberne. 1967. Dose-response characteristics of aflatoxin B_1 carcinogenesis in the rat. Cancer Res. 27:2370-2376.

Wong, J. J., and D. P. H. Hsieh. 1976. Mutagenicity of aflatoxins related to their metabolism and carcinogenic potential. Proc. Natl. Acad. Sci. U.S.A. 73:2241-2244.

Würzner, H.-P., E. Lindström, L. Vuataz, and H. Luginbühl. 1977. A 2-year feeding study of instant coffees in rats. II. Incidence and types of neoplasms. Food Cosmet. Toxicol. 15:289-296.

Wynder, E. L., and R. Goldsmith. 1977. The epidemiology of bladder cancer. A second look. Cancer 40:1246-1268.

Wynder, E. L., J. Onderdonk, and N. Mantel. 1963. An epidemiological investigation of cancer of the bladder. Cancer 16:1388-1407.

Wynder, E. L., K. Mabuchi, and W. F. Whitmore, Jr. 1974. Epidemiology of adenocarcinoma of the kidney. J. Natl. Cancer Inst. 53:1619-1634.

Yamanaka, H., M. Nagao, and T. Sugimura. 1979. Mutagenicity of pyrrolizidine alkaloids in the Salmonella/mammalian-microsome test. Mutat. Res. 68:211-216.

Yang, C. S. 1980. Research on esophageal cancer in China: A review. Cancer Res. 40:2633-2644.

Zeitlin, B. R. 1972. Letter to the Editor: Coffee and bladder cancer. Lancet 1:1066.

Zimmerman, F. K. 1977. Genetic effects of nitrous acid. Mutat. Res. 39:127-147.

13 Mutagens in Food

As interest in the possible relationship between diet and cancer has increased in recent years, so have attempts to determine whether chemical carcinogens may be present in our foods. The foods that we eat contain a vast number of separate chemical entities: several thousand as additives and many times this number as natural constituents. Of course, most of these chemicals are present in relatively low concentrations, but if potent carcinogens exist, even at low concentrations in commonly consumed foods, they may warrant concern. The problem, therefore, is how to test the very large number of chemicals present in the complex mixtures we call food to determine whether or not they may be contributing to our risk for cancer. An adequately performed chronic feeding study in rodents to determine whether a chemical is a carcinogen takes several years to complete and analyze and can cost more than $500,000. Therefore, the use of simpler and less expensive tests may be considered, at least to help us determine which chemicals to subject to long-term studies.

As discussed elsewhere in this report, initiation of the carcinogenic process may involve an alteration in the genetic material of a cell. Therefore, it is reasonable to suppose that chemicals that alter DNA (e.g., cause mutations) will have a high probability of being initiators of carcinogenesis. The fact that DNA is chemically similar in all living organisms means that even chemicals that cause mutations in bacteria can be suspected as potential carcinogens in humans. In several extensive studies conducted in independent laboratories, the correlations between mutagenic activity in bacteria and carcinogenicity in mammals have been analyzed (McCann and Ames, 1976; McCann et al., 1975; Purchase et al., 1978; Simmon, 1979; Sugimura et al., 1976). It is clear from these and other studies that a chemical found to be mutagenic in any living system should be suspected of being carcinogenic. However, it is impossible to provide a single number to express the degree of confidence with which a mutagen can be considered to be a carcinogen or with which a nonmutagen can be regarded as a noncarcinogen. This uncertainty arises from several sources, the most important of which is that the correlation between mutagenicity and carcinogenicity is highly dependent upon the class of chemical being investigated. For some classes of chemical carcinogens, such as aromatic amines, polycyclic hydrocarbons, and direct alkylating agents, there appears to be a high degree of correlation. However, it is difficult to detect the mutagenic activity of some types of carcinogens, especially highly chlorinated compounds. Therefore, judgment must be exercised, including a careful consideration of the structure and likely metabolites of the chemical under test, when the significance of a positive or negative mutagenicity test is being evaluated.

The utility of mutagenicity tests in identifying chemical carcinogens and the subsequent removal of these compounds from products to which humans are exposed can be illustrated by several historical examples. These would include the food preservatives 2-(2-furyl)-3-(5-nitrofuryl)acrylamide (AF-2), which was extensively used in Japan, the flame retardant chemical tris(2,3-dibromopropyl)phosphate, which was widely used in children's sleepwear in the United States, and the hair dye ingredient 2,4-diaminoanisole. The fact that simple mutagenicity tests correctly predicted the carcinogenic potential of these chemicals adds to our confidence that correctly interpreted mutagenicity data can assist us in identifying environmental carcinogens.

The most widely used of the mutagenicity assays is the Salmonella plate incorporation test, commonly known as the Ames test. In this assay, a chemical is tested for its ability to induce mutations in different strains of a bacterium (Salmonella typhimurium). Most chemical carcinogens and mutagens do not interact directly with DNA. They require alteration by enzymes in order to become activated. This process of "metabolic activation" cannot usually be accomplished by enzymes present in bacteria. Therefore, in the Salmonella test, an extract of mammalian liver (usually from the rat) is added to provide the enzymes necessary for metabolic activation.

Many mutagenic test systems other than S. typhimurium have been used to test chemicals (see review by Hollstein and McCann, 1979). In the discussion that follows, however, most of the studies discussed involve S. typhimurium. Mutagenicity assays have also been used to investigate the interactions between chemicals. This has resulted in the discovery of both comutagens, which enhance mutagenic activity of other chemicals, and inhibitors of mutagenesis. The knowledge that a chemical is a comutagen or an inhibitor of mutagenesis can provide us with a useful tool for investigating the metabolic fate and genetic interactions of chemicals. Modification of mutagenic activity, particularly as determined in in vitro test systems, frequently has no relevance to in vivo effects. Specific in vitro effects of modifiers of mutagenesis, such as inhibition of a particular metabolizing enzyme, for example, may not operate or may even have the opposite effect in living organisms. However, where modification of mutagenesis is observed, the mechanism should be elucidated.

MUTAGENS RESULTING FROM COOKING OF FOODS

Benzo[a]pyrene and Other Polynuclear Aromatic Hydrocarbons

Almost 20 years ago Lijinsky and Shubik (1964) and Seppilli and Sforzolini (1963) reported that beef grilled over a gas or charcoal fire contained a variety of polycyclic aromatic hydrocarbons (PAH's). Benzo[a]pyrene was found in charcoal-broiled steak in levels up to 8 μg/kg (Lijinsky and Shubik, 1964). The source of the PAH's resulting

from charcoal broiling was the smoke generated when pyrolyzed fat
dripped from the meat onto the hot coals. Thus, meats with the highest
fat content acquired the highest levels of these chemicals (Lijinsky
and Ross, 1967). When meat was cooked in a manner that prevented exposure to the smoke generated by the dripping fat, this source of contamination was either reduced or eliminated (Lijinsky and Ross, 1967;
Lintas et al., 1979; Masuda et al., 1966).

PAH's have also been found in a variety of smoked foods and in
roasted coffee (Howard and Fazio, 1980). Vegetables can easily become
contaminated by PAH's from air, soil, or water; fish and shellfish can
assimilate such chemicals from their marine environments (Howard and
Fazio, 1980). However, unless vegetables or seafood are obtained from
highly contaminated environments, the major source of PAH will probably
be the smoking or cooking of food.

Mutagens from Pyrolyzed Proteins and Amino Acids

During the past few years, it has become clear that PAH's account
for only a small fraction of the mutagenic (and, therefore, potentially
carcinogenic) activity that occurs in foods during cooking. Nagao et
al. (1977a) used dimethylsulfoxide to prepare extracts of the charred
surfaces of broiled fish and meat. They found that the mutagenic activities of these extracts for histidine-requiring strains of S. typhimurium were hundreds or thousands of times greater than could be
accounted for by the reported benzo[a]pyrene contents of these cooked
foods. For example, the mutagenic activity of charcoal-broiled beef-
steak was the equivalent to that of approximately 4,500 µg of benzo[a]-
pyrene per kilogram of steak, even though Lijinsky and Shubik (1964)
had reported that charcoal-broiled steak contained no more than
8 µg of this chemical per kilogram.

The mutagenic activity in the broiled fish and beef could also be
detected in S. typhimurium strain TA98, implying that the agent could
induce frameshift mutations (Nagao et al., 1977a; Sugimura et al.,
1977). Positive results in these assays depended on the presence of
an in vitro metabolic activation system utilizing the postmitochon-
drial supernatant from homogenized livers of rats pretreated with
polychlorinated biphenyls. Bjeldanes et al. (in press, a, b) have recently completed a series of detailed studies on the cooking conditions under which mutagenic activity is produced in various types of
fish, meats (including organ meats), as well as eggs, milk, cheese,
and tofu.

To determine what constituent or constituents of fish and meat
contribute to the mutagenic activity produced by cooking, studies have
been conducted to examine the mutagenicity of smoke condensates from
various substances. Smoke obtained from pyrolyzed proteins, such as
lysozyme and histone, was found to be highly mutagenic to S. typhimurium, whereas smoke condensates from pyrolyzed DNA, RNA, starch, or
vegetable oil were only slightly mutagenic (Nagao et al., 1977b).

Pyrolysis of tryptophan resulted in more mutagenic activity than did any other common amino acid, but almost all of the amino acids tested yielded some mutagenic activity when pyrolyzed (Matsumoto et al., 1977; Nagao et al., 1977c).

Purification of the mutagenic products resulting from pyrolysis of tryptophan resulted in the isolation of two previously unknown amino-γ-carbolines that are potent mutagens: 3-amino-1,4,-dimethyl-5H-pyrido-[4,3-b]indole (referred to as Trp-P-1, for "Tryptophan Pyrolysate 1") and 3-amino-1-methyl-5H-pyrido[4,3-b]indole (Trp-P-2) (Akimoto et al., 1977; Sugimura et al., 1977; Takeda et al., 1977).

The mutagenic activity resulting from pyrolysis of L-glutamic acid was shown to be due to the formation of 2-amino-6-methyldipyrido-[1,2-a:3'2'-d]imidazole (Glu-P-1) and 2-aminodipyrido[1,2-a:3',2'-d]-imidazole (Glu-P-2) (Yamamoto et al., 1978). The structural similarity between these products of glutamic acid pyrolysate and Trp-P-1 and Trp-P-2 is evident from Figure 13-1.

Wakabayashi et al. (1978) isolated a different, but structurally related, heterocyclic mutagen from pyrolyzed lysine. This compound was 3,4-cyclopentenopyrido[3,2-a]carbazole (Lys-P-1). Pyrolysis of phenylalanine resulted in the formation of the mutagen 2-amino-5-phenylpyridine (Phe-P-1) (Sugimura et al., 1977).

When soybean globulin was pyrolyzed, the substances that contributed to the mutagenic activity were compounds not previously identified as pyrolysis products of any individual amino acid. These compounds, 2-amino-9H-pyrido[2,3-b]indole (AαC) and 2-amino-3-methyl-9H-pyrido-[2,3-b]indole (MeAαC), are quite closely related to the γ-carboline compounds Trp-P-1 and Trp-P-2 (Yoshida et al., 1978).

Uyeta et al. (1979) found that both Trp-P-1 and Trp-P-2 were present in pyrolysates of casein and gluten. Yamaguchi et al. (1979) identified Glu-P-2 in the tar resulting from pyrolysis of casein. These investigators estimated that Glu-P-2 and Glu-P-1 accounted for approximately 10% of the total mutagenic activity of the pyrolysate.

Analyses have confirmed that at least some of the mutagenic pyrolysis products of amino acids are present in cooked foods. For example, Trp-P-1 has been found in "very well done" broiled beef and Glu-P-2 in broiled cuttlefish, although they account for less than 10% of the total mutagenic activity in extracts of these foods (Yamaguchi et al., 1980a,b). Similarly, sardines broiled to a dark brown color contain Trp-P-1, Trp-P-2, and Phe-P-1, although most of the mutagenic activity in these fish was due to the presence of other compounds (Yamaizumi et al., 1980) (Table 13-1). Pieces of beef or chicken grilled in a high gas flame contained AαC and MeAαC (Matsumoto et al., 1981). Similarly, AαC could be identified in grilled onions.

From Amino Acids:

Tryptophan pyrolysates

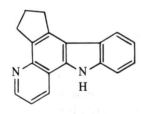

Trp-P-1   Trp-P-2

Glutamic acid pyrolysates

Glu-P-1   Glu-P-2

Lysine pyrolysate   Phenylalanine pyrolysate

Lys-P-1   Phe-P-1

From Proteins:

Soybean globulin pyrolysates

AαC   MeAαC

FIGURE 13-1.   Some mutagens from pyrolysates and from cooked foods. (Figure continued on next page.)

Figure 13-1 (continued): Some mutagens from pyrolysates and from cooked foods.

From Broiled Sardines:

Protein pyrolysates

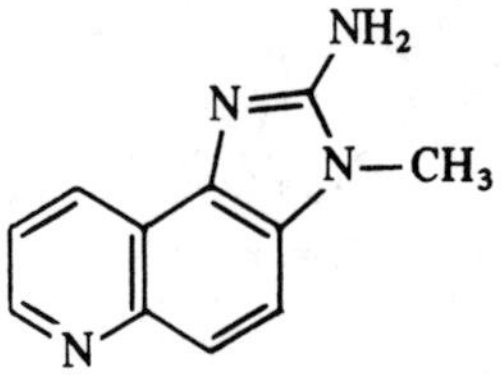

IQ

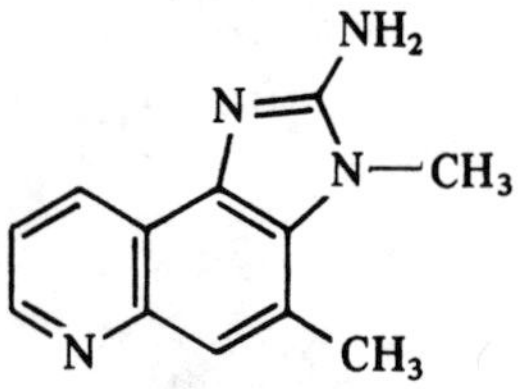

MeIQ

From Broiled Beef:

Protein pyrolysate

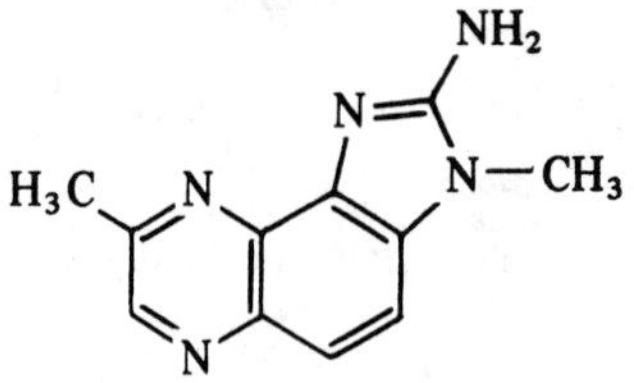

MeIQx

Two previously unknown mutagens were isolated from broiled sardines (Kasai et al., 1979). These were 2-amino-3-methylimidazo[4,5-f]quinoline (IQ) and 2-amino-3,4-dimethylimidazo[4,5-f]quinoline (MeIQ), which are extraordinarily potent mutagens to S. typhimurium strain TA98 (Kasai et al., 1980a,b,c). Except for the beef that contained IQ and possibly that containing MeIQ and 2-amino-3,8-dimethylimidazo-[4,5-f]-quinoxaline (MeIQx), the foods listed as sources of mutagens in Table 13-1 appear to have been very well cooked and even charred on the surfaces to produce the mutagenic compounds identified in the table. Information on mutagens formed by cooking foods at lower temperatures is discussed in the next section.

As discussed in Chapter 3, the mutagenic activity of a chemical in bacteria indicates potential genotoxicity and possible carcinogenicity in mammals. To test for carcinogenic activity, it is necessary to use mammalian cell systems and intact mammals. Whenever other test systems also indicate genotoxic activity, it is more likely that a bacterial mutagen can act as a carcinogen.

TABLE 13-1

Mutagenic Activities of the Mutagens Isolated from Cooked Foods[a]

Abbreviation	Chemical Name	Mutagenicity (revertants/μg)		Source of Mutagen	Concentration of Mutagen in Heated Material (ng/g)	Reference
		TA98	TA100			
Trp-P-1	3-Amino-1,4-dimethyl-5H-pyrido[4,3-b]indole	39,000	1,650	Broiled sun-dried sardine Broiled beef	13.3 53 (in raw beef)	Yamaizumi et al., 1980 Yamaguchi et al., 1980a
Trp-P-2	3-Amino-1-methyl-5H-pyrido[4,3-b]indole	104,200	1,750	Broiled sun-dried sardine	13.1	Yamaizumi et al., 1980
Glu-P-2	2-Aminodipyrido[1,2-a:3',2'-d]imidazole	1,900	1,200	Broiled sun-dried cuttlefish	280	Yamaguchi et al., 1980b
Phe-P-1	2-Amino-5-phenylpyridine	41	23	Broiled sun-dried sardine	8.6	Yamaizumi et al., 1980
AαC	2-Amino-9H-pyrido-[2,3-b]indole	300	20	Grilled beef Grilled chicken Grilled onion	650 180 1.5	Matsumoto et al., 1981 Matsumoto et al., 1981 Matsumoto et al., 1981
MeAαC	2-Amino-3-methyl-9H-pyrido[2,3-b]indole	200	120	Grilled beef Grilled chicken	64 15	Matsumoto et al., 1981 Matsumoto et al., 1981
IQ	2-Amino-3-methylimid-azo[4,5-f]quinoline	433,000	7,000	Broiled sun-dried sardine Broiled beef	158 0.59	Yamaizumi et al., 1981 Sugimura et al., 1981
MeIQ	2-Amino-3,4-dimethyl-imidazo[4,5-f]quinoline	661,000	30,000	Broiled sun-dried sardine	72	Yamaizumi et al., 1981
MeIQx	2-Amino-3,8-dimethyl-imidazo[4,5-f]quinoxa-line	145,000	14,000	Fried beef	No information available.	Kasai et al., 1981

aAdapted from Sugimura and Nagao, in press.

Four of the mutagenic pyrolysates derived from amino acids or protein--Trp-P-1, Trp-P-2, Glu-P-1, and AαC--have been shown to induce sister chromatid exchanges in a permanent line of human lymphoblastoid cells (Tohda et al., 1980). In addition, the basic fraction extracted from pyrolyzed tryptophan was found to cause mutations resulting in resistance to ouabain or 8-azaguanine in cultured Chinese hamster lung cells (Inui et al., 1980). Trp-P-1, Trp-P-2, and Glu-P-1 can transform primary Syrian golden hamster embryo cells (Takayama et al., 1977, 1979). The cells transformed by Trp-P-2 have been shown to grow in soft agar and to result in tumors when inoculated into the cheek pouches of young hamsters with unimpaired immunocompetence (Takayama et al., 1978). Although these findings support the potential carcinogenicity of these chemicals, a definitive determination of carcinogenicity must be made in whole animals.

Several of the mutagenic pyrolysates of amino acids or proteins have been tested for carcinogenicity in vivo. Neoplastic nodules, which are presumed to be precancerous changes, were found in the livers of Wistar rats given the basic fraction from pyrolyzed tryptophan at 0.2% in the diet (Matsukura et al., 1981b). Neither neoplastic nodules nor liver tumors had previously been observed in this strain of rats in this laboratory. Subcutaneous injection of Trp-P-1 (1.5 mg once a week for 20 weeks) induced sarcomas in Syrian golden hamsters and in Fischer rats (Ishikawa et al., 1979). Trp-P-2 did not induce tumors in either hamsters or rats under the same experimental conditions (Ishikawa et al., 1979). Trp-P-1 and Trp-P-2 produced liver tumors in CDF$_1$ (BALB/c x DBA) mice that were fed a diet containing 0.02% of either of these chemicals (Matsukura et al., 1981a). Some of these liver tumors metastasized to the lung. Female mice were more susceptible to these carcinogens than were the males. Six of nine female ACI rats fed 0.1% Trp-P-2 in their diet developed neoplastic nodules of the liver, and one of the six developed a hemangioendothelial sarcoma of the liver (Hosaka et al., 1981). None of the control animals developed such nodules or tumors. Glu-P-1, Glu-P-2, AαC, and MeAαC induced hepatomas in mice. Glu-P-1 and Glu-P-2 also induced hemangioendotheliomas between the scapulae of mice fed diets containing 0.05% of either of these chemicals (Sugimura, in press). Thus, it appears that the identification of several of the mutagenic compounds found in pyrolysates of proteins and amino acids was an accurate predictor of carcinogenicity. However, the presence of a carcinogenic chemical in a pyrolyzed amino acid or protein mixture does not necessarily imply that the carcinogen will also be present in normally cooked, uncharred food.

Mutagens Formed from Meat at Lower Temperatures

In the experiments concerning the formation of mutagenic pyrolysis products from amino acids and proteins, temperatures of 250°C or greater were used (Matsumoto et al., 1977; 1978; Uyeta et al., 1979). However, it is now known that simply boiling beef stock at temperatures of approximately 100°C results in the formation of bacterial mutagens (Commoner et al., 1978; Vithayathil et al., 1978). In fact, the formation of mutagens in beef stock has been detected at temperatures as low as 68°C (Dolara et al., 1979). Frying of fish at 190°C produces mutagenic activity (Krone and Iwaoka, 1981). Mutagenic activity also results when hamburgers are broiled, even when the surface temperature does not exceed 130°C (Weisburger and Spingarn, 1979). A portion of the mutagenic activity formed from heated beef extract or from fried beef was found to be due to a chemical with a molecular weight of 198 (Spingarn et al., 1980a), which has now been shown to be IQ (Kasai et al., 1980a). MeIQx, another heterocyclic mutagenic compound that has not been identified as an amino acid or protein pyrolysate, has also been found in fried beef (Kasai et al., 1981). However, the frying temperature was not specified. Weisburger and Spingarn (1979) suggested that this mutagen, formed in beef at moderate temperatures, may result from a browning reaction between sugars and amines rather than from the pyrolysis of proteins.

Mutagen Formation Involving Carbohydrates

If the formation of IQ during the cooking of beef results from a browning reaction, it might be expected that the browning of starchy foods could also result in the formation of mutagens. Spingarn et al. (1980b) have observed that the frying of potatoes and the toasting of bread result in the formation of mutagenic activity, but the chemical(s) responsible for this activity and their source during the cooking process remain to be determined.

Browning of foods results from the reaction of amines with sugars. Using a model system for the browning reaction, Spingarn and Garvie (1979) found that mutagenic activity occurred when any of six different sugars, including glucose, were refluxed with ammonium hydroxide. Several laboratories have found that heating a mixture of the amino acid lysine with glucose at temperatures between 100°C and 121°C results in products that are mutagenic (Powrie et al., 1981; Shinohara et al., 1980; Yoshida and Okamoto, 1980). The increase in mutagenic activity with time paralleled the increase in browning (Shinohara et al., 1980). Mutagenic activity could also be produced by using certain amino acids other than lysine (Powrie et al., 1981; Yoshida and Okamoto, 1980) or by using fructose rather than glucose (Powrie et al., 1981).

Chromosome aberrations are alterations in the structures of chromosomes that can be observed through a microscope. Such aberrations are not likely to be heritable. The significance of their induction in cells in vitro is not clear, particularly for chemicals unable to induce heritable mutations or in vivo chromosome aberrations.

Pyrazine and four of its alkyl derivatives—compounds formed by heating mixtures of sugars and amino acids (Koehler et al., 1969)—were found to be nonmutagenic to S. typhimurium but capable of inducing chromosome aberrations in cultured Chinese hamster ovary (CHO) cells (Stich et al., 1980). Commercial caramel and caramelized samples of several sugars prepared by heating sugar solutions also caused chromosome aberrations in CHO cells (Stich et al., 1981b). Similarly, furan and six of its derivatives, which can be produced in foods by heating carbohydrates (Maga, 1979), were found to cause chromosome aberrations in CHO cells but to be nonmutagenic to bacteria (Stich et al., 1981a).

PLANT FLAVONOIDS

Among the most widespread of the known naturally occurring mutagens (possible carcinogens) that are normal constituents of many foods are the mutagenic flavonoids. Among the flavonol aglycones that have been shown to be mutagenic to S. typhimurium are quercetin, kaempferol, and galangin (Bjeldanes and Chang, 1977; Brown, 1980; Hardigree and Epler, 1978; MacGregor and Jurd, 1978). Quercetin has also been reported to induce gene conversion in yeast (Hardigree and Epler, 1978), transformation of both hamster embryo cells (Umezawa et al., 1977) and BALB/c 3T3 mouse cells (Meltz and MacGregor, 1981), and mutations and single-stranded DNA breaks in L5178Y mouse cells (Meltz and MacGregor, 1981). Both quercetin and kaempferol have been reported to cause mutations in V79 Chinese hamster cells (Maruta et al., 1979) and heritable mutations (sex-linked recessive lethals) in the fruit fly Drosophila melanogaster (Watson, 1982).

In some mutagenic plant products consumed by humans, the mutagenic substances isolated were identified as flavonoids. For example, most of the mutagenic activity of an acid hydrolysate of green tea could be accounted for by three flavonoids: kaempferol, quercetin, and myricetin (Uyeta et al., 1981). The flavonoids kaempferol and isorhamnetin were found to be responsible for most of the mutagenic activity found in Japanese pickles (Takahashi et al., 1979). The mutagen in the spice of sumac was found to be quercetin (Seino et al., 1978). Isorhamnetin and quercetin were the major mutagens in a methanol extract of dill weed (Fukouka et al., 1980).

Brown (1980) reported that the edible portions of most food plants contain flavonoid glycosides, especially quercetin and kaempferol. He estimated that the average daily intake of flavonoids in the U.S. diet is approximately 1 g and that the daily intake of mutagenic flavonoid glycosides may be equivalent to approximately 50 mg of quercetin. Approximately 25% of the flavonoid intake is derived from tea, coffee, cocoa, fruit jams, red wine, beer, and vinegar (Brown, 1980).

In view of the mutagenic activity and widespread distribution of certain flavonoids, particularly quercetin, it is important to determine the carcinogenic potential of these chemicals. At present, the data concerning the carcinogenicity of quercetin are contradictory. Pamukcu et al. (1980) reported that adding 0.1% quercetin to the diet of albino Norwegian rats for 58 weeks resulted in the induction of tumors in the epithelium of the intestine and urinary bladder. However, when Saito et al. (1980) fed 2% quercetin to ddY mice throughout the lives of the animals, they found no significant increase in tumor incidence. At doses as high as 10% quercetin in the diet fed throughout life, no significant increase in tumor incidence was observed in ACI rats (Hirono et al., 1981) or in hamsters (Morino et al., 1982). The reason for the discrepancy between the findings of Pamukcu et al. and the other investigators is not clear, but may relate to differences in sensitivity among the species and strain tested.

Flavonols often exist in plants in the form of glycosides. For example, rutin is a glycoside of quercetin that can be hydrolyzed to release quercetin by enzymatic or chemical treatment. Such hydrolysis, mediated by intestinal bacteria, occurs when glycosides are consumed in foods. Rutin and other glycosides of mutagenic flavonoids have been shown to be mutagenic to S. typhimurium following treatment with glycosidase-containing extracts of the mold Aspergillus niger (Nagao et al., 1981), the snail Helix pomatia (Brown and Dietrich, 1979), rat cecal contents (Brown and Dietrich, 1979), or human feces (Tamura et al., 1980). Mutagenic activity of rutin has also been reported in S. typhimurium in the absence of glycosidase treatment, but only at doses higher than those required when such treatment is used (Hardigree and Epler, 1978).

MUTAGENIC ACTIVITY IN EXTRACTS OF FOODS AND BEVERAGES

Several food substances have been reported to contain mutagenic activity, although the specific chemicals responsible for this activity have not yet been identified. For example, coffee is mutagenic to Salmonella typhimurium strain TA100, whether it is brewed, instant, or decaffeinated (Aeschbacher and Würzner, 1980; Aeschbacher et al., 1980; Nagao et al., 1979). Although caffeine has been reported to be mutagenic to bacteria (Clarke and Wade, 1975; Demerec et al., 1948, 1951; Gezelius and Fries, 1952; Glass and Novick, 1959; Johnson and Bach, 1965; Kubitschek and Bendigkeit, 1958, 1964; Novick, 1956), it could not have been responsible for the mutagenicity of coffee observed in these reports, since decaffeinated coffee was as mutagenic as regular coffee and caffeine itself was not detected as a mutagen under the test conditions used (Aeschbacher et al., 1980; Nagao et al., 1979). Studies examining the possible carcinogenicity of coffee are discussed in Chapter 12.

Black tea, green tea, and roasted tea were mutagenic to S. typhimurium strain TA100 in the absence of added enzymes (Nagao et al., 1979). When extracts of Aspergillus niger or human feces containing enzymes capable of hydrolyzing glycosides were added, tea became mutagenic to S. typhimurium strain TA98 (Nagao et al., 1979; Tamura et al., 1980). Acid hydrolysis of green or black tea also caused mutagenic activity to be released (Uyeta et al., 1981). The flavonols quercetin, kaempferol, and myricetin have recently been shown to account for most of the mutagenic activity of an acid hydrolysate of green tea (Uyeta et al., 1981). Grape juice was also found to be mutagenic to strain TA98, although only when tested with fecal extracts containing glycosidases (Tamura et al., 1980).

Mutagenic activity has also been detected in concentrates of 17 out of 27 commonly consumed Chinese alcoholic beverages, mostly fermented from rice, glutinous rice, and barley (Lee and Fong, 1979). The mutagenic spirits were those that had been distilled only once or to which herbs or meat had been added. Evaporated residues from 12 out of 13 Japanese, Scotch, and North American whiskies were found to contain mutagenic activity (Nagao et al., 1981). This activity did not require the addition of glycosidases or mammalian enzymes. It was mutagenic to S. typhimurium strain TA100, but not to TA98, indicating that it was inducing base-pair substitution rather than frameshift mutations. Some French brandies and apple brandies were also mutagenic when concentrated or fractionated (Loquet et al., 1981; Nagao et al., 1981).

Extracts of relatively few fruits, vegetables, and beverages are mutagenic. When Stoltz et al. (in press, a,b) fractionated extracts of 28 beverages and 40 fruits and vegetables, only 3 beverages and 5 fruits and vegetables showed reproducible mutagenic activity. The activity of three of the fruits (strawberries, raspberries, and peaches) was due to residues of the fungicide captan. Quercetin accounted for the mutagenicity of the remaining fruit and vegetable (raisins and onions) as well as two of the beverages (red wine and grape juice). The mutagen in coffee was not identified. This extensive survey of fractionated extracts of 68 foods did not reveal the presence of any mutagenic chemicals or foods that had not been previously reported. Similarly, Bjeldanes et al. (in press, a,b) found no significant mutagenic activity in extracts of eggs, milk, cheese, or tofu unless they had been cooked at high temperatures or to the point of darkening. Thus, with the exception of mutagens produced by cooking, it seems unlikely that large numbers of mutagens remain to be discovered in common foods.

MODIFIERS OF MUTAGENIC ACTIVITY

A number of substances in food have been reported either to enhance or to diminish the mutagenic activity of other substances. Most of these effects have been observed in in vitro test systems, and their relevance to effects in intact mammals is unknown. Modifiers of mutagenicity can be either comutagens or antimutagens. A comutagen is a substance that enhances the mutagenic activity of a chemical although it is not in itself mutagenic. This enhancement may take one of two forms: it may strengthen the mutagenic response of chemicals that are themselves mutagenic or may create a mutagenic response from nonmutagens. Similarly, an antimutagen is a substance that reduces or eliminates the mutagenic activity of a mutagen.

Harman and Norharman

Among the more interesting comutagens discovered in recent years are harman (1-methyl-β-carboline) and norharman (β-carboline). Norharman is present in tobacco tar (Poindexter and Carpenter, 1962) as well as in toasted bread, broiled beef, and broiled sardines (Yasuda et al., 1978). Harman is found in these same sources as well as in mushrooms and in Japanese sake (Takase and Murakami, 1966; Takeuchi et al., 1973).

These compounds were identified as comutagens when fractionation of pyrolyzed tryptophan resulted in a significant loss of mutagenic activity on S. typhimurium. Mixing the fraction containing harman and norharman with the fraction containing Trp-P-1 and Trp-P-2 restored the mutagenic activity of these mutagens (Nagao et al., 1977d). Norharman, which is at most marginally mutagenic, has been shown to be comutagenic when mixed with a variety of chemicals, including 4-dimethylaminoazobenzene, (Nagao et al., 1977d), aniline, o-toluidine (but not m- or p-toluidine) (Nagao et al., 1977e), nitrosodiphenylamine (Wakabayashi et al., 1981), 3-aminopyridine, 2-amino-3-methylpyridine (Sugimura et al., 1982), 2-acetylaminofluorene, 2-aminofluorene, and N-hydroxy-2-acetylamino-fluorene (Umezawa et al., 1978). These chemicals all require an in vitro mammalian metabolic activation system for mutagenic activity. In addition, norharman is comutagenic with N-acetoxy-2-acetylaminofluorene in the absence of any metabolic activation system (Umezawa et al., 1978).

Aniline, which is nonmutagenic in the absence of norharman, was believed for many years to be noncarcinogenic. Its weak carcinogenic activity has only recently been demonstrated (National Cancer Institute, 1978). Although the mutagenic activity of a number of chemical carcino-gens can only be observed in the presence of norharman, data are insuffi-cient to justify recommending the inclusion of norharman in routine screening. The possibility that many "false positive" results might be obtained with norharman has not yet been ruled out.

The mechanism of the comutagenic action of harman and norharman is still unclear. Although these comutagens are generally believed to exert their activity by affecting the metabolic activation of the test compounds, they may act through other mechanisms as well. For example, the mutagenicity of N-acetoxy-2-acetylaminofluorene, which does not require activation, was enhanced by the addition of harman and/or nor-harman (Umezawa et al., 1978).

A number of substances in foods can reduce the activity of certain mutagens in in vitro test systems. For example, Morita et al. (1978) reported that juices prepared from some common vegetables, fruits, and spices, including cabbage, broccoli, green pepper, eggplant, apple, shallot, ginger, pineapple, and mint leaf, reduced the mutagenic acti-vity of tryptophan pyrolysates. Lai (1979) and Lai et al. (1980) have also found antimutagenic activity in extracts of wheat sprouts, leaf lettuce, parsley, brussels sprouts, mustard greens, spinach, cabbage, broccoli, and other vegetables. Although they concluded that the anti-mutagenic substance in these vegetables is chlorophyll, certain food substances without chlorophyll, such as apples, also inhibit mutagenic activity (Morita et al., 1978), indicating that some factor in foods other than chlorophyll can be antimutagenic.

Hemin

Certain pigments derived from animal systems have also been reported to have antimutagenic activity. For example, hemin inhibited the activity of a number of polycyclic mutagens including benzo[a]pyrene, 3-methylcholanthrene, 2-acetylaminofluorene, 2-nitrofluorene, and alfatoxin B_1 as well as several mutagenic amino acid pyrolysates, such as Trp-P-1 and Trp-P-2 (Arimoto et al., 1980a,b). The heme metabolites biliverdin and bilirubin also interfered with the mutagenic activity of some of these compounds. The mechanism of these antimutagenic effects awaits complete elucidation. Hemin interfered with the mutagenic activity of 2-nitrofluorene and the activated forms of Trp-P-1 and Glu-P-1, all of which are mutagenic to S. typhimurium in the absence of a mammalian metabolic activation system. Therefore, at least some of the anti-mutagenic activity of hemin must be unrelated to such activation.

Fatty Acids

Other chemicals in foods have also been reported to inhibit mutagenic activity. For example, the unsaturated fatty acids oleic acid and linoleic acid (but not the saturated fatty acids stearic acid and palmitic acid) inhibited the mutagenic activity of a number of chemicals for S. typhimurium (Hayatsu et al., 1981a,b). The mechanism for this inhibition is unknown.

Nitrite

Yoshida and Matsumoto (1978) reported that when pyrolyzed casein (a mutagenic extract of roasted chicken meat), tobacco-smoke condensate, and certain aromatic amines were treated with nitrite under acidic conditions, there was a decrease in the mutagenic activity of these substances when tested on Salmonella typhimurium. Concentrations of sodium nitrite as low as 3 mg/liter were sufficient to cause a loss of most of the mutagenic activity of casein pyrolysate. Similarly, Tsuda et al. (1980) found that acidic treatment with 2.3 mg/liter solution of sodium nitrite resulted in the loss of mutagenic activity of Trp-P-1, Trp-P-2, and Glu-P-1.

A more complex situation has been found to exist for the interaction of nitrite with 2-amino-α-carboline (Tsuda et al., 1981). At pH of approximately 4, the reaction results in a loss of mutagenic activity through the conversion of 2-amino-α-carboline to the nonmutagen 2-hydroxy-α-carboline. However, when the pH was below 3.5, a new, direct-acting mutagen was formed: 2-hydroxy-3-nitroso-α-carboline. Thus, nitrite can either neutralize mutagens or result in the formation of new mutagens. The ability of nitrite to interact with dietary amines to form mutagenic and carcinogenic N-nitrosamines is discussed in Chapter 12.

Antioxidants

A number of antioxidants have been shown to inhibit the mutagenicity of a variety of chemicals. For example, McKee and Tometsko (1979) found that butylated hydroxyanisole (BHA) and butylated hydroxytoluene (BHT) were antimutagenic in the presence of a series of mutagens that require in vitro metabolic activation, but not in the presence of mutagens that are directly mutagenic to S. typhimurium without an added metabolic activation system. Similarly, Katoh et al. (1980) found that BHA inhibits the mutagenicity of benzo[a]pyrene in Chinese hamster V-79 cells, but not the mutagenicity of the direct-acting compound N-acetoxy-2-acetylaminofluorene. These findings are consistent with the hypothesis that these antioxidants interfere with the in vitro metabolic activation of the mutagens, rather than reacting with them or their active metabolites directly. Further evidence that a metabolism-modifying mechanism is related to the ability of certain chemicals to exert anticarcinogenic activity is discussed in Chapter 15.

The observation that some antioxidant antimutagens appear to act by interfering with metabolic activation does not exclude the possibility that, in some cases, direct reaction with a mutagen may be an important mechanism of action. For example, Shamberger et al. (1979) have found that BHT, ascorbic acid, vitamin E, and selenium can interfere with the mutagenicity of β-propiolactone and, in some strains of S. typhimurium, malonaldehyde. These two chemicals do not require a mammalian-derived metabolic activation system for activity. Similarly, Guttenplan (1978) attributes the ability of ascorbic acid to inhibit the mutagenic activity of the direct-acting mutagen N-methyl-N'-nitro-N-nitrosoguanidine (MNNG) to a direct reaction between ascorbate and the mutagen.

Rosin and Stich (1979) reported that some antioxidants, including sodium bisulfite and sodium ascorbate, inhibit the mutagenicity of MNNG in S. typhimurium, but not that of another direct-acting mutagen, N-acetoxy-2-acetylaminofluorene. Other antioxidants tested inhibited both or neither of these mutagens. These findings probably reflect an underlying complex mechanism concerning the inhibition by antioxidants of the mutagenicity of even direct-acting mutagens.

Retinol (vitamin A alcohol) inhibits the mutagenic activity of 2-aminofluorene and aflatoxin B_1, both of which require metabolic activation, but not that of the direct-acting mutagens adriamycin and diepoxybutane (Baird and Birnbaum, 1979; Busk and Ahlborg, 1980). Similar to the antioxidants discussed above, these results may indicate that retinol inhibits mutagenesis by interfering with metabolic activation rather than by acting as a scavenger of mutagenic chemicals. However, more experimental evidence is needed to clarify this point.

SUMMARY AND CONCLUSIONS

Considerable attention has recently been directed toward the presence of mutagenic activity in foods. Many vegetables contain mutagenic flavonoids such as quercetin, kaempferol, and their glycosides. Furthermore, some substances found in foods can enhance or inhibit the mutagenic activity of other compounds. Mutagens in charred meat and fish are produced during the pyrolysis of proteins that occurs when foods are cooked at very high temperatures. Normal cooking of meat at lower temperatures can also result in the production of mutagens. Smoking of foods as well as charcoal broiling results in the deposition of mutagenic and carcinogenic polynuclear aromatic compounds such as benzo[a]pyrene on the surface of the food.

The production of mutations in bacterial or other tests is an indication that a chemical may be carcinogenic in animals. However, many mutagens detected in foods have not been adequately tested for carcinogenicity. Of those that have been tested, the data on the carcinogenicity of the mutagenic flavonol quercetin are conflicting, and several mutagens isolated from pyrolyzed proteins or amino acids appear to be carcinogenic. It is not yet clear to what extent the mutagens produced by pyrolyzing proteins or amino acids are found in normally cooked foods. The finding that some constituents of food can enhance or inhibit the in vitro mutagenicity of other compounds should not be interpreted as meaning that these compounds would produce the same effects in living animals or humans.

If mutagens that are widely distributed in common foods are consistently found to cause cancer in animals, many factors should be considered before action is taken to reduce exposure. For example, cooking of meat and fish produces mutagens, but it also destroys pathogenic microorganisms and parasites. Furthermore, some foods contain mutagenic flavonoids but also have high nutritional value.

REFERENCES

Aeschbacher, H. U., and H. P. Würzner. 1980. An evaluation of instant and regular coffee in the Ames mutagenicity test. Toxicol. Lett. 5:139-145.

Aeschbacher, H. U., C. Chappuis, and H. P. Würzner. 1980. Mutagenicity testing of coffee: A study of problems encountered with the Ames Salmonella test system. Food Cosmet. Toxicol. 18:605-613.

Akimoto, H., A. Kawai, H. Nomura, M. Nagao, T. Kawachi, and T. Sugimura. 1977. Syntheses of potent mutagens in tryptophan pyrolysates. Chem. Lett. 9:1061-1064.

Arimoto, S., T. Negishi, and H. Hayatsu. 1980a. Inhibitory effect of hemin on the mutagenic activities of carcinogens. Cancer Lett. 11:29-33.

Arimoto, S., Y. Ohara, T. Namba, T. Negishi, and H. Hayatsu. 1980b. Inhibition of the mutagenicity of amino acid pyrolysis products by hemin and other biological pyrrole pigments. Biochem. Biophys. Res. Commun. 92:662-668.

Baird, M. B., and L. S. Birnbaum. 1979. Inhibition of 2-fluorenamine-induced mutagenesis in Salmonella typhimurium by vitamin A. J. Natl. Cancer Inst. 63:1093-1096.

Bjeldanes, L. F., and G. W. Chang. 1977. Mutagenic activity of quercetin and related compounds. Science 197:577-578.

Bjeldanes, L. F., M. M. Morris, J. S. Felton, S. Healy, D. Stuermer, P. Berry, H. Timourian, and F. T. Hatch. In press a. Mutagens from the cooking of food. II. Survey by Ames/Salmonella test of mutagen formation in the major protein-rich foods of the American diet. Food Chem. Toxicol.

Bjeldanes, L. F., M. M. Morris, J. S. Felton, S. Healy, D. Stuermer, P. Berry, H. Timourian, and F. T. Hatch. In press b. Mutagens from the cooking of food. III. Secondary sources of cooked dietary protein. Food Chem. Toxicol.

Brown, J. P. 1980. A review of the genetic effects of naturally occurring flavonoids, anthraquinones and related compounds. Mutat. Res. 75:243-277.

Brown, J. P., and P. S. Dietrich. 1979. Mutagenicity of plant flavonols in the Salmonella/mammalian microsome test. Activation of flavonol glycosides by mixed glycosidases from rat cecal bacteria and other sources. Mutat. Res. 66:223-240.

Busk, L., and U. G. Ahlborg. 1980. Retinol (vitamin A) as an inhibitor of the mutagenicity of aflatoxin B_1. Toxicol. Lett. 6:243-249.

Clarke, C. H., and M. J. Wade. 1975. Evidence that caffeine, 8-methoxy-psoralen and steroidal diamines are frameshift mutagens for E. coli K-12. Mutat. Res. 28:123-125.

Commoner, B., A. J. Vithayathil, P. Dolara, S. Nair, P. Madyastha, and G. C. Cuca. 1978. Formation of mutagens in beef and beef extract during cooking. Science 201:913-916.

Demerec, M., B. Wallace, and E. M. Witkin. 1948. The gene. Carnegie Inst. Washington Yearb. 47:169-176.

Demerec, M., G. Bertani, and J. Flint. 1951. A survey of chemicals for mutagenic action on E. coli. Am. Nat. 85:119-136.

Dolara, P., B. Commoner, A. Vithayathil, G. Cuca, E. Tuley, P. Madyastha, S. Nair, and D. Kriebel. 1979. The effect of temperature on the formation of mutagens in heated beef stock and cooked ground beef. Mutat. Res. 60:231-237.

Fukuoka, M., K. Yoshihira, S. Natori, K. Sakamoto, S. Iwahara, S. Hosaka, and I. Hirono. 1980. Characterization of mutagenic principles and carcinogenicity test of dill weed and seeds. J. Pharmacobio-Dyn. 3:236-244.

Gezelius, K., and N. Fries. 1952. Phage resistant mutants induced in Escherichia coli by caffeine. Hereditas 38:112-114.

Glass, E. A., and A. Novick. 1959. Induction of mutation in chlor-amphenicol-inhibited bacteria. J. Bacteriol. 77:10-16.

Guttenplan, J. B. 1978. Mechanisms of inhibition by ascorbate of microbial mutagenesis induced by N-nitroso compounds. Cancer Res. 38:2018-2022.

Hardigree, A. A., and J. L. Epler. 1978. Comparative mutagenesis of plant flavonoids in microbial systems. Mutat. Res. 58:231-239.

Hayatsu, H., S. Arimoto, K. Togawa, and M. Makita. 1981a. Inhibitory effect of the ether extract of human feces on activities of mutagens: Inhibition by oleic and linoleic acids. Mutat. Res. 81:287-293.

Hayatsu, H., K. Inoue, H. Ohta, T. Namba, K. Togawa, T. Hayatsu, M. Makita, and Y. Wataya. 1981b. Inhibition of the mutagenicity of cooked-beef basic fraction by its acidic fraction. Mutat. Res. 91:437-442.

Hirono, I., I. Ueno, S. Hosaka, H. Takanashi, T. Matsushima, T. Sugimura, and S. Natori. 1981. Carcinogenicity examination of quercetin and rutin in ACI rats. Cancer Lett. 13:15-21.

Hollstein, M., and J. McCann. 1979. Short-term tests for carcinogens and mutagens. Mutat. Res. 65:133-226.

Hosaka, S., T. Matsushima, I. Hirono, and T. Sugimura. 1981. Carcinogenic activity of 3-amino-1-methyl-5H-pyrido[4,3-b]indole (TRP-P-2), a pyrolysis product of tryptophan. Cancer Lett. 13:23-28.

Howard, J. W., and T. Fazio. 1980. Analytical methodology and reported findings of polycyclic aromatic hydrocarbons in foods. J. Assoc. Off. Anal. Chem. 63:1077-1104.

Inui, N., Y. Nishi, M. M. Hasegawa, and T. Kawachi. 1980. Induction of 8-azaguanine or ouabain resistant somatic mutation of Chinese hamster lung cells by treatment with tryptophan pyrolysis products. Cancer Lett. 9:185-189.

Ishikawa, T., S. Takayama, T. Kitagawa, T. Kawachi, M. Kinebuchi, N. Matsukura, E. Uchida, and T. Sugimura. 1979. In vivo experiments on tryptophan pyrolysis products. Pp. 159-167 in E. C. Miller, J. A. Miller, I. Hirono, T. Sugimura, and S. Takayama, eds. Naturally Occurring Carcinogens-Mutagens and Modulators of Carcinogenesis. Japan Scientific Societies Press, Tokyo; University Park Press, Baltimore, Md.

Johnson, H. G., and M. K. Bach. 1965. Apparent suppression of mutation rates in bacteria by spermine. Nature 208:408-409.

Kasai, H., S. Nishimura, M. Nagao, Y. Takahashi, and T. Sugimura. 1979. Fractionation of a mutagenic principle from broiled fish by high-pressure liquid chromatography. Cancer Lett. 7:343-348.

Kasai, H., Z. Yamaizumi, K. Wakabayashi, M. Nagao, T. Sugimura, S. Yokoyama, T. Miyazawa, N. E. Spingarn, J. H. Weisburger, and S. Nishimura. 1980a. Potent novel mutagens produced by broiling fish under normal conditions. Proc. Jpn. Acad. 56(B):278-283.

Kasai, H., Z. Yamaizumi, K. Wakabayashi, M. Nagao, T. Sugimura, S. Yokoyama, T. Miyazawa, and S. Nishimura. 1980b. Structure and chemical synthesis of Me-IQ, a potent mutagen isolated from broiled fish. Chem. Lett. 11:1391-1394.

Kasai, H., S. Nishimura, K. Wakabayashi, M. Nagao, and T. Sugimura. 1980c. Chemical synthesis of 2-amino-3-methylimidazo[4,5-f]quinoline (IQ), a potent mutagen isolated from broiled fish. Proc. Jpn. Acad. 56(B):382-384.

Kasai, H., Z. Yamaizumi, T. Shiomi, S. Yokoyama, T. Miyazawa, K. Wakabayashi, M. Nagao, T. Sugimura, and S. Nishimura. 1981. Structure of a potent mutagen isolated from fried beef. Chem. Lett. 4: 485-488.

Katoh, Y., M. Tanaka, K. Umezawa, and S. Takayama. 1980. Inhibition of mutagenesis in Chinese hamster V-79 cells by antioxidants. Toxicol. Lett. 7:125-130.

Koehler, P. E., M. E. Mason, and J. A. Newell. 1969. Formation of pyrazine compounds in sugar-amino acid model systems. J. Agric. Food Chem. 17:393-396.

Krone, C. A., and W. T. Iwaoka. 1981. Mutagen formation during the cooking of fish. Cancer Lett. 14:93-99.

Kubitschek, H. E., and H. E. Bendigkeit. 1958. Delay in the appearance of caffeine-induced T5 resistance in Escherichia coli. Genetics 43:647-661.

Kubitschek, H. E., and H. E. Bendigkeit. 1964. Mutation in continuous cultures. I. Dependence of mutational response upon growth-limiting factors. Mutat. Res. 1:113-120.

Lai, C.-N. 1979. Chlorophyll: The active factor in wheat sprout extract inhibiting the metabolic activation of carcinogens in vitro. Nutr. Cancer 1(3):19-21.

Lai, C.-N., M. A. Butler, and T. S. Matney. 1980. Antimutagenic activities of common vegetables and their chlorophyll content. Mutat. Res. 77:245-250.

Lee, J. S. K., and L. Y. Y. Fong. 1979. Mutagenicity of Chinese alcoholic spirits. Food Cosmet. Toxicol. 17:575-578.

Lijinsky, W., and A. E. Ross. 1967. Production of carcinogenic polynuclear hydrocarbons in the cooking of food. Food Cosmet. Toxicol. 5:343-347.

Lijinsky, W., and P. Shubik. 1964. Benzo(a)pyrene and other polynuclear hydrocarbons in charcoal-broiled meat. Science 145:53-55.

Lintas, C., M. C. De Matthaeis, and F. Merli. 1979. Determination of benzo(a)pyrene in smoked, cooked and toasted food products. Food Cosmet. Toxicol. 17:325-328.

Loquet, C., G. Toussaint, and J. Y. LeTalaer. 1981. Studies on mutagenic constituents of apple brandy and various alcoholic beverages collected in Western France, a high incidence area for oesophageal cancer. Mutat. Res. 88:155-164.

MacGregor, J. T., and L. Jurd. 1978. Mutagenicity of plant flavonoids: Structural requirements for mutagenic activity in Salmonella typhimurium. Mutat. Res. 54:297-309.

Maga, J. A. 1979. Furans in foods. CRC Crit. Rev. Food Sci. Nutr. 11:355-400.

Maruta, A., K. Enaka, and M. Umeda. 1979. Mutagenicity of quercetin and kaempferol on cultured mammalian cells. Gann 70:273-276.

Masuda, Y., K. Mori, and M. Kuratsune. 1966. Polycyclic aromatic hydrocarbons in common Japanese foods. I. Broiled fish, roasted barley, shoyu, and caramel. Gann 57:133-142.

Matsukura, N., T. Kawachi, K. Morino, H. Ohgaki, T. Sugimura, and S. Takayama. 1981a. Carcinogenicity in mice of mutagenic compounds from a tryptophan pyrolyzate. Science 213:346-347.

Matsukura, N., T. Kawachi, K. Wakabayashi, H. Ohgaki, K. Morino, T. Sugimura, H. Nukaya, and T. Kosuge. 1981b. Liver cancer and precancerous changes in rats induced by the basic fraction of tryptophan pyrolysate. Cancer Lett. 13:181-186.

Matsumoto, T., D. Yoshida, S. Mizusaki, and H. Okamoto. 1977. Mutagenic activity of amino acid pyrolyzates in Salmonella typhimurium TA 98. Mutat. Res. 48:279-286.

Matsumoto, T., D. Yoshida, S. Mizusaki, and H. Okamoto. 1978. Mutagenicities of the pyrolyzates of peptides and proteins. Mutat. Res. 56:281-288.

Matsumoto, T., D. Yoshida, and H. Tomita. 1981. Determination of mutagens, amino-α-carbolines in grilled foods and cigarette smoke condensate. Cancer Lett. 12:105-110.

McCann, J., and B. N. Ames. 1976. Detection of carcinogens as mutagens in the Salmonella/microsome test: Assay of 300 chemicals: Discussion. Proc. Natl. Acad. Sci. U.S.A. 73:950-954.

McCann, J., E. Choi, E. Yamasaki, and B. N. Ames. 1975. Detection of carcinogens as mutagens in the Salmonella/microsome test: Assay of 300 chemicals. Proc. Natl. Acad. Sci. U.S.A. 72:5135-5139.

McKee, R. H., and A. M. Tometsko. 1979. Inhibition of promutagen activation by the antioxidants butylated hydroxyanisole and butylated hydroxytoluene. J. Natl. Cancer Inst. 63:473-477.

Meltz, M. L., and J. T. MacGregor. 1981. Activity of the plant flavanol quercetin in the mouse lymphoma L5178Y TK$^{+/-}$ mutation, DNA single-strand break, and Balb/c 3T3 chemical transformation assays. Mutat. Res. 88:317-324.

Morino, K., N. Matsukura, T. Kawachi, H. Ohgaki, T. Sugimura, and I. Hirono. 1982. Carcinogenicity test of quercetin and rutin in golden hamsters by oral administration. Carcinogenesis 3:93-97.

Morita, K., M. Hara, and T. Kada. 1978. Studies on natural desmutagens: Screening for vegetable and fruit factors active in inactivation of mutagenic pyrolysis products from amino acids. Agric. Biol. Chem. 42:1235-1238.

National Cancer Institute. 1978. Bioassay of Aniline Hydrochloride for Carcinogenicity. Carcinogenesis Technical Report Series No. 130. DHEW Publication No. (NIH)78-1385. Carcinogenesis Testing Program, National Cancer Institute, Bethesda, Md. 109 pp.

Nagao, M., M. Honda, Y. Seino, T. Yahagi, and T. Sugimura. 1977a. Mutagenicities of smoke condensates and the charred surface of fish and meat. Cancer Lett. 2:221-226.

Nagao, M., M. Honda, Y. Seino, T. Yahagi, T. Kawachi, and T. Sugimura. 1977b. Mutagenicities of protein pyrolysates. Cancer Lett. 2: 335-340.

Nagao, M., T. Yahagi, T. Kawachi, Y. Seino, M. Honda, N. Matsukura, T. Sugimura, K. Wakabayashi, K. Tsuji, and T. Kosuge. 1977c. Mutagens in foods, and especially pyrolysis products of protein. Pp. 259-264 in D. Scott, B. A. Bridges, and F. H. Sobels, eds. Progress in Genetic Toxicology. Elsevier/North-Holland, New York, Amsterdam, and Oxford.

Nagao, M., T. Yahagi, T. Sugimura, T. Kosuge, K. Tsuji, K. Wakabayashi, S. Mizusakai, and T. Matsumoto. 1977d. Comutagenic action of norharman and harman. Proc. Jpn. Acad. 53(2):95-98.

Nagao, M., T. Yahagi, M. Honda, Y. Seino, T. Matsushima, and T. Sugimura. 1977e. Demonstration of mutagenicity of aniline and o-toluidine by norharman. Proc. Jpn. Acad. 53(B)):34-37.

Nagao, M., Y. Takahashi, H. Yamanaka, and T. Sugimura. 1979. Mutagens in coffee and tea. Mutat. Res. 68:101-106.

Nagao, M., Y. Takahashi, K. Wakabayashi, and T. Sugimura. 1981. Mutagenicity of alcoholic beverages. Mutat. Res. 88:147-154.

Novick, A. 1956. Mutagens and antimutagens. Brookhaven Symp. Biol. 8:201-215.

Pamuckcu, A. M., Ş. Yalçiner, J. F. Hatcher, and G. T. Bryan. 1980. Quercetin, a rat intestinal and bladder carcinogen present in bracken fern (Pteridium aquilinum). Cancer Res. 40:3468-3472.

Poindexter, E. H., Jr., and R. D. Carpenter. 1962. The isolation of harmane and norharmane from tobacco and cigaret smoke. Phytochemistry 1:215-221.

Powrie, W. D., C. H. Wu, M. P. Rosin, and H. F. Stich. 1981. Clastogenic and mutagenic activities of Maillard reaction model systems. J. Food Sci. 46:1433-1438, 1445.

Purchase, I. F. H., E. Longstaff, J. Ashby, J. A. Styles, D. Anderson, P. A. Lefevre, and F. R. Westwood. 1978. An evaluation of 6 shortterm tests for detecting organic chemical carcinogens. Br. J. Cancer 37:873-959.

Rosin, M. P., and H. F. Stich. 1979. Assessment of the use of the Salmonella mutagenesis assay to determine the influence of antioxidants on carcinogen-induced mutagenesis. Int. J. Cancer 23:722-727.

Saito, D., A. Shirai, T. Matsushima, and I. Hirono. 1980. Test of carcinogenicity of quercetin, a widely distributed mutagen in food. Teratog., Carcinog., Mutagen. 1:213-221.

Seino, Y., M. Nagao, T. Yahagi, T. Sugimura, T. Yasuda, and S. Nishimura. 1978. Identification of a mutagenic substance in a spice, sumac, as quercetin. Mutat. Res. 58:225-229.

Seppilli, A., and G. S. Sforzolini. 1963. [In Italian.] Sulla presenza di idrocarburi policiclici cancerigeni nelle carni cotte alla graticola. Boll. Soc. Ital. Biol. Sper. 39:110-111.

Shamberger, R. J., C. L. Corlett, K. D. Beaman, and B. L. Kasten. 1979. Antioxidants reduce the mutagenic effect of malonaldehyde and β-propiolactone. Part IX, Antioxidants and cancer. Mutat. Res. 66:349-355.

Shinohara, K., R.-T. Wu, N. Jahan, M. Tanaka, N. Morinaga, H. Murakami, and H. Omura. 1980. Mutagenicity of the browning mixtures by aminocarbonyl reactions on Salmonella typhimurium TA 100. Agric. Biol. Chem. 44:671-672.

Simmon, V. F. 1979. In vitro mutagenicity assays of chemical carcinogens and related compounds with Salmonella typhimurium. J. Natl. Cancer Inst. 62:893-899.

Spingarn, N. E., and C. T. Garvie. 1979. Formation of mutagens in sugar-ammonia model systems. J. Agric. Food Chem. 27:1319-1321.

Spingarn, N., E., L. A. Slocum, and J. H. Weisburger. 1980a. Formation of mutagens in cooked foods. II. Foods with high starch content. Cancer Lett. 9:7-12.

Spingarn, N. E., H. Kasai, L. L. Vuolo, S. Nishimura, Z. Yamaizumi, T. Sugimura, T. Matsushima, and J. H. Weisburger. 1980b. Formation of mutagens in cooked foods. III. Isolation of a potent mutagen from beef. Cancer Lett. 9:177-183.

Stich, H. F., W. Stich, M. P. Rosin, and W. D. Powrie. 1980. Mutagenic activity of pyrazine derivatives: A comparative study with Salmonella typhimurium, Saccharomyces cerevisiae, and Chinese hamster ovary cells. Food Cosmet. Toxicol. 18:581-584.

Stich, H. F., M. P. Rosin, C. H. Wu, and W. D. Powrie. 1981a. Clastogenicity of furans found in food. Cancer Lett. 13:89-95.

Stich, H. F., W. Stich, M. P. Rosin, and W. D Powrie. 1981b. Clastogenic activity of caramel and caramelized sugars. Mutat. Res. 91:129-136.

Stoltz, D. R., B. Stavric, R. Klassen, and T. Muise. In press a. The health significance of mutagens in foods. In H. F. Stich, ed. Carcinogens and Mutagens in the Environment. Volume 1, Food Products. CRC Press, Boca Raton, Fla.

Stoltz, D. R., B. Stavric, D. Krewski, R. Klassen, R. Bendall, and B. Junkins. In press b. Mutagenicity screening of foods. I. Results with beverages. Environ. Mutagen.

Sugimura, T. In press. Food-born genotoxins. In R. Fleck and A. Hollaender, eds. Genetic Toxicology: An Agricultural Perspective. Plenum Press, New York.

Sugimura, T., and M. Nagao. In press. The use of mutagenicity to evaluate carcinogenic hazards in our daily lives. In J. A. Haddle, ed. Mutagenicity: New Horizons in Genetic Toxicology. Academic Press, New York.

Sugimura, T., S. Sato, M. Nagao, T. Yahagi, T. Matsushima, Y. Seino, M. Takeuchi, and T. Kawachi. 1976. Overlapping of carcinogens and mutagens. Pp. 191-213 in P. N. Magee, S. Takayama, T. Sugimura, and T. Matsuhima, eds. Fundamentals in Cancer Prevention. University Park Press, Baltimore, London, and Tokyo.

Sugimura, T., T. Kawachi, M. Nagao, T. Yahagi, Y. Seino, T. Okamoto, K. Shudo, T. Kosuge, K. Tsuji, K. Wakabayashi, Y. Iitaka, and A. Itai. 1977. Mutagenic principle(s) in tryptophan and phenylalanine pyrolysis products. Proc. Jpn. Acad. 53(1):58-61.

Sugimura, T., M. Nagao, and K. Wakabayashi. 1982. The metabolic aspects of the comutagenic action of norharman. Pp. 1011-1025 in R. Synder, D. Parke, J. J. Kocsis, D. J. Jollow, C. G. Gibson, and C. M. Witmer, eds. Biological Reactive Intermediates 2. Part B. Plenum Press, New York.

Takahashi, Y., M. Nagao, T. Fujino, Z. Yamaizumi, and T. Sugimura. 1979. Mutagens in Japanese pickle identified as flavonoids. Mutat. Res. 68:117-123.

Takase, S., and H. Murakami. 1966. Fluorescence of sake. I. Fluorescence spectrum of sake and identification of harman. Agric. Biol. Chem. 30:869-876.

Takayama, S., Y. Katoh, M. Tanaka, M. Nagao, K. Wakabayashi, and T. Sugimura. 1977. In vitro transformation of hamster embryo cells with tryptophan pyrolysis products. Proc. Jpn. Acad. 53(B):126-129.

Takayama, S., T. Hirakawa, and T. Sugimura. 1978. Malignant transformation in vitro by tryptophan pyrolysis products. Proc. Jpn. Acad. 54(B):418-422.

Takayama, S., T. Hirakawa, M. Tanaka, T. Kawachi, and T. Sugimura. 1979. In vitro transformation of hamster embryo cells with a glutamic acid pyrolysis product. Toxicol. Lett. 4:281-284.

Takeda, K., T. Ohta, K. Shudo, T. Okamoto, K. Tsuji, and T. Kosuge. 1977. Synthesis of a mutagenic principle isolated from tryptophan pyrolyzate. Chem. Pharm. Bull. 25:2145-2146.

Takeuchi, T., K. Ogawa, H. Iinuma, H. Suda, K. Ukita, T. Nagatsu, M. Kato, and H. Umezawa. 1973. Monoamine oxidase inhibitors isolated from fermented broths. J. Antibiot. 26:162-167.

Tamura, G., C. Gold, A. Ferro-Luzzi, and B. N. Ames. 1980. Fecalase: A model for activation of dietary glycosides to mutagens by intestinal flora. Proc. Natl. Acad. Sci. U.S.A. 77:4961-4965.

Tohda, H., A. Oikawa, T. Kawachi, and T. Sugimura. 1980. Induction of sister-chromatid exchanges by mutagens from amino acid and protein pyrolysates. Mutat. Res. 77:65-69.

Tsuda, M., Y. Takahashi, M. Nagao, T. Hirayama, and T. Sugimura. 1980. Inactivation of mutagens from pyrolysates of tryptophan and glutamic acid by nitrite in acidic solution. Mutat. Res. 78:331-339.

Tsuda, M., M. Nagao, T. Hirayama, and T. Sugimura. 1981. Nitrite con-converts 2-amino-α-carboline, an indirect mutagen, into 2-hydroxy-α-carboline, a non-mutagen, and 2-hydroxy-3-nitroso-α-carboline, a direct mutagen. Mutat. Res. 83:61-68.

Umezawa, K., A. Shirai, T. Matsushima, and T. Sugimura. 1978. Comu-tagenic effect of norharman and harman with 2-acetylaminofluorene derivatives. Proc. Natl. Acad. Sci. U.S.A. 75:928-930.

Uyeta, M., T. Kanada, M. Mazaki, S. Taue, and S. Takahashi. 1979. Assaying mutagenicity of food pyrolysis products using the Ames test. Pp. 169-176 in E. C. Miller, J. A. Miller, I. Hirono, T. Sugimura, and S. Takayama, eds. Naturally Occurring Carcinogens-Mutagens and Modulators of Carcinogenesis. Japan Scientific Societies Press, Tokyo; University Park Press, Baltimore, Md.

Uyeta, M., S. Taue, and M. Mazaki. 1981. Mutagenicity of hydrolysates of tea infusions. Mutat. Res. 88:233-240.

Vithayathil, A. J., B. Commoner, S. Nair, and P. Madyastha. 1978. Isola-tion of mutagens from bacterial nutrients containing beef extract. J. Toxicol. Environ. Health 4:189-202.

Wakabayashi, K., K. Tsuji, T. Kosuge, K. Takeda, K. Yamaguchi, K. Shudo, Y. Iitaka, T. Okamoto, T. Yahagi, M. Nagao, and T. Sugimura. 1978. Isolation and structure determination of a mutagenic substance in L-lysine pyrolysate. Proc. Jpn. Acad. 54(B):569-571.

Wakabayashi, K., M. Nagao, T. Kawachi, and T. Sugimura. 1981. Co-muta-genic effect of norharman with N-nitrosamine derivatives. Mutat. Res. 80:1-7.

Watson, W. A. F. 1982. The mutagenic activity of quercetin and kaempferol in Drosophila melanogaster. Mutat. Res. 103:145-147.

Weisburger, J. H., and N. E. Spingarn. 1979. Mutagens as a function of mode of cooking of meats. Pp. 177-184 in E. C. Miller, J. A. Miller, I. Hirono, T. Sugimura, and S. Takayama, eds. Naturally Occurring Carcinogens-Mutagens and Modulators of Carcinogenesis. Japan Scien-tific Societies Press, Tokyo; University Park Press, Baltimore, Md.

Yamaguchi, K., H. Zenda, K. Shudo, T. Kosuge, T. Okamoto, and T. Sugimura. 1979. Presence of 2-aminodipyrido[1,2-a:3',2'-d]imidazole in casein pyrolysate. Gann 70:849-850.

Yamaguchi, K., K. Shudo, T. Okamoto, T. Sugimura, and T. Kosuge. 1980a. Presence of 3-amino-1,4-dimethyl-5H-pyrido[4,3-b]indole in broiled beef. Gann 71:745-746.

Yamaguchi, K., K. Shudo, T. Okamoto, T. Sugimura, and T. Kosuge. 1980b. Presence of 2-aminodipyrido[1,2-a:3'2'-d]imidazole in broiled cuttlefish. Gann 71:743-744.

Yamaizumi, Z., T. Shiomi, H. Kasai, S. Nishimura, Y. Takahashi, M. Nagao, and T. Sugimura. 1980. Detection of potent mutagens, Trp-P-1 and Trp-P-2, in broiled fish. Cancer Lett. 9:75-83.

Yamamoto, T., K. Sutji, T. Kosuge, T. Okamoto, K. Shudo, K. Takeda, Y. Iitaka, K. Yamaguchi, Y. Seino, T. Yahagi, M. Nagao, and T. Sugimura. 1978. Isolation and structure determination of mutagenic substances in L-glutamic acid pyrolysate. Proc. Jpn. Acad. 54(B):248-250.

Yasuda, T., Z. Yamaizumi, S. Nishimura, M. Nagao, Y. Takahashi, H. Fujiki, T. Sugimura, and K. Tsuji. 1978. Detection of comutagenic compounds, harman and norharman in pyrolysis product of proteins and food by gas chromatograph-mass spectrometry. Nippon Gan Gakkai Sokai Kiji 37:6). Abstract 41.

Yoshida, D., and T. Matsumoto. 1978. Changes in mutagenicity of protein pyrolyzates by reaction with nitrite. Mutat. Res. 58:35-40.

Yoshida, D., and H. Okamoto. 1980. Formation of mutagens by heating the aqueous solution of amino acids and some nitrogenous compounds with addition of glucose. Agric. Biol. Chem. 44:2521-2522.

Yoshida, D., T. Matsumoto, R. Yoshimura, and T. Matsuzaki. 1978. Mutagenicity of amino-α-carbolines in pyrolysis products of soybean globulin. Biochem. Biophys. Res. Commun. 83:915-920.

14 Additives and Contaminants

This section contains summaries of data on a few selected compounds that are added directly to foods, as well as for processing aids and some compounds that may migrate into foods in small amounts as a result of their use in packaging.

Saccharin

Saccharin has been used as a nonnutritive sweetener since 1907. In 1977, an estimated 2.2 million kilograms of saccharin and sodium saccharin were produced in the United States and an additional 1.3 million kilograms were imported (National Academy of Sciences, 1978). During that year, approximately 2.9 million kilograms ($\sim$83% of the domestic and imported saccharin) were used in foods (U.S. Department of Agriculture, 1978).

Epidemiological Studies. The use of nonnutritive sweeteners has been studied primarily to determine their relationship to bladder cancer. Results from studies of diabetics did not indicate that there is a direct association between saccharin use and bladder cancer (Armstrong and Doll, 1975; Armstrong et al., 1976; Kessler, 1970); however, diabetics are not generally representative of the general population in epidemiological studies of cancer incidence and mortality since they differ in several important respects. For example, diabetics as a group smoke less, and since smoking is associated with bladder cancer, less cancer at that site might be anticipated among these subjects (Armstrong and Doll, 1975; Christiansen, 1978).

Burbank and Fraumeni (1970) found no increase in mortality from bladder cancer in the United States following the widespread introduction of nonnutritive sweeteners. They examined mortality rates for this cancer after saccharin was introduced early in this century and after a 10:1 mixture of cyclamate:saccharin came into use during 1962. In England and Wales a cohort analysis of bladder cancer mortality from 1911 to 1970 provided no evidence of any disruption of mortality trends for either men or women corresponding to the introduction of saccharin (Armstrong and Doll, 1974). However, time-trend studies generally cannot detect weak effects and can detect no effects for diseases with long latency periods, if only a short time has elapsed between exposure to the substances and the observation.

The consumption of saccharin by bladder cancer patients and healthy controls has been compared in several case-control studies, although

most of these studies were not originally designed to investigate the relationship between nonnutritive sweeteners and bladder cancer.
In a case-control study based on responses to questionnaires from 74 female cases, 158 male cases, and an equal number of matched controls, Morgan and Jain (1974) observed that prolonged use of any nonnutritive sweetener was not associated with an increased risk in males and was associated with a reduced risk for females. In another study based on mailed questionnaires, Simon et al. (1975) studied women only, and found no differences between the cases and controls in either saccharin or cyclamate use.

Howe et al. (1977) conducted a case-control study of 480 male and 152 female sex-matched pairs. They observed that men who used nonnutritive sweeteners had a 60% increase in risk of bladder cancer and provided evidence of a dose-response relationship. On the other hand, there was no significant increase in risk for women. These preliminary findings were confirmed in a later study by the same investigators, who reanalyzed the data, controlling for potential confounding factors such as smoking and using a logistic regression model (Howe et al., 1980).

In a case-control study of 519 bladder cancer patients and twice as many controls, Kessler and Clark (1978) found no evidence of a link between nonnutritive sweetener consumption and bladder cancer. Miller et al. (1978) studied 265 bladder cancer patients and 530 matched controls. They also found no significant risk associated with the regular use of nonnutritive sweeteners. Morrison (1979) found no association between current use of nonnutritive sweeteners and bladder cancer in 13 cases and 10,874 controls.

Morrison and Buring (1980) evaluated the relationship between cancer of the lower urinary tract and the consumption of nonnutritive sweeteners in a case-control study of 592 patients and 596 controls. Overall, there was no increase in risk for lower urinary tract cancer among users of nonnutritive sweeteners. However, in a subgroup of nonsmoking women, there were elevated risks of 2.1 for use of sugar substitutes and 2.6 for use of dietetic beverages.

Wynder and Stellman (1980) conducted a case-control study of 302 men and 65 women with bladder cancer and an equal number of matched controls. They also found no association between bladder cancer and the consumption of nonnutritive sweeteners or dietetic beverages.

The National Cancer Institute (NCI) and the Food and Drug Administration (FDA) jointly sponsored a large scale case-control study in which 3,010 bladder cancer patients and 5,783 population controls were interviewed. This investigation was designed specifically to evaluate the relationship between nonnutritive sweetener consumption and bladder cancer. Subjects who reported ever having used nonnutritive sweeteners or artificially sweetened foods or beverages were found to have no increase in the risk of bladder cancer. However, white nonsmoking women who had not been exposed to known bladder carcinogens such as azo dyes were found to have an increased risk of bladder cancer with increased nonnutritive sweetener consumption (relative risk of 2.7-3.0 in heavy users for at least 10 years and a suggested dose-response relationship). Users of both tabletop sweeteners and diet drinks,with a heavy use of at least one of the two, showed a relative risk of 1.5 (Hoover and Strasser, 1980).

The International Agency for Research on Cancer (1980) concluded, "Although a small increase in the risk of urinary bladder cancer in the general population or a larger increase in some individuals consuming very high doses of saccharin cannot be excluded, the epidemiological data provide no clear evidence that saccharin alone, or in combination with cyclamates, causes urinary bladder cancer."

There have also been some observations concerning consumption of saccharin and cancer at other sites, for example, pancreatic cancer. An increase in deaths from pancreatic cancer was found in cohort studies of diabetics (Armstrong et al., 1976; Kessler, 1970). Blot et al. (1978) found a direct correlation of pancreatic cancer mortality by county in the United States with diabetes mellitus in women, but not in men, who consumed saccharin. In a case-control study, Wynder et al. (1973) found a direct association of pancreatic cancer with early-onset diabetes in women who used saccharin.

Experimental Evidence: Carcinogenicity. The carcinogenicity of saccharin has been reviewed extensively (National Academy of Sciences, 1978). The following discussion focuses on some recent data.

There was no evidence of saccharin-induced carcinogenesis in a number of single-generation studies in which various doses of saccharin were fed to several strains of mice and rats (Furuya et al., 1975; Homburger, 1978; National Institute of Hygienic Sciences, 1973; Roe et al., 1970; Schmähl, 1973) and to hamsters and rhesus monkeys (Althoff et al., 1975; McChesney et al., 1977).

In a single-generation study, Wistar specific-pathogen-free (SPF) rats were fed saccharin at either 4 g/kg body weight (bw) daily in the diet for 2 years or saccharin containing 698 mg/kg o-toluenesulfonamide (OTS) at 2 g/kg bw in drinking water daily for the same period. The treated males in both groups developed more tumors than did the untreated controls, but there was no significant difference in the females (Chowaniec and Hicks, 1979).

In another single-generation study, Charles River CD rats fed 5% sodium saccharin (free of OTS) for their lifetime had a higher incidence of benign and malignant bladder tumors than observed in the untreated controls (D. L. Arnold et al., 1977, 1980).

Saccharin has also been tested in two-generation carcinogenicity bioassays in which parent animals (the F_0 generation) are fed saccharin from weaning through pregnancy until their offspring are weaned. The offspring (F_1 generation), already exposed to saccharin in utero, are given the same diet as their parents for the rest of their lives.

In one such study, there was no difference in the incidence of tumors in treated or control Swiss SPF mice in either generation (Kroes et al., 1977). In three two-generation studies with Charles River and Sprague-Dawley rats (D. L. Arnold et al., 1977, 1980; Taylor and Friedman, 1974; Tisdel et al., 1974; U.S. Department of Health, Education, and Welfare, 1973a,b), the incidence of bladder tumors in treated male rats of the F_1 generations given the highest dose was significantly higher than that in controls in all three studies and in the F_0 males in one study (D. L. Arnold et al., 1977, 1980).

Saccharin (2 or 4 g/kg bw/day in diet) increased the incidence of and decreased the latent period for tumor development in animals treated with N-nitroso-N-methylurea (NMU) (Chowaniec and Hicks, 1979; Hicks et al., 1978) or with N-[4(5-nitro-2-furyl)-2-thiazolyl]formamide (FANFT) (Cohen et al., 1979). In several in vitro cell culture systems, saccharin also exhibited an activity similar to the tumor-promoting activity of tetradecanoylphorbol acetate (Trosko et al., 1980).

Experimental Evidence: Mutagenicity. Efforts to test saccharin for mutagenicity have produced conflicting results. In the Ames Salmonella reverse mutation assay, saccharin of various degrees of purity was not mutagenic (Ashby et al., 1978; McCann, 1977; Poncelot et al., 1979). Batzinger et al. (1977) reported that saccharin was weakly mutagenic to S. typhimurium TA98 and TA100 strains in a modified plate assay and that the urine of animals fed saccharin contained mutagens for TA98 and TA100 strains.

Weak mutagenic effects were observed in the mouse lymphoma assay (Clive et al., 1979). Dominant lethal mutations were found in animals fed 1.72% sodium saccharin in the diet (Rao and Qureshi, 1972), and a dose-dependent increase in unscheduled DNA synthesis in fibroblasts from humans was reported by Ochi and Tonomura (1978).

Continuous exposure to saccharin following treatment of C3H/10T1/2 cells with 3-methylcholanthrene led to a significant increase in the number of transformed colonies (Mondal et al., 1978). Saccharin also induces chromosome aberrations in mammalian cells (Abe and Sasaki, 1977; McCann, 1977; Yoshida et al., 1978) and sister chromatid exchanges in cells from humans (Wolff and Rodin, 1978).

Summary and Conclusions. The epidemiological data do not provide a clear indication of an association between the use of nonnutritive sweeteners and cancer, and the results of most studies of bladder cancer have shown no association. Exceptions are the study by Howe et al. (1977), which showed a direct association in men, and those by Hoover and Strasser (1980) and Morrison and Buring (1980), whose results suggested a possible effect in certain subgroups. Since the data regarding saccharin and pancreatic cancer are based on studies of diabetics, who as a group are not representative of the general population, no firm conclusions can be drawn.

Experimental studies have provided sufficient evidence that saccharin alone, given at high doses, produces tumors of the urinary tract in male rats and can promote the action of known carcinogens in the bladder of rats. There is limited evidence of its carcinogenicity in mice.

Cyclamates

Until 1970, when cyclamates were banned from use in the United States (U.S. Food and Drug Administration, 1970), cyclamic acid, sodium cyclamate, and calcium cyclamate were used as nonnutritive sweeteners in carbonated beverages, in dry beverage bases, in diet foods, and in sweetener formulations. Sodium and calcium cyclamates were used primarily as a 10:1 cyclamate:saccharin salt mixture (Wiegand, 1978).

Epidemiological Evidence. Epidemiological data on cyclamates alone are not adequate, because cyclamates were rarely used without saccharin. Thus, it was not usually possible to distinguish the consumption of cyclamate-containing mixtures from the consumption of saccharin.

Experimental Evidence: Carcinogenicity. Swiss and Charles River CD mice receiving up to 5% sodium cyclamate for 18 months or 24 months, respectively, did not yield evidence that cyclamates are carcinogenic (Homburger, 1978; Roe et al., 1970). When sodium cyclamate (99.5% pure) was administered in drinking water (6 g/liter, or 20-25 mg/mouse) to mice for their lifetime, there was no evidence of carcinogenesis in male and female C3H mice, but there was an increased incidence of lung tumors in RIII male and XVII female mice and of hepatocellular carcinomas in (C3H x RIII)F_1 male mice (Rudali et al., 1969). Female SPF mice fed diets containing up to 7% sodium cyclamate for 80 weeks had a higher, but statistically insignificant increase in the incidence of lymphosarcomas than did the controls (Brantom et al., 1973).

Osborne Mendel rats fed sodium cyclamate at 0.4%, 2%, or 10% in their diet for 101 weeks had an increased incidence of transitional cell papillomas of the urinary bladder, although the number of animals examined histopathologically was small (Friedman et al., 1972). Cyclamate (1.0 g/kg bw/day) fed for 2 years led to a slight increase in the incidence of bladder tumors in Sprague-Dawley rats (Hicks and Chowaniec, 1977; Hicks et al., 1978).

Lifetime studies in one generation of Syrian golden hamsters (Althoff et al., 1975) and rhesus monkeys (Coulston et al., 1977) and a six-generation study of Swiss SPF mice (Kroes et al., 1977) produced no evidence that sodium cyclamate is carcinogenic.

Female Wistar SPF rats treated with 1.5 mg NMU and subsequently fed sodium cyclamate (containing 13 mg/kg cyclohexylamine) in diets at doses of 1, 1.5, or 2.0 g/kg bw/day for their lifetime or up to 2 years had a significantly higher incidence of bladder cancer and a significant decrease in latent period (8 weeks vs. 87 weeks) compared to animals treated with NMU only and the untreated controls (Hicks et al., 1978).

In another study, a single 2 mg dose of NMU was instilled into the urinary bladder of female Wistar rats before giving them a diet containing sodium cyclamate at 2% for 10 weeks and then at 4% for the rest of their lives. The overall incidence of urinary tract tumors was 70% in those given NMU and sodium cyclamate, 57% in animals receiving NMU alone, and 65% in another control group given NMU and calcium carbonate (Mohr et al., 1978).

Wistar weanling rats were fed a 10:1 mixture of sodium cyclamate: saccharin in the diet at doses of 0, 500, 1,120, or 2,500 mg/kg bw/day for 2 years. After the 79th week, 50% of the survivors from all three treated groups were also fed cyclohexylamine hydrochloride, in addition to the cyclamate:saccharin diet. The animals consuming the diet containing the highest levels of cyclamate:saccharin (with and without added cyclohexylamine hydrochloride) were found to have a significantly higher number of urinary bladder cancers (9/25 males and 3/35 females) compared to the controls (0/35 males and 0/45 females). Of the tumor-bearing animals, three males and two females had received cyclohexylamine, indicating that cyclohexylamine hydrochloride is not carcinogenic (Oser et al., 1975).

Experimental Evidence: Mutagenicity. There are no published data on the ability of cyclamates alone to induce point mutations in microbial and mammalian cells. In two studies, cyclamates induced chromosome breaks in leukocytes from humans (Ebenezer and Sadasivan, 1970; Tokumitsu, 1971).

No increase in chromosome aberrations was observed in hamsters given oral doses of sodium cyclamate or cyclohexylamine sulfate (Machemer and Lorke, 1976).

Summary and Conclusions. There are no adequate epidemiological data on the effect of cyclamate alone since it was rarely consumed by humans in the absence of saccharin.

The experimental data provide limited evidence for the carcinogenicity of cyclamates in mice and rats. In addition, there is evidence that cyclamates can promote the action of known carcinogens in the bladder.

Aspartame

Aspartame, the methyl ester of the amino acids phenylalanine and aspartic acid, is approximately 180 times sweeter than sugar (Mazur, 1976). In July 1981 the FDA approved its use as a sweetener or flavoring agent in certain foods (U.S. Food and Drug Administration, 1981). Aspartame cannot be used in soft drinks because of its instability in liquids during storage.

Epidemiological Evidence. Since aspartame has been on the market only since 1981 and in only a few countries (e.g., Belgium, France, and Canada), there are no epidemiological data regarding its association with cancer in humans.

Experimental Evidence: Carcinogenicity. A number of feeding studies have been conducted on mice and rats under the sponsorship of the G. D. Searle Co. to test the carcinogenicity of aspartame. In one of these studies, male and female Charles River mice received aspartame at 0 (control), 1.0, 2.0, or 4.0 g/kg bw/day in their diet for 2 years. No tumors attributable to aspartame ingestion were reported (G. D. Searle and Co., 1974a). In another study, no statistically significant differences in the incidence of neoplasms were observed in the urinary bladders of control and treated mice 26 weeks after implantation of cholesterol pellets containing aspartame or its breakdown product diketopiperazine (DKP) (G. D. Searle and Co., 1973a).

Male and female Sprague-Dawley rats fed aspartame in the diet at various levels for up to 2 years were observed for the incidence of brain tumors (G. D. Searle and Co., 1973b). After the study was completed, the FDA appointed an independent board of inquiry to review the data. The board concluded that aspartame was a possible carcinogen, based on three of the study's findings: The incidence of brain neoplasms in aspartame-fed rats was greater than that in controls, a possible dose response was observed when tumor incidence in the controls was compared with the two lower dose and the two higher dose treatment groups combined, and there was a decrease in the latent period for gliomas (U.S. Food and Drug Administration, 1980a).

Investigators at the G. D. Searle Co. interpreted these data differently. They contended that statistical analysis using concurrent instead of historical controls indicates that there was no significant increase in tumor incidence, that more appropriate statistical tests show no dose response, and that the board of inquiry made errors concerning the time of death of certain rats (U.S. Food and Drug Administration, 1980a).

In a follow-up study by the Searle group, rats were exposed in utero to aspartame at 0 (control), 2, and 4 g/kg bw and maintained on this diet for the duration of their lives (G. D. Searle and Co., 1974b).

The incidence of brain tumors was: 4/115 (3.4%), 3/75 (4.0%), and 1/80 (1.3%), respectively, which indicated no statistically significant difference between the control and treated groups.

Recently, Ishii et al. (1981) also found no evidence for carcinogenicity in chronic feeding studies with Wistar rats given aspartame or a mixture of aspartame and DKP. The FDA concluded that this study provides additional evidence favoring the safety of aspartame (U.S. Food and Drug Administration, 1981).

Groups of five male and female beagle dogs were fed aspartame at 0 (control), 1.0, 2.0, and 4.0 g/kg bw in their diet for more than 106 weeks. No evidence of neoplasia was observed in any of the treated or control groups (G. D. Searle and Co., 1973c).

Experimental Evidence: Mutagenicity. Aspartame and DKP were negative in the Ames test with and without using the S9 fraction from rats (G. D. Searle and Co., 1978a,b,c). Similarly, no evidence of the mutagenicity of these compounds was observed in the host-mediated assay in rats and mice at doses ranging from 0.25 to 8.0 g/kg/day (G. D. Searle and Co., 1972a,b, 1974c). Aspartame and DKP (1 or 2 g/kg bw/day) were also negative in the in vivo dominant lethal assay in rats (G. D. Searle and Co., 1973d).

Summary and Conclusions. Aspartame has been used as a sweetener in Belgium and France only since 1981. It has recently been approved for use in Canada and the United States. Consequently, there are no epidemiological data pertaining to its effects on human health.

Aspartame appears to be negative in in vitro bacterial mutagenicity tests, in the host-mediated assay, and in dominant lethal tests in rats. It has been reported to be noncarcinogenic in chronic feeding studies in mice and dogs, most of which were conducted by G. D. Searle and Company. Although a board of inquiry appointed by the FDA concluded that aspartame may be neurooncogenic in rats, additional evidence led the FDA to conclude that aspartame is not carcinogenic in animals.

Butylated Hydroxytoluene (BHT) and Butylated Hydroxyanisole (BHA)

Butylated hydroxytoluene (BHT) and butylated hydroxyanisole (BHA) are widely used as food additives, mainly because of their preservative and antioxidant properties. These compounds are included in the FDA's list of substances generally recognized as safe (GRAS). Many studies have been conducted to test them for acute and chronic toxicity under a variety of experimental conditions, ranging from in vitro studies to in vivo studies in animals (U.S. Food and Drug Administration, 1977a). Based on the evidence from these studies, the FDA in 1977 recommended that BHT be removed from the GRAS list and proposed interim regulations pending future studies.

Epidemiological Evidence. There are no epidemiological studies concerning the effects of BHT and BHA on human health.

Experimental Evidence for BHT: Carcinogenicity. Male and female B6C3F$_1$ mice were fed 0, 0.3%, or 0.6% BHT in the diet for 107 to 108 weeks. In female mice receiving the low dose, the incidence of alveolar/bronchiolar adenomas or carcinomas was significantly higher than in the controls, but there was no dose response (National Cancer Institute, 1979a). In a similar study of male and female Fischer 344 rats, the incidence of tumors in treated animals was not statisically different from that in controls (National Cancer Institute, 1979a).

Experimental Evidence for BHT: Promoting Effects. Three groups of A/J mice were injected with urethan, 3-methylcholanthrene, or nitrosodimethylamine and then given repeated injections of BHT. The treatment with BHT significantly increased the multiplicity of lung tumors induced by all three carcinogens (Witschi et al., 1981).

BHT administered orally increased the incidence of lung tumors in A/J mice pretreated with a single dose of urethan (Witschi, 1981). When injections were begun as late as 5 months after the urethan was administered, they still produced an increase in the incidence of lung tumors. BHT does not appear to enhance lung tumor formation, even if given repeatedly prior to urethan administration. This suggests that BHT may be a tumor promoter (Witschi, 1981; Witschi et al., 1977). BHT also appears to have some promoting activity in BALB/c mice (Clapp et al., 1974) and in male Sprague-Dawley rats treated with 2-aminoacetyl-fluorene (2-AAF) (Peraino et al., 1977).

Experimental Evidence for BHT: Mutagenicity. BHT inhibited cell-to-cell communication of mammalian cells in vitro--an indication of promoting activity (Trosko et al., 1982). When BHT in concentrations of 0-50 μg/ml were added to phytohemagglutinin-stimulated cultures of leukocytes from humans, it resulted in a dose-dependent decrease in cell survival, as well as in an uncoiling of the chromosomes (Sciorra et al., 1974). In the sister chromatid exchange assay, BHT was negative and it did not induce chromosome aberrations (Abe and Sasaki, 1977).

Experimental Evidence for BHA: Carcinogenicity. The administration of BHA had no significant effect on the tumor yield or tumor multiplicity in Swiss Webster mice injected with urethan and then given BHA in the diet (Witschi, 1981). In other experiments, repeated intraperitoneal injections of BHA at high doses produced a slight, although not statistically significant, increase in lung tumors in male A/J mice (Witschi et al., 1981). Under different experimental conditions, BHA has been shown to inhibit the activity of a wide variety of carcinogens (see Chapter 15).

Experimental Evidence for BHA: Mutagenicity. BHA was positive in the sister chromatid exchange assay with Chinese hamster cells as indicator organisms; however, it did not induce chromosome aberrations in these cells (Abe and Sasaki, 1977).

Summary and Conclusions. BHT and BHA are used as antioxidants and
preservatives in many types of foods. There are no epidemiological
studies concerning their effect on human health.

At least one adequate bioassay to test the carcinogenicity of
BHT has been conducted in each of two species, the mouse and the
rat, without clear evidence of carcinogenicity under the conditions
of the tests. Evidence for the enhancement of tumorigenesis by BHT
is restricted to two experimental systems—carcinogen-induced lung
tumors in mice and liver tumors in rats. The studies in mice have
been repeated several times with other carcinogenic initiators.
These studies provide evidence that BHT has a tumor-promoting effect,
especially for urethan and 2-AAF. On the other hand, as discussed in
Chapter 15, large amounts of BHT can inhibit neoplasia induced by a
number of chemicals.

There is no indication that BHA has any carcinogenic or tumor-
promoting activity. Its ability to inhibit neoplasia is discussed
in Chapter 15.

Vinyl Chloride

Containers made of polyvinyl chloride (PVC) are widely used for
packaging and storing foods. Since the appearance of reports linking
several fatal cases of a rare form of liver tumor with prolonged
industrial exposure to vinyl chloride, considerable attention has been
paid to the possible carcinogenicity and other toxic effects of the
monomer vinyl chloride, of which PVC is composed (Creech and Johnson,
1974; Nicholson et al., 1975).

PVC is classified as an indirect food additive by the FDA, whereas
the monomer, which may be present at low levels as a residue in PVC, is
regarded as a contaminant (U.S. Consumer Product Safety Commission,
1974).

Vinyl chloride has been detected in a variety of alcoholic drinks
at levels ranging from 0.2 to 1 mg/liter (Williams, 1976a,b) and in
vinegars at levels as high as 9.4 mg/liter (Williams and Miles, 1975).
It has also been found in products packaged and stored in polyvinyl
chloride containers. For example, concentrations ranging from 0.05 to
14.8 mg/kg have been detected in edible oils (Rösli et al., 1975),
0.05 mg/kg has been detected in margarine and butter (Fuchs et al.,
1975), and 10.0 µg/liter is the highest concentration found in finished
drinking water in the United States (U.S. Environmental Protection
Agency, 1975a).

Epidemiological Evidence. There have been no epidemiological
studies on exposure to vinyl chloride as a food contaminant; however,

several investigators have studied the effect of occupational exposure. In the United States, Creech and Johnson (1974) were the first to report an association between inhalation exposure to vinyl chloride and hepatic angiosarcomas. In a cohort study of males who had been occupationally exposed to vinyl chloride for at least 1 year, Tabershaw and Gaffey (1974) observed an excess of cancer of the digestive system, liver (mainly angiosarcoma), respiratory tract, and brain, as well as lymphomas. Nicholson et al. (1975) noted a 2.3-fold excess of cancer mortality among workers exposed for at least 5 years. Monson et al. (1974) reported a 50% excess of deaths due to all cancers in workers producing and polymerizing vinyl chloride. Several other studies have indicated an association between exposure to vinyl chloride and increased mortality from cancer at various sites (Duck and Carter, 1976; Fox and Collier, 1977; Waxweiler et al., 1976).

Experimental Evidence: Carcinogenicity. Male and female Sprague-Dawley rats receiving gastric intubations of vinyl chloride in doses up to 50 mg/kg bw developed mainly angiosarcomas and cancers of Zymbal's gland (Maltoni, 1977; Maltoni et al., 1975).

In lifetime feeding studies with Wistar rats, Feron et al. (1975, 1981) observed that vinyl chloride monomer in doses ranging from 1.7 to 14.1 mg/kg bw induced hepatocellular carcinomas, hepatic angiosarcomas, pulmonary angiosarcomas, extrahepatic abdominal angiosarcomas, tumors of Zymbal's gland, abdominal mesotheliomas, and adenocarcinomas of mammary glands.

Inhalation exposures to vinyl chloride produced cancers of the lung, mammary gland, and liver in mice (Maltoni, 1977); cancers of Zymbal's gland, the liver, kidney, and brain in Sprague-Dawley rats (Maltoni et al., 1974); and cancers of the liver, skin, and stomach in hamsters (Maltoni, 1977; Maltoni et al., 1974).

Experimental Evidence: Mutagenicity Tests and Other Short-Term Tests. Vinyl chloride vapors induced mutations in Ames Salmonella strains (Andrews et al., 1976; Bartsch et al., 1979), Escherichia coli (Greim et al., 1975), Schizosaccharomyces pombe (Loprieno et al., 1976), Drosophila melanogaster (Verburgt and Vogel, 1977), and mammalian cells (Huberman et al., 1975). They also induced gene conversions in yeast (Eckardt et al., 1981).

Male workers occupationally exposed to vinyl chloride were reported to have more chromosome aberrations than were observed in unexposed cohorts (Funes-Cravioto et al., 1975; Heath et al., 1977; Purchase et al., 1975).

Summary and Conclusions. Occupational exposure to vinyl chloride is associated with increased incidence of cancer of the liver, brain, respiratory tract, and lymphatic system, but this evidence has been derived from studies of groups occupationally exposed to high doses of vinyl chloride. Similar carcinogenic effects were demonstrated in rats that ingested or inhaled large amounts of vinyl chloride. These results were later confirmed in mice and hamsters.

Vinyl chloride is mutagenic in bacteria, yeast, Drosophila, and mammalian cells. It also has clastogenic effects on humans.

Acrylonitrile

Acrylonitrile is produced on a large scale in industry. Its occurrence in foods as an "indirect" additive or contaminant may be attributed to its use in food packaging and the migratory quality of the monomer, which is present in small amounts in the polymer. For example, in a preliminary analysis of three foods wrapped in acrylonitrile-based packaging materials (margarine, olive oil, and bologna), C. V. Breder (U.S. Food and Drug Administration, personal communication, 1980) detected acrylonitrile in concentrations ranging from 13 to 49 ng/kg.

Epidemiological Evidence. Exposure of the general public to acrylonitrile could occur through migration of the residual monomer in polymeric products in contact with food or potable water. The significance of such exposure has not yet been evaluated. However, a retrospective cohort study of 1,345 male employees possibly exposed to acrylonitrile at a DuPont textile plant indicated that there was a trend toward increased risk of cancer at all sites, especially the lung. The risk was greater as the duration and amount of exposure increased (O'Berg, 1980).

Experimental Evidence: Carcinogenicity. Rats receiving acrylonitrile in drinking water in doses of 100 or 300 mg/liter for 12 months developed stomach papillomas, tumors of the central nervous system, and carcinomas of Zymbal's gland (Norris, 1977). In an inhalation study with acrylonitrile, rats developed tumors of the central nervous system and ear duct, as well as masses in the mammary region (Norris, 1977).

Experimental Evidence: Mutagenicity. Acrylonitrile induced mutations in the Ames test in Salmonella strains TA1535, TA1538, and TA78 (Milvy, 1978; Milvy and Wolff, 1977) and in E. coli (Venitt et al., 1977). But chromosome aberrations in workers exposed to acrylonitrile for an average of 15.3 years did not exceed those in unexposed controls (Thiess and Fleig, 1978).

Summary and Conclusions. There is no information on the health effects resulting from the ingestion of small amounts of acrylonitrile monomer in the diet. Humans potentially exposed to acrylonitrile in a synthetic fiber plant were found to be at an increased risk of cancer, particularly of the lung, but there is no further information on this subject. In experiments in rats, ingestion or inhalation of large amounts of acrylonitrile enhanced tumors at several sites. This limited evidence, combined with the finding that acrylonitrile is mutagenic, suggests that acrylonitrile may be carcinogenic in humans.

Diethylstilbestrol (DES)

Considerable attention has centered on the public health consequences of drug residues in animal tissues consumed by humans. Among the approximately 20 growth hormones commonly used in animal feed, attention has mainly focused on diethylstilbestrol (DES), whose residues have been monitored for many years following reports that DES was carcinogenic in animals (Fitzhugh, 1964; Jukes, 1974). Until June 1978, DES was permitted for use by humans as a control for functional menstrual disorders; for prevention of postpartum breast engorgement; as therapy for estrogen deficiencies associated with the climacteric and other hormone-related conditions; as a "morning-after pill"; and as chemotherapy for prostate cancer and for breast cancer in postmenopausal women.

Until 1979, when the use of DES was terminated, it was also permitted as a growth promoter for cattle and sheep under certain conditions delineated by the FDA (Code of Federal Regulations, 1978; U.S. Food and Drug Administration, 1979).

In 1972 and 1973, the U.S. Department of Agriculture detected DES residues in beef liver at levels of 2 and 0.5 µg/kg, respectively (Jukes, 1976; Mussman, 1975). Since 1973 no residues of DES have been detected in 99.4% of a small number of beef livers sampled by methods that have a detection limit of 0.5 µg/liter (Rurainski et al., 1977).

Epidemiological Evidence. There are no reports of epidemiological studies concerning the health effects of DES residues in food. Therapeutic doses of DES during pregnancy have been associated with an increase in vaginal and cervical adenocarcinoma among the daughters of DES users, primarily in those between the ages of 10 and 30 years (Greenwald et al., 1973; Herbst and Cole, 1978; Herbst et al., 1972; Hill, 1973).

Cases of breast cancer in men treated with DES for prostate cancer have been observed after the start of the treatment (Bülow et al., 1973). Of 24 female patients treated with DES for 5 years or more for gonadal dysgenesis (Turner's syndrome), two developed endometrial carcinoma (Cutler et al., 1972), but the risk of endometrial carcinoma in untreated patients is not known.

Experimental Evidence: Carcinogenicity. DES fed to C3H female mice in concentrations ranging from 6.26 to 1,000 µg/kg diet produced mammary carcinomas in increasing incidence with increased doses (Gass et al., 1964). At the highest doses (500 and 1,000 µg/kg diet), the latent period was reduced from 49 weeks to 31 weeks. Male C3H mice developed mammary carcinomas when fed DES at doses of 500 µg/kg diet or more (Gass et al., 1964).

In C3H/An mice fed DES at 0 and 250 µg/kg diet for 18 months, the incidence of mammary cancers was significantly higher than in the controls (Gass et al., 1974).

Sprague-Dawley rats fed DES at 0.02 or 0.2 mg/kg bw in the diet daily for 2 years developed pituitary tumors (males only), some hepatomas (females only), and mammary tumors (males and females) (Gibson et al., 1967). In the progeny of pregnant Syrian golden hamsters administered DES by intragastric tube, there was a high incidence of metaplastic, dysplastic, and neoplastic lesions in the genital tract (Rustia, 1979; Rustia and Shubik, 1976).

Experimental Evidence: Mutagenicity and Other Short-Term Tests. DES was not mutagenic in the Ames test with and without metabolic activation (Glatt et al., 1979; McCann and Ames, 1976) and in E. coli (Fluck et al., 1976). It induced chromosome aberrations in Chinese hamster fibroblasts (Ishidate and Odashima, 1977) and in murine bone marrow cells in vivo (Ivett and Tice, 1981). In other studies, DES induced mutations in mouse lymphoma cells (Clive, 1977), unscheduled DNA synthesis in HeLa cells (Martin et al., 1978), and aneuploidy in vivo in several strains of mice (Chrisman, 1974).

Summary and Conclusions. There is sufficient evidence that DES used in therapeutic doses produces vaginal and cervical cancer in the female offspring of treated women. In animals, it produces mainly mammary tumors in various species.

ENVIRONMENTAL CONTAMINANTS

Environmental contaminants in food can be loosely divided into three categories: some trace metals and organometallic compounds, some natural and synthetic radioactive substances, and some natural and synthetic organic compounds. Only a few pesticides, two industrial chemicals, and some contaminants falling into the third category are discussed in this section.

Pesticides

Residues of pesticides often remain on agricultural commodities after they have been harvested and prepared for consumer purchase. They are also found in processed foods derived from these commodities.

Despite extensive exposure of the general population to low levels of pesticides from numerous sources, especially foods and drinking water, very little reliable information is available about their effects on human health. Nevertheless, since many pesticides whose residues are present in food are known or suspected of being carcinogenic in some animal species, there is a basis for concern about their potential effects on human health. Although the use of several organochlorine compounds has been gradually suspended by the Environmental Protection Agency, some concern is still warranted because they have a propensity to persist in the environment, to accumulate in foods commonly consumed by humans (U.S. Department of Health, Education, and Welfare, 1969; U.S. Food and Drug Administration, 1980b), and to concentrate in body tissues (International Agency for Research on Cancer, 1979).

The general population is exposed to these compounds principally through food and drinking water (International Agency for Research on Cancer, 1979). As demonstrated by the Market Basket Surveys conducted since the early 1960s by the FDA, the levels of pesticides in food are very low and they vary only slightly from region to region. The organochlorine compounds tend to accumulate in fat-containing foods such as meat, fish, poultry, and dairy products, whereas the organophosphates are generally more common in cereal products (U.S. Food and Drug Administration, 1980b).

This section focuses on only a few pesticides—primarily, the organochlorine insecticides and miticides, some organophosphates, and two carbamate insecticides. These compounds have been selected because most of them are monitored regularly through the Market Basket Surveys (U.S. Food and Drug Administration, 1980b), because they were or are used widely and, therefore, present a greater probability for human exposure, and because many of them, especially the cyclodienes and their epoxides, are believed to be potentially hazardous to human health (International Agency for Research on Cancer, 1974, 1979; National Academy of Sciences, 1977).

Epidemiological Evidence. Two cross-sectional studies were conducted on workers engaged in the manufacture of dichlorodiphenyltrichloroethane (DDT). In one, 40 men exposed to an estimated 10 to 40 mg DDT daily, mainly through inhalation or dermal contact over 1 to 8 years, showed no evidence of neoplasia (Ortelee, 1958). In the second, no cases of cancer or blood dyscrasia were reported among 35 workers exposed to 3 to 18 mg DDT daily for 11 to 19 years (Laws et al., 1967).

More than 30 cases of aplastic anemia associated with exposure to toxaphene, lindane, or benzene hexachloride have been reported (International Agency for Research on Cancer, 1974; West, 1967; U.S. Environmental Protection Agency, 1980). Jedlička et al. (1958) described a family with two boys who developed leukemia 8 months after exposure to lindane in an agricultural distribution center. Infante et al. (1978) reported 14 cases of neuroblastoma over a 16-month period. Of these, five were in children who were unintentionally exposed pre- and postnatally to chlordane formulations.

Wang and MacMahon (1979) reported that there was no overall excess in mortality from cancer and no significant excess in deaths due to lung cancer among 7,403 workers employed for 3 or more months in plants manufacturing chlordane and heptachlor. However, no definitive conclusions can be drawn because the population was small, and the period of follow-up was short.

In a case-control study of 60 subjects and 120 controls, Wang and Grufferman (1981) found no correlation between the disappearance data for various chlorinated hydrocarbons and mortality (during 1950-1975) from aplastic anemia among workers engaged in occupations associated with such exposure.

Jager (1970) and Versteeg and Jager (1973) reported a follow-up study of 233 workers who were exposed to aldrin and dieldrin for as long as 17.5 years (average, 7.6 years). One death due to stomach cancer was reported among the 181 workers still employed by the firm at the time of the study in 1968.

The EPA conducted a survey of 199 workers exposed to toxaphene for an average of 5.23 years between 1949 and 1977 (U.S. Department of Agriculture, 1977). Among the 20 deaths that occurred, one was due to stomach cancer.

Barthel (1976) reported a high incidence of lung cancer (11 cases versus 0.54 expected) among 316 farm workers exposed to various pesticides including DDT, toxaphene, lindane (γ-benzene hexachloride), hexachlorobenzene (HCB), and parathion for 6 to 23 years. Whether cancer was associated with exposure to individual pesticides is difficult to determine because the investigator did not control for smoking, and the workers were exposed to various chemicals simultaneously or alternately.

Experimental Evidence. Tables 14-1, 14-2, and 14-3 present the results of carcinogenicity and mutagenicity tests for some organochlorine compounds, some organophosphates, and two carbamates. Only studies in which the chemical was administered orally have been included in the evaluation for carcinogenicity.

For most organochlorine pesticides, the evidence for carcinogenicity is based on the production of parenchymal liver-cell tumors in mice. With the exception of methoxychlor, which has not been found to be mutagenic or carcinogenic, all other organochlorine compounds listed in Table 14-1 appear to be weakly carcinogenic in mice. Results from tests in rats indicate that toxaphene and Kepone (chlordecone) are carcinogenic and that heptachlor (with chlordane), hexachlorobenzene, and lindane may be carcinogenic. Hexachlorobenzene also causes cancer in hamsters.

In bioassays conducted by the National Cancer Institute (1978a, 1979b,c,d,e), the organophosphates malathion, methyl parathion, and diazinon did not lead to an increase in tumor incidence in rats or mice (Table 14-2). However, parathion resulted in an increased incidence of cortical tumors of the adrenal gland in Osborne Mendel rats (National Cancer Institute, 1979f). Parathion and diazinon were not mutagenic in bacterial tests, but studies have indicated that parathion induces chromosome abnormalities in guinea pigs (Dikshith, 1973) and that diazinon induces them in the lymphocytes of humans (Huang, 1973). Aldicarb is a highly toxic compound, as indicated in Table 14-3, but it does not appear

14-16

TABLE 14-1

Carcinogenicity of Some Organochlorine Pesticides

Pesticide	ADI[a] (μg/kg bw)	Daily Dietary Intake (μg/kg bw), by year[b]	Mutagenicity and Related Tests	Carcinogenicity (Oral Administration Only)[c]
Dieldrin	0.1 (Total, including aldrin)	1975 - 0.0387 1977 - 0.0405 1979 - 0.0156	Negative in Ames test (McCann et al., 1975)	Significant increase in hepatocellular carcinoma in mice (National Cancer Institute, 1978b; Thorpe and Walker, 1973), but not in rats (National Cancer Institute, 1978c)
DDT	5.0 (Total, including dichlorodiphenyl-dichloroethylene [DDE] and trichlorodiphenyl-dichloroethylene [TDE])	1975 - 0.0152 1977 - 0.0057 1979 - 0.0041	Negative in Ames test (Bartsch et al., 1980; Marshall et al., 1976) and in host-mediated assay and dominant lethal tests in mice (Buselmaier et al., 1973)	Significant increase in hepatocellular carcinoma in several strains of mice (Innes et al., 1969; Terracini et al., 1973; Thorpe and Walker, 1973; World Health Organization, 1973); negative in mice and rats (National Cancer Institute, 1978d)
Captan	10.0	1975 - ND[d] 1977 - 0.0305 1979 - 0.0294	Positive in Ames test (McCann et al., 1975; Simmon et al., 1979), E. coli, S. cerevisiae, and B. subtilis (Simmon et al., 1979)	Significant increase in duodenal tumors in B6C3F1 mice; inconclusive in rats (National Cancer Institute, 1977a)
Heptachlor and heptachlor epoxide	0.5 (total for both)	1975 - 0.0072 1977 - 0.0074 1979 - 0.0058	Negative in Salmonella with or without metabolic activation (Marshall et al., 1976) and in dominant lethal tests in mice (D. W. Arnold et al., 1977)	Significant increase in hepatocellular carcinoma in mice and in multiple tumors in female rats (Epstein, 1976; National Cancer Institute, 1977b)
Pentachloronitrobenzene (PCNB)	7.0	1975 - 0.0004 1977 - 0.0010 1979 - 0.0006	Negative in reversion tests in Salmonella, yeast, E. coli, and B. subtilis (Simmon et al., 1976)	Significant increase in hepatomas in one strain of male mice (Innes et al., 1969), but not in Osborne Mendel rats or B6C3F1 mice (National Cancer Institute, 1978e)
Hexachlorobenzene	NE[e]	1975 - 0.0046 1977 - 0.0019 1979 - 0.0032	Negative in yeast and in dominant lethal test in rats (Guerzoni et al., 1976; Khera, 1974)	Significant increase in liver cell tumors in mice (Cabral et al., 1979) and in hepatomas, liver hemangiotheliomas, and thyroid adenomas in hamsters (Cabral et al., 1977)

Pesticide	ADI[a]	Residue levels[b]	Mutagenicity	Carcinogenicity
Methoxychlor	100[f]	1975 – 0.0037 1977 – 0.0078 1979 – 0.0032	Negative in Salmonella with or without metabolic activation, and in E. coli (Simmon et al., 1979)	No significant increase in tumors or decrease in age at which tumors occurred in mice (Deichmann et al., 1967) or rats (National Cancer Institute, 1978f)
Toxaphene	NE	1975 – 0.0072 1977 – 0.0802 1979 – 0.0035	Positive in Salmonella (Hooper et al., 1979); negative for dominant lethals in mice (Epstein et al., 1972)	Dose-related increase in hepatocellular carcinoma in mice and thyroid tumors in rats (National Cancer Institute, 1979g)
Lindane	10	1975 – 0.0031 1977 – 0.0038 1979 – 0.0038	Positive for chromosome aberrations, polyploidy and mitotic arrest in plant systems, and chromatid breaks in human lymphocytes in vitro (International Agency for Research on Cancer, 1979)	Significant increase in liver tumors in two studies in mice (Nagasaki et al., 1971; Thorpe and Walker, 1973); inconclusive in rats (National Cancer Institute, 1977c)
Chlordane	1	Oxychlordane 1975 – 0.0017 1977 – 0.0025 1979 – 0.0041 Trans-monachlor 1975 – 0.0004 1977 – 0.0020 1979 – 0.0004	Not mutagenic in Ames test (Tardiff et al., 1976) and negative in dominant lethal tests in mice (D. W. Arnold et al., 1977); induced mutations in mammalian cells in culture (Ahmed et al., 1977)	Significant increase in hepatocellular carcinomas in CD-1 mice (Epstein, 1976) and in B6C3F1 mice (National Cancer Institute, 1977d); inconclusive in Osborne Mendel rats (National Cancer Institute, 1977d)
Kepone (chlordecone)	NE	Not monitored in the Market Basket Surveys	Not mutagenic in dominant lethal assay in rats (Simon et al., 1978)	Significant dose-related increase in hepatocellular carcinomas in B6C3F1 mice and Osborne Mendel rats (National Cancer Institute, 1976)

[a]ADI = Acceptable Daily Intake of pesticide residues in diet established periodically by the World Health Organization, based on standards established by the FAO/WHO Expert Committee on Food Additives (World Health Organization, 1958).
[b]Data from FDA Market Basket Surveys (U.S. Food and Drug Administration, 1980b).
[c]Doses used in these studies were many times higher (usually 100 times or more) than the amounts to which humans are exposed in the average U.S. diet.
[d]ND = Not detected.
[e]NE = ADI not established.
[f]Data from Food and Agriculture Organization, 1978.

14-19

TABLE 14-2

Carcinogenicity of Some Organophosphate Pesticides

Pesticide	ADI[a] (μg/kg bw)	Daily Dietary Intake (μg/kg bw), by Year[b]	Mutagenicity and Related Tests	Carcinogenicity (Oral Administration Only)[c]
Malathion	20	1975 - 0.1340 1977 - 0.1540 1979 - 0.2644	Negative in E. coli, Salmonella, and in dominant lethal tests in mice (Degraeve et al., 1980; Simmon et al., 1979)	No significant increase in tumors in Fischer 344 rats (National Cancer Institute, 1979d), negative in Osborne Mendel rats, and inconclusive in B6C3F1 mice (National Cancer Institute, 1978a)
Parathion	1.0	1975 - 0.0010 1977 - 0.0016 1979 - 0.0022	Negative in Salmonella and dominant lethal tests in mice (Bartsch et al., 1980; Degraeve et al., 1980); chromosome aberrations in guinea pigs given 0.05 mg intratesticularly (Dikshith, 1973)	Increased incidence of tumors of the adrenal gland in Osborne Mendel rats, but not in B6C3F1 mice (National Cancer Institute, 1979f)
Methyl parathion	1.0	1975 - 0.0007 1977 - 0.0006 1979 - ND[d]	Weakly positive in E. coli (Mohn, 1973); at low doses, no increase in chromosome aberrations in mice (Huang, 1973)	Negative in bioassay in Fischer 344 rats and B6C3F1 mice (National Cancer Institute, 1979e)
Diazinon	2.0	1975 - 0.0087 1977 - 0.0061 1979 - 0.0102	Negative in E. coli and Salmonella (Simmon et al., 1979); increase in chromosome aberrations in human lymphocytes at doses of 0.5-2.5 mg/ml (Coneva-Maneva et al., 1969)	Negative in Fischer 344 rats and B6C3F1 mice (National Cancer Institute, 1979c)

[a]ADI = Acceptable Daily Intake of pesticide residues in the diet established periodically by the World Health Organization, based on standards established by the FAO/WHO Expert Committee on Food Additives (World Health Organization, 1958).
[b]Data from FDA Market Basket Surveys (U.S. Food and Drug Administration, 1980b).
[c]Doses used in these studies were many times higher (usually 100 times or more) than the amounts to which humans are exposed in the average U.S. diet.
[d]ND = Not detected.

TABLE 14-3

Carcinogenicity of Some Carbamate Pesticides

Pesticide	ADI[a] (μg/kg bw)	Daily Dietary Intake (μg/kg bw)[b]	Mutagenicity and Related Tests	Carcinogenicity (Oral Administration Only)[c]
Carbaryl	10	Average intake from 1964 to 1970 was 0.5; maximum was 2.1 (Duggan and Corneliussen, 1972)	Negative in dominant lethal assay in mice (Epstein et al., 1972); negative in E. coli (Ashwood-Smith et al., 1972), in B. subtilis (DeGiovanni-Donnelly et al., 1968), and in Ames test (McCann et al., 1975); positive in D. melanogaster (Brzhesky, 1972)	No significant increase in incidence of tumors in rats, dogs, and CD-1 mice (U.S. Enviromental Protection Agency, 1975b), in CFE rats (Weil and Carpenter, 1965), and in (C57BL/6 x C3H/Anf)F_1 and (C57BL/6 x AKR)F_1 mice (Innes et al., 1969); increased incidence of sarcomas in random-bred rats at doses that reduced survival (Andrianova and Alekseev, 1970)
Aldicarb	1	Not routinely included in the Market Basket Survey	Negative in dominant lethal assay in rats (Weil and Carpenter, 1974)	No significant increase in the incidence of tumors in B6C3F_1 mice and Osborne Mendel rats (National Cancer Institute, 1979b)

[a]ADI = Acceptable Daily Intake of pesticide residues in diet established periodically by the World Health Organization based on standards established by the FAO/WHO Expert Committee on Food Additives (World Health Organization, 1958).
[b]Data from FDA Market Basket Surveys (U.S. Food and Drug Administration, 1980b).
[c]Doses used in these studies were many times higher (usually 100 times or more) than the amounts to which humans are exposed in the average U.S. diet.

to be carcinogenic in rats and mice. The data for carbaryl are inconclusive and do not permit an assessment of carcinogenicity. However, carbaryl
is capable of reacting with nitrite under mildly acidic conditions (similar
to those present in the human stomach) to produce N-nitrosocarbaryl, which
is known to induce cancer in rats (Eisenbrand et al., 1976; Lijinsky and
Taylor, 1976). Although Ohshima and Bartsch (1981) have provided direct
evidence that nitrosamines can be formed in the human stomach, such information should be interpreted with caution because the extent to which this
reaction could occur endogenously would depend on a number of factors,
including the differences in the concentration of the reactants, pH, and
the presence of catalysts and blocking agents.

The results of mutagenicity and related short-term tests for some
organochlorine pesticides did not coincide with data from experiments to
study carcinogenicity in animals. This disparity may indicate the limited
value of mutagenicity tests for screening organochlorine compounds for
potential adverse effects.

Summary and Conclusions. Residues of a few organochlorine, organophosphate, and carbamate pesticides are commonly detected in the diet,
generally at levels that are one to two orders of magnitude below their
Acceptable Daily Intake (ADI). Unlike the organophosphates and carbamates, most of the organochlorine compounds are metabolized slowly and
tend to accumulate in body tissues. The organochlorine compounds and the
organophosphates have the potential to modify the activity of microsomal
enzymes and to engage in synergistic interactions.

Data from the few epidemiological studies that have been conducted
permit no conclusion to be drawn about the carcinogenic risk to humans
exposed to pesticides.

The experimental data reviewed in this section indicate the following:

• A number of the common organochlorine pesticides to which the
general population is exposed cause cancer in mice and some in other
animal species.

• With the exception of parathion, the organophosphate pesticides
discussed herein have not been found to be carcinogenic in laboratory
animals.

• Of the two carbamates, aldicarb does not appear to be carcingenic
in rats or mice, and the data on the carcinogenicity of carbaryl are
inconclusive. Carbaryl is capable of reacting with nitrite under mildly
acidic conditions to produce carcinogenic N-nitroso compounds. Such
nitrosation reactions have been shown to occur in the human stomach, but
the degree of risk they pose to human health is not known.

On the basis of studies in animals, and in the absence of adequate
data from epidemiological studies, it appears that Kepone (chlordecone),

toxaphene, hexachlorobenzene, and, perhaps, heptachlor (with chlordane) and lindane present a carcinogenic risk to humans. However, it is reasonable to assume that the amounts present in the average U.S. diet do not make a major contribution to the overall risk of cancer for humans.

Polychlorinated Biphenyls (PCB's)

Polychlorinated biphenyls (PCB's), which are complex mixtures of chlorinated hydrocarbons, have been used for industrial purposes for the past half century. With rare exceptions, commercial PCB's are contaminated with low levels of toxic impurities such as polychlorinated dibenzofurans and chlorinated naphthalenes.

The effects of PCB's on health have been reviewed recently by the International Agency for Research on Cancer (1978) and the Subcommittee on the Health Effects of Polychlorinated Biphenyls and Polybrominated Biphenyls (1978). Initial concern about the adverse health effects of various commercial PCB mixtures originated when chloracne and hepatic changes were observed among workers engaged in the production of these compounds (Schwartz, 1943). The gradual realization that PCB's are highly toxic and exceedingly persistent in the environment led the U.S. Environmental Protection Agency (1979) to suspend their manufacture and use in commerce. Because of the extreme stability and high potential of PCB's for assimilation in the food chain, the FDA has established limits for their levels in different foods (U.S. Food and Drug Administration, 1977b).

For humans, the major source of exposure to low levels of PCB's is diet. Generally, PCB's have been found only in the flesh or products of animals (e.g., fish, milk, eggs, and cheese) and in animal feed derived from animal products (e.g., fish meal) (Jelinek, 1981; Jelinek and Corneliussen, 1976). Between 1969 and 1975 the levels of PCB's declined in all foods examined, except fish. Daily dietary intakes measured between 1974 and 1977 indicated that PCB's had dropped to levels well below the tolerance levels in individual foods (U.S. Food and Drug Administration, 1980b). PCB's also tend to accumulate in the adipose tissue of humans, in milk, and in blood (Kutz and Strassman, 1976).

Epidemiological Evidence. During a 9-year period in Japan (1968-1975), there were reports of more than 1,200 cases of Yusho disease (a disorder involving ocular, dermatological, and nervous symptoms) in humans who had consumed rice oil accidentally contaminated with Kanechlor 400 (a PCB) (Higuchi, 1976; Kuratsune et al., 1976). Nine out of 22 (41%) of the deaths, which were reported as long as 5.5 years after the initial exposure, were due to malignant neoplasms (Kuratsune, 1976; Urabe, 1974). However, the investigators did not compare this incidence with the rate of expected deaths from various neoplasms in the population.

Bahn et al. (1976, 1977) reported two malignant melanomas among 31 workers (20 times the expected incidence) who had been heavily exposed to

Aroclor 1254 (a PCB) and possibly other chemicals, and one melanoma among 41 others who had been less heavily exposed. Three other workers in the heavily exposed group were diagnosed as having four cancers at other sites, including two in the pancreas.

Brown and Jones (1981) reported a retrospective study of 2,567 workers employed for at least 3 months in plants using PCB's. The total mortality from all causes and mortality from cancers were lower than expected, but were slightly, although not significantly, excessive (3 vs. 1.07 expected) for liver cancer.

Experimental Evidence. A number of experiments have been conducted in laboratory animals to test the carcinogenicity of various PCB's. Table 14-4 summarizes the results of some experiments in which various compounds were administered orally to study their carcinogenicity, mutagenicity, or their ability to act as tumor-promoting agents.

On the basis of data from the five experiments examined, it appears that Kanechlor 500 and Aroclor 1254 induce cancer in mice and that Aroclor 1260 is carcinogenic in rats. All three compounds have induced benign and malignant liver cell tumors in laboratory animals. From experiments in which PCB's were tested as promoting agents, it appears that Kanechlor 400 and 500 enhance hepatocarcinogenicity of 3-methyl-4-aminoazobenzene (3'-DMAB) and N-nitrosodiethylamine (NDEA) in rats and of lindane in mice, whereas Kanechlor 500 when administered to rats simultaneously with the carcinogen inhibited the hepatocarcinogenicity of 3'-DMAB, 2-AAF, and NDEA (Makiura et al., 1974).

Aroclor 1221 and 1268 are mutagenic, and have been shown to induce microsomal activation in the Ames test (Wyndham et al., 1976). A number of other PCB's, e.g., Aroclor 1254 (see Table 14-4), are negative in the dominant lethal assay in rats and do not induce chromosome aberrations in cultures of lymphocytes from humans. These findings are difficult to interpret for Aroclor 1254, which induces dose-related hepatocellular carcinoma in female rats and enhances NDEA-induced hepatocellular carcinoma in rats (Preston et al., 1981).

Summary and Conclusions. PCB's are highly persistent in the environment and have been detected in human tissues. They occur in fish, meat, and dairy foods in amounts that are well below the tolerance levels established by the FDA.

Limited data from epidemiological studies suggest that exposure to high levels of PCB's may be associated with the development of malignant melanomas, but no conclusion can be drawn about the risk to humans from exposure to PCB-contaminated foods. Results of laboratory experiments indicate that some PCB's are carcinogenic in rodents, producing mostly tumors of the liver at doses much higher than those generally present in the average U.S. diet. Recent evidence indicates that some PCB's may act primarily as tumor-promoting agents.

TABLE 14-4

Carcinogenicity of Polychlorinated Biphenyls (PCB's)[a]

Compound	Mutagenicity and Related Tests	Carcinogenicity (Oral Administration Only)
Aroclor 1221 and 1268	Mutagenic to S. typhimurium (Wyndham et al., 1976)	
Aroclor 1242	Did not induce chromosome aberrations in bone marrow (Green et al., 1973, 1975a)	
Aroclor 1254	Did not induce chromosome aberrations in bone marrow of rats (Green et al., 1973, 1975a); negative in dominant lethal assay in rats (Green et al., 1975b); did not induce chromosome aberrations in human lymphocytes in culture (Hoopingarner et al., 1972)	Increased the incidence of hepatomas in BALB/cJ mice (Kimbrough and Linder, 1974); promoted hepatocellular carcinomas induced by NDEA in rats (Preston et al., 1981)
Aroclor 1260		Induced dose-related increase in hepatocellular carcinomas in female Sherman rats (Kimbrough et al., 1975)
Kanechlor 300		Increased the incidence of hepatocellular carcinomas in dd mice (Ito et al., 1973)
Kanechlor 400		Increased the incidence of hepatocellular carcinomas in dd mice (Ito et al., 1973); enhanced hepatomas in rats when fed after 3'-DMAB (Kimura et al., 1976); enhanced hepatocarcinogenicity of lindane in mice (Nagasaki et al., 1975)
Kanechlor 500		Increased the incidence of hepatocellular carcinomas in dd mice (Ito et al., 1973); enhanced liver tumors in rats when fed after NDEA (Nishizumi, 1976), but when fed in combination with 3'-DMAB, 2-AAF, and NDEA, it inhibited hepatocarcinomas in rats (Makiura et al., 1974); enhanced hepatocarcinogenicity of lindane in mice (Nagasaki et al., 1975).

[a]The tolerance levels for PCB's in various food products range from 0.2 to 5 μg/g fat (U.S. Food and Drug Administration, 1977b). From 1974 to 1977, daily dietary intake ranged from 0 to 0.0164 μg/kg bw (U.S. Food and Drug Administration, 1980b).

Polybrominated Biphenyls (PBB's)

Polybrominated biphenyls (PBB's), which are chemically related to the PCB's, have been used as flame retardants in industrial processes. Like PCB's, PBB's persist in the environment and can accumulate in body fat.

Epidemiological Evidence. Studies of a population accidentally exposed to PBB's in Michigan in 1973 indicated that the exposure was associated with a number of adverse effects on health (Kay, 1977; Office of Technology Assessment, 1979); however, because of the short interval between the time of exposure and the measurement of effects, these studies could provide no definitive information about the relationship between PBB's and cancer.

Experimental Evidence. Sherman rats given a single oral dose of PBB's by gavage developed neoplastic liver nodules after 6 months (Kimbrough et al., 1978). In a follow-up study, Sherman rats were given a single large dose of PBB's or 12 divided doses by gavage. Both treatments resulted in a high incidence of hepatocellular carcinomas. In the rats given multiple high doses, the incidence of tumors was higher and some of the liver carcinomas were less differentiated than in rats given the single dose (Kimbrough et al., 1981).

Recently, Aust has shown that PBB's are tumor promoters in rats (S. D. Aust, Michigan State University, personal communication, 1981). The doses given in this in vivo assay ranged from 1 to 100 mg/kg diet.

PBB's did not induce mutations in the Ames test and in Chinese hamster uterine cells (Aust, personal communication, 1981). When administered orally to mice at doses ranging from 50 to 500 mg/kg bw, they did not induce chromosome aberrations in bone marrow cells (Wertz and Ficsor, 1978).

Summary and Conclusions. These studies indicate that single doses or short-term treatment with PBB's can induce liver tumors in rats. There is some indication that the effect is dose-dependent, but the number of rats given the lower doses was small. Because of the lack of data from epidemiological studies, it is difficult to determine the significance of these findings for human health.

Polycyclic Aromatic Hydrocarbons (PAH's)

Polycyclic aromatic hydrocarbons (PAH's) are organic compounds containing two or more benzene rings. To date, more than 100 of these compounds have been identified in the environment and in foods (Lo and Sandi, 1978; U.S. Environmental Protection Agency, 1975c). Of these, less than 20 have been shown to cause cancer in laboratory animals, and only five of these have induced cancer following oral administration: benzo[a]pyrene (BaP), dibenz[a,h]anthracene (DBA), benz[a]anthracene

(BA), 3-methylcholanthrene (3-MCA), and 7,12-dimethylbenz[a]anthracene (7,12-DMBA). Of these, 3-MCA and 7,12-DMBA are synthetic chemicals that do not occur normally in the diet.

The major sources of the PAH contamination of food are curing smokes, contaminated soils, polluted air and water, and endogenous biosynthesis by plants and microorganisms. The methods with which foods are cooked or processed also affect the PAH content of the foods (Howard and Fazio, 1980; Lo and Sandi, 1978).

The contamination of foods by PAH's is widespread. These compounds have been detected in fresh meats, smoked fish and meats, grilled and roasted foods, leafy and root vegetables, vegetable oils, grains, plants, fruits, seafoods, whiskies, etc. Smoking of meat increases the total PAH burden (Howard and Fazio, 1980). Similarly, hot air drying and roasting are potential sources of contamination of grain and coffee (Fritz, 1969). Most foods contain very low levels of PAH's, but shellfish seem to concentrate these compounds and are unable to metabolize them. Various PAH's, including BaP, benzanthracene, and chrysene, have been detected in Scotch, bourbon, and Japanese whiskies at extremely low levels, ranging from 0.03 to 0.08 µg/liter (Masuda et al., 1966). Leafy plants such as spinach, kale, and tobacco contain higher levels of BaP (Grimmer, 1968), and only a small fraction (∿10%) appears to be removed by washing (Grimmer, 1968).

Although BaP constitutes only between 1% and 20% of the total amount of carcinogenic PAH's in the environment, there is a great deal of information on the levels of that compound in various foods (Suess, 1976). In contrast, the information on the levels of other carcinogenic PAH's is still fragmentary. Fritz (1971) estimated that the average annual intake of BaP in the German Democratic Republic ranged from 340 to 1,200 µg per person annually. In Hungary, it was calculated to be 290 to 612 µg/person annually (Soós, 1980). The main sources of ingested BaP were vegetables and fruits, whereas the smoked foods contributed only a minor fraction of the total BaP intake. Although there is information concerning the levels of BaP in specific foods, such as oils and smoked meats, the total intake of BaP from all sources in the United States has not been reported.

Epidemiological Evidence. Evidence concerning the association between cancer in humans (mainly cancer of the skin and lung) and exposure to PAH's derives from studies of humans exposed occupationally to PAH's in soot from chimneys, coal tar, creasote oil, and other petroleum products (Butlin, 1892; Doll et al., 1972; Heller, 1930; Kennaway and Kennaway, 1947; Pott, 1775).

There is little information concerning the relationship between ingestion of PAH-contaminated food and cancer in humans. In one study, Hajdu (1974) observed that the incidence of stomach cancer among the Vend population living in West Hungary is significantly higher than the incidence for the general Hungarian population. The Vend population routinely consumes home-smoked meat products that contain substantially higher BaP levels than found in samples of smoked food consumed in other parts of Hungary (Soós, 1980). In another report, Dungal (1961) speculated that the high incidence of gastric cancer in the northwestern part of Iceland may be associated with the frequent consumption of smoked trout and smoked mutton, which were found to contain relatively high concentrations of PAH's. In Latvia, Voitalovich et al. (1957) reported that the incidence of gastrointestinal cancer over a 5-year period was significantly higher in a coastal region than in a nearby inland region. They attributed this difference to occupational exposures in the fishing industry (e.g., during the smoking of fish), frequent consumption of smoked fish, and poorly balanced diet. However, these investigators (Dungal, 1961; Soós, 1980; Voitalovich et al., 1957) did not take into consideration the potential effect of nitrite or N-nitroso compounds, which may also be present in such foods and which are also believed to be associated with gastric cancer.

Experimental Evidence: Carcinogenicity and Mutagenicity. The PAH's exert their toxic, carcinogenic, and mutagenic effects only after being metabolized by the mixed-function oxidases of various tissues (Freudenthal and Jones, 1976). Their carcinogenic activity varies from very weak to potent. Some of the PAH's have been shown to be carcinogenic to mice, rats, hamsters, rabbits, and monkeys when administered topically, orally, or parenterally (Freudenthal and Jones, 1976). Many PAH's have also been found to be mutagenic. The discussion below is limited to those PAH's generally detected in foods and found to be carcinogenic when administered orally.

Benzo[a]pyrene

The carcinogenicity of BaP in various animal species has been well established. A single 0.2 mg dose of BaP administered intragastrically produced forestomach tumors in mice (Peirce, 1961). In other studies, mice fed a diet containing BaP at 250 mg/kg developed an increasing number of forestomach tumors as the duration of the experiment was extended (Neal and Rigdon, 1967), and mice exposed for 140 days developed lung tumors and leukemia in addition to forestomach tumors (Rigdon and Neal, 1969).

In Sprague-Dawley rats, a single dose of 100 mg BaP resulted in the induction of mammary tumors (Huggins and Yang, 1962). Hamsters fed BaP at 500 mg/kg diet 4 days/week for up to 14 months developed esophageal, intestinal, and stomach tumors (Chu and Malmgren, 1965).

BaP has been also shown to be mutagenic to Ames Salmonella strains (Hollstein et al., 1979; Nagao and Sugimura, 1978), to be genotoxic in the hepatocyte primary culture-DNA repair test (Tong et al., 1981), to induce mutations in the epithelial cells of the liver of rats (Tong et al., 1981), and to induce transformations in Syrian golden hamster embryo cells (Casto, 1979).

Dibenz[a,h]anthracene

Dietary administration of DBA for 5 to 7 months (total dose, 9-19 mg/animal) resulted in the appearance of forestomach tumors in mice after 1 year (Larionov and Soboleva, 1938). Mice receiving the compound at 0.2 mg/ml in an olive oil emulsion, which was substituted for their drinking water, received an average dose of 0.76 to 0.85 mg/day. Pulmonary adenomatosis developed in these animals after 200 days. In addition, females in this group developed mammary carcinomas (Snell and Stewart, 1962). Administration of DBA by stomach tube to several strains of mice (total dose, 15 mg/mouse administered over 15 weeks) resulted in a significant increase in mammary carcinomas (Biancifiori and Caschera, 1962).

DBA was positive in the Ames test (McCann et al., 1975). Treatment of hamster embryo cells with DBA increased the frequency of transformations induced by the simian adenovirus SA7 (Casto, 1979).

Benz[a]anthracene

Administration of 0.5 mg BA in mineral oil by stomach tube at intervals of 3 to 7 days induced papillomas of the forestomach in mice (Bock and King, 1959). Mice receiving 15 doses of 1.5 mg BA each for 15 weeks by stomach tube developed lung adenomas, hepatomas, and forestomach papillomas (Klein, 1963).

BA has been shown to be mutagenic in the Ames test (Hollstein et al., 1979; McCann et al., 1975). It was also positive in the prophage induction test (Morreau et al., 1976) and genotoxic in the hepatocyte primary culture-DNA repair test (Tong et al., 1981).

Summary and Conclusions. Low levels of many PAH's are present as contaminants in a variety of foods. Smoking and broiling of foods and the use of curing smokes contributes to the PAH content of foods. Of the more than 100 PAH's found in the environment, approximately 20 are carcinogenic in laboratory animals. Of the five PAH's found to be carcinogenic when administered orally, three (BaP, DBA, and BA) occur in the average U.S. diet.

Occupational exposure of humans to PAH's is associated with an increased incidence of skin and lung cancer. There is no reliable information about the consumption of foods contaminated with low levels of PAH's and the development of human cancer. Some investigators have speculated that a high incidence of stomach cancer in Hungary and Iceland could be associated with consumption of smoked meat and fish, which are potential sources of PAH's and/or nitrosamines and their precursors, but this has not been conclusively demonstrated. However, since studies in animals have shown that PAH's are carcinogenic when administered orally, and occupational exposure to substances containing PAH's has been associated with skin and lung cancer, it would be prudent to minimize the dietary exposure to PAH's.

14-28

OVERALL SUMMARY AND CONCLUSIONS

Food Additives

Nearly 3,000 substances are intentionally added to process foods in the United States. Another estimated 12,000 chemicals, such as vinyl chloride and acrylonitrile, which are used in food-packaging, are classified as indirect additives. Some additives, such as sugar, are consumed in large amounts by the general population. However, the annual per capita exposure to most of these substances constitutes a minute portion of the diet. Although the Food Safety Provisions and, in many cases, the Delaney Clause of the Federal Food, Drug, and Cosmetic Act prohibit the addition of known carcinogens to foods, only a small proportion of substances added to foods have been tested for carcinogenicity according to protocols that are considered acceptable by current standards. Moreover, except for the studies on nonnutritive sweeteners, very few epidemiological studies have been conducted to examine the effect of food additives on cancer incidence.

Of the few direct food additives that have been tested and found to be carcinogenic in animals, all except saccharin have been banned from use in the food supply. Minute residues of a few indirect additives that are known either to produce cancer in animals, e.g., vinyl chloride and acrylonitrile, or to be carcinogenic in humans, e.g., vinyl chloride, are occasionally detected in foods. There is no evidence suggesting that the increasing use of food additives has contributed significantly to the overall risk of cancer for humans. However, the lack of detectable effect may be due to the relatively recent use of these substances, to their lack of carcinogenicity, or to the inability of epidemiological techniques to detect the effects of additives against the background of common cancers from other causes. Therefore, no definitive conclusion can be reached until more data become available.

Environmental Contaminants

Very low levels of a large and chemically diverse group of substances—environmental contaminants—may be present in a variety of foods. The dietary levels of some of these substances are monitored by the FDA Market Basket Surveys. Many of these contaminants have been extensively tested for carcinogenicity.

The results of standard chronic toxicity tests indicate that a number of environmental contaminants (e.g., some organochlorine pesticides, polychlorinated biphenyls, and polycyclic aromatic hydrocarbons) cause cancer in laboratory animals. There is no epidemiological evidence to suggest that these compounds individually make a major contribution to the risk of human cancer. However, the possibility that they may act synergistically and may thereby create a greater carcinogenic risk cannot be excluded.

REFERENCES

Abe, S., and M. Sasaki. 1977. Chromosome aberrations and sister chromatid exchanges in Chinese hamster cells exposed to various chemicals. J. Natl. Cancer Inst. 58:1635-1641.

Ahmed, F. E., R. W. Hart, and N. J. Lewis. 1977. Pesticide induced DNA damage and its repair in cultured human cells. Mutat. Res. 42:161-173.

Althoff, J., A. Cardesa, P. Pour, and P. Shubik. 1975. A chronic study of artificial sweeteners in Syrian golden hamsters. Cancer Lett. 1:21-24.

Andrews, A. W., E. S. Zawistowski, and C. R. Valentine. 1976. A comparison of the mutagenic properties of vinyl chloride and methyl chloride. Mutat. Res. 40:273-275.

Andrianova, M. M., and I. V. Alekseev. 1970. [In Russian; English Summary.] On the carcinogenous properties of the pesticides Sevine, Maneb, Ciram and Cineb. Vopr. Pitan. 29(6):71-74.

Armstrong, B., and R. Doll. 1974. Bladder cancer mortality in England and Wales in relation to cigarette smoking and saccharin consumption. Br. J. Prev. Soc. Med. 28:233-240.

Armstrong, B., and R. Doll. 1975. Bladder cancer mortality in diabetics in relation to saccharin consumption and smoking habits. Br. J. Prev. Soc. Med. 29:73-81.

Armstrong, B., A. J. Lea, A. M. Adelstein, J. W. Donovan, G. C. White, and S. Ruttle. 1976. Cancer mortality and saccharin consumption in diabetics. Br. J. Prev. Soc. Med. 30:151-157.

Arnold, D. L., C. A. Moodie, B. Stavric, D. R. Stoltz, H. C. Grice, and I. C. Munro. 1977. Letter to the Editor: Canadian saccharin study. Science 197:320.

Arnold, D. L., C. A. Moodie, H. C. Grice, S. M. Charbonneau, B. Stavric, B. T. Collins, P. F. McGuire, Z. Z. Zawidzka, and I. C. Munro. 1980. Long-term toxicity of ortho-toluenesulfonamide and sodium saccharin in the rat. Toxicol. Appl. Pharmacol. 52:113-152.

Arnold, D. W., G. L. Kennedy, Jr., M. L. Keplinger, J. C. Calandra, and C. J. Galo. 1977. Dominant lethal studies with technical chlordane, HCS-3260, and heptachlor:heptachlor epoxide. J. Toxicol. Environ. Health 2:547-555.

Ashby, J., J. A. Styles, D. Anderson, and D. Paton. 1978. Saccharin: An epigenetic carcinogen/mutagen? Food Cosmet. Toxicol. 16:95-103.

Ashwood-Smith, M. J., J. Trevino, and R. Ring. 1972. Mutagenicity of dichlorvos. Nature 240:418-420.

Bahn, A. K., I. Rosenwaike, N. Herrmann, P. Grover, J. Stellman, and K. O'Leary. 1976. Letter to the Editor: Melanoma after exposure to PCB's. N. Engl. J. Med. 295:450.

Bahn, A. K., P. Grover, I. Rosenwaike, K. O'Leary, and J. Stellman. 1977. Letter to the Editor: A reply to PCB's and melanoma. N. Engl. J. Med. 296:108.

Barthel, E. 1976. [In German; English Summary.] High incidence of lung cancer in persons with chronic professional exposure to pesticides in agriculture. Z. Erkr. Atmungsorgane 146:266-274.

Bartsch, H., C. Malaveille, A. Barbin, and G. Planche. 1979. Mutagenic and alkylating metabolites of halo-ethylenes, chlorobutadienes and dichlorobutenes produced by rodent or human liver tissues. Evidence for oxirane formation by P450-linked microsomal mono-oxygenases. Arch. Toxicol. 41:249-277.

Bartsch, H., C. Malaveille, A.-M. Camus, G. Martel-Planche, G. Brun, A. Hautefeuille, N. Sabadie, and A. Barbin. 1980. Validation and comparative studies on 180 chemicals with S. typhimurium strains and V79 Chinese hamster cells in the presence of various metabolizing systems. Mutat. Res. 76:1-50.

Batzinger, R. P., S.-Y. L. Ou, and E. Bueding. 1977. Saccharin and other sweeteners: Mutagenic properties. Science 198:944-946.

Biancifiori, C., and F. Caschera. 1962. The relation between pseudopregnancy and the chemical induction by four carcinogens of mammary and ovarian tumours in BALB/c mice. Brit. J. Cancer 16:722-730.

Blot, W. J., J. F. Fraumeni, and B. J. Stone. 1978. Geographic correlates of pancreas cancer in the United States. Cancer 42:373-380.

Bock, F. G., and D. W. King. 1959. A study of the sensitivity of the mouse forestomach toward certain polycyclic hydrocarbons. J. Natl. Cancer Inst. 23:833-840.

Brantom, P. B., I. F. Gaunt, and P. Grasso. 1973. Long-term toxicity of sodium cyclamate in mice. Food Cosmet. Toxicol. 11:735-746.

Brown, D. P., and M. Jones. 1981. Mortality and industrial hygiene study of workers exposed to polychlorinated biphenyls. Arch. Environ. Health 36:120-129.

Brzhesky, V. V. 1972. [In Russian; English Summary.] Study of mutagenic properties of Sevin, a carbamate insecticide. Genetika 8(6):151-153.

Bülow, H., H.-K. Wullstein, G. Böttger, and F. H. Schröder. 1973. [In German; English Summary.] Carcinomas of the breast under estrogen-treatment for prostatic carcinoma. Urologe A 12:249-153.

Burbank, F., and J. F. Fraumeni, Jr. 1970. Synthetic sweetener consumption and bladder cancer trends in the United States. Nature 227: 296-297.

Buselmaier, W., G. Röhrborn, and P. Propping. 1973. Comparative investigations on the mutagenicity of pesticides in mammalian test systems. Mutat. Res. 21:25-26. Abstract 9.

Butlin, H. T. 1892. Three lectures on cancer of the scrotum in chimney sweeps and others. Lecture III.--Tar and paraffin cancer. Br. Med. J. 2:66-71.

Cabral, J. R. P., P. Shubik, T. Mollner, and F. Raitano. 1977. Letter to the Editor: Carcinogenic activity of hexachlorobenzene in hamsters. Nature 269:510-511.

Cabral, J. R. P., T. Mollner, F. Raitano, and P. Shubik. 1979. Carcinogenesis of hexachlorobenzene in mice. Int. J. Cancer 23:47-51.

Casto, B. C. 1979. Polycyclic hydrocarbons and Syrian hamster embryo cells: Cell transformation, enhancement of viral transformation and analysis of DNA damage. Pp. 51-66 in P. W. Jones and P. Leber, eds. Polynuclear Aromatic Hydrocarbons. Ann Arbor Science Publishers, Ann Arbor, Mich.

Chowaniec, J., and R. M. Hicks. 1979. Response of the rat to saccharin with particular reference to the urinary bladder. Br. J. Cancer 39: 355-375.

Chrisman, C. L. 1974. Aneuploidy in mouse in embryos induced by diethylstilbestrol diphosphate. Teratology 9:229-232.

Christiansen, J. S. 1978. Cigarette smoking and prevalence of microangiopathy in juvenile-onset insulin-independent diabetes mellitus. Diabetes Care 1:146-149.

Chu, E. W., and R. A. Malmgren. 1965. An inhibitory effect of vitamin A on the induction of tumors of forestomach and cervix in the Syrian hamster by carcinogenic polycyclic hydrocarbons. Cancer Res. 25:884-895.

Clapp, N. K., R. L. Tyndall, R. B. Cumming, and J. A. Otten. 1974. Effects of butylated hydroxytoluene alone or with diethylnitrosamine in mice. Food Cosmet. Toxicol. 12:367-371.

Clive, D. 1977. A linear relationship between tumorigenic potency in vivo and mutagenic potency at the heterozygous thymidine kinase $(TK^{+/-})$ locus of L5178Y mouse lymphoma cells coupled with mammalian metabolism. Pp. 241-247 in D. Scott, B. A. Bridges, and F. H. Sobels, eds. Progress in Genetic Toxicology. Proceedings of the Second International Conference on Environmental Mutagens, Edinburgh. Elsevier/North-Holland Biomedical Press, Amsterdam, New York, and Oxford.

Clive, D., K. O. Johnson, J. F. S. Spector, A. G. Batson, and M. M. M. Brown. 1979. Validation and characterization of the L5178Y/$TK^{+/-}$ mouse lymphoma mutagen assay system. Mutat. Res. 59:61-108.

Code of Federal Regulations. 1978. Title 21, Section 556.190. Office of the Federal Register, National Archives and Records Service, General Services Administration, Washington, D.C.

Cohen, S. M., M. Arai, J. B. Jacobs, and G. H. Friedell. 1979. Promoting effect of saccharin and DL-tryptophan in urinary bladder carcinogenesis. Cancer Res. 39:1207-1217.

Coneva-Maneva, M., F. Kaloyanova, and A. Georgieva. 1969. [In Russian; English Summary.] Mutation action of Diazinone on lymphocytes of the human peripheral blood in vitro. Eksp. Med. Morfol. 8:132-136.

Coulston, F., E. W. McChesney, and K.-F. Benitz. 1977. Eight-year study of cyclamate in rhesus monkeys. Toxicol. Appl. Pharmacol. 41:164-165. Abstract 80.

Creech, J. L., Jr., and M. N. Johnson. 1974. Angiosarcoma of liver in the manufacture of polyvinyl chloride. J. Occup. Med. 16:150-151.

Cutler, B. S., A. P. Forbes, F. M. Ingersoll, and R. E. Scully. 1972. Endometrial carcinoma after stilbestrol therapy in gonadal dysgenesis. N. Engl. J. Med. 287:628-631.

DeGiovanni-Donnelly, R., S. M. Kolbye, and P. D. Greeves. 1968. The effects of IPC, CIPC, Sevin and Zectran on Bacillus subtilis. Experientia 24:80-81.

Degraeve, N., J. Gilot-Delhalle, J. Moutschen, M. Moutschen-Dahmen, A. Colizzi, M. Chollet, and N. Houbrechts. 1980. Comparison of the mutagenic activity of organophosphorous insecticides in mouse and in the yeast Schizosaccharomyces pombe. Mutat. Res. 74:201-202. Abstract 65.

Deichmann, W. B., M. Keplinger, F. Sala, and E. Glass. 1967. Synergism among oral carcinogens. IV. The simultaneous feeding of four tumorigens to rats. Toxicol. Appl. Pharmacol. 11:88-103.

Dikshith, T. S. S. 1973. In vivo effects of parathion on guinea pig chromosomes. Environ. Physiol. Biochem. 3:161-168.

Doll, R., M. P. Vessey, R. W. R. Beasley, A. R. Buckley, E. C. Fear, R. E. W. Fisher, E. J. Gammon, W. Gunn, G. O. Hughes, K. Lee, and B. Norman-Smith. 1972. Mortality of gas-workers--Final report of a prospective study. Br. J. Ind. Med. 29:394-406.

Duck, B. W., and J. T. Carter. 1976. Response to letter. Lancet 2:195.

Duggan, R. E., and P. E. Corneliussen. 1972. Dietary intake of pesticide chemicals in the United States (III), June 1968-April 1970. Pestic. Monit. J. 5:331-341.

Dungal, N. 1961. The special problem of stomach cancer in Iceland. With particular reference to dietary factors. J. Am. Med. Assoc. 176: 789-798.

Ebenezer, L. N., and G. Sadasivan. 1970. In vitro effect of cyclamates on human chromosomes. Q. J. Surg. Sci. 6:116-118.

Eckardt, F., H. Muliawan, N. de Ruiter, and H. Kappus. 1981. Rat hepatic vinyl chloride metabolites induce gene conversion in the yeast strain D7RAD in vitro and in vivo. Mutat. Res. 91:381-390.

Eisenbrand, G., D. Schmähl, and R. Preussmann. 1976. Carcinogenicity in rats of high oral doses of N-nitrosocarbaryl, a nitrosated pesticide. Cancer Lett. 1:281-284.

Epstein, S. S. 1976. Carcinogenicity of heptachlor and chlordane. Sci. Total Environ. 6:103-154.

Epstein, S. S., E. Arnold, J. Andrea, W. Bass, and Y. Bishop. 1972. Detection of chemical mutagens by the dominant lethal assay in the mouse. Toxicol. Appl. Pharmacol. 23:288-325.

Feron, V. J., A. J. Speek, M. I. Willems, D. van Battum, and A. P. de Groot. 1975. Observations on the oral administration and toxicity of vinyl chloride in rats. Food Cosmet. Toxicol. 13:633-638.

Feron, V. J., C. F. M. Hendriksen, A. J. Speek, H. P. Til, and B. J. Spit. 1981. Lifespan oral toxicity study of vinyl chloride in rats. Food Cosmet. Toxicol. 19:317-333.

Fitzhugh, O. G. 1964. Appraisal of the safety of residues of veterinary drugs and their metabolites in edible animal tissues. Ann. N.Y. Acad. Sci. 111:665-670.

Fluck, E. R., L. A. Poirier, and H. W. Ruelius. 1976. Evaluation of a DNA polymerase-deficient mutant of E. coli for the rapid detection of carcinogens. Chem.-Biol. Interact. 15:219-231.

Food and Agriculture Organization. 1978. Pesticide residues in food-- 1977. FAO Plant Prod. Prot. Paper 10 Rev.:41-42.

Fox, A. J., and P. F. Collier. 1977. Mortality experience of workers to vinyl chloride monomer in the manufacture of polyvinyl chloride in Great Britain. Br. J. Ind. Med. 34:1-10.

Freudenthal, R., and P. W. Jones, eds. 1976. Carcinogenesis--A comprehensive survey. Volume 1. Polynuclear Aromatic Hydrocarbons. Chemistry, Metabolism, and Carcinogenesis. Raven Press, New York. 450 pp.

Friedman, L., H. L. Richardson, M. E. Richardson, E. J. Lethco, W. C. Wallace, and F. M. Sauro. 1972. Toxic response of rats to cyclamates in chow and semisynthetic diets. J. Natl. Cancer Inst. 49:751-764.

Fritz, W. 1969. [In German.] Zum Lösungsverhalten der Polyaromaten beim Kochen von Kaffee-Ersatzstoffen und Bohnenkaffee. Dtsch. Lebensm. Rundsch. 65:83-85.

Fritz, W. 1971. [In German.] Umfang und Quellen der Kontamination unserer Lebensmittel mit krebserzeugenden Kohlenwasserstoffen. Ernaehrungsforschung 16:547-557.

Fuchs, G., B.-M. Gawell, L. Albanus, and S. Slorach. 1975. [In Swedish; English Summary.] Vinyl chloride monomer levels in edible fats. Var Foeda 17:134-145.

Funes-Cravioto, F., B. Lambert, J. Lindsten, L. Ehrenberg, A. T. Natarajan, and S. Osterman-Golkar. 1975. Letter to the Editor: Chromosome aberrations in workers exposed to vinyl chloride. Lancet 1:459.

Furuya, T., K. Kawamata, T. Kaneko, O. Uchida, S. Horiuchi, and Y. Ikeda. 1975. Long-term toxicity study of sodium cyclamate and saccharin sodium in rats. Jpn. J. Pharmacol. 25(Suppl.):55P-56P. Abstract.

Gass, G. H., D. Coats, and N. Graham. 1964. Carcinogenic dose-response curve to oral diethylstilbestrol. J. Natl. Cancer Inst. 33:971-977.

Gass, G. H., J. Brown, and A. B. Okey. 1974. Carcinogenic effects of oral diethylstilbestrol on C3H mice with and without the mammary tumor virus. J. Natl. Cancer Inst. 53:1369-1370.

Gibson, J. P., J. W. Newberne, W. L. Kuhn, and J. R. Elsen. 1967. Comparative chronic toxicity of three oral estrogens in rats. Toxicol. Appl. Pharmacol. 11:489-510.

Glatt, H. R., Metzler, and F. Oesch. 1979. Diethylstilbestrol and 11 derivatives. A mutagenicity study with Salmonella typhimurium. Mutat. Res. 67:113-121.

Green, S., K. A. Palmer, and E. J. Oswald. 1973. Cytogenetic effects of the polychlorinated biphenyls (Aroclor 1242) on rat bone marrow and spermatogonial cells. Toxicol. Appl. Pharmacol. 25:482. Abstract 113.

Green, S., J.V. Carr, K. A. Palmer, and E. J. Oswald. 1975a. Lack of cytogenetic effects in bone marrow and spermatogonial cells in rats treated with polychlorinated biphenyls (Aroclors 1242 and 1254). Bull. Environ. Contam. Toxicol. 13:14-22.

Green, S., F. M. Sauro, and L. Friedman. 1975b. Lack of dominant lethality in rats treated with polychlorinated biphenyls (Aroclors 1242 and 1254). Food Cosmet. Toxicol. 13:507-510.

Greenwald, P., P. C. Nasca, W. S. Burnett, and A. Polan. 1973. Prenatal stilbestrol experience in mothers of young cancer patients. Cancer 31:568-572.

Greim, H., G. Bonse, Z. Radwan, D. Reichert, and D. Henschler. 1975. Mutagenicity in vitro and potential carcinogenicity of chlorinated ethylenes as a function of metabolic oxirane formation. Biochem. Pharmacol. 24:2013-2017.

Grimmer, G. 1968. [In German.] Cancerogene Kohlenwasserstoffe in der Umgebung des Menschen. Dtsch. Apoth. Ztg.108:529-533.

Guerzoni, M. E., L. Del Cupolo, and I. Ponti. 1976. [In Italian; English Summary.] Mutagenic activity of pesticides. Riv. Sci. Tecnol. Alimenti Nutr. Um. 6:161-165.

Hajdu, G. 1974. [In Magyar.] A "Vendvidéken" előforduló gyomorrák és a Különleges füstölési mód összefüggése. Medicus Universalis 7(6):278-289.

Heath, C. W., Jr., C. R. Dumont, and R. J. Waxweiller. 1977. Chromosomal damage in men occupationally exposed to vinyl chloride monomer and other chemicals. Environ. Res. 14:68-72.

Heller, I. 1930. Occupational cancers. J. Ind. Hyg. 12(5):169–197.

Herbst, A. L., and P. Cole. 1978. Epidemiologic and clinical aspects of clear cell adenocarcinoma in young women. Pp. 2–7 in A. L. Herbst, ed. Intrauterine Exposure to Diethylstilbestrol in the Human. American College of Obstetricians and Gynecologists, Chicago, Ill.

Herbst, A. L., R. J. Kurman, R. E. Scully, and D. C. Poskanzer. 1972. Clear-cell adenocarcinoma of the genital tract in young females. Registry Report. N. Engl. J. Med. 287:1259–1264.

Hicks, R. M., and J. Chowaniec. 1977. The importance of synergy between weak carcinogens in the induction of bladder cancer in experimental animals and humans. Cancer Res. 37:2943–2949.

Hicks, R.M., J. Chowaniec, and J. St.J. Wakefield. 1978. Experimental induction of bladder tumors by a two-stage system. Pp. 475–489 in T. J. Slaga, A. Sivak, and R. K. Boutwell, eds. Carcinogenesis—A Comprehensive Survey. Volume 2. Mechanisms of Tumor Promotion and Cocarcinogenesis. Raven Press, New York.

Higuchi, K. 1976. Outline. Pp. 3–7 in K. Higuchi, ed. PCB Poisoning and Pollution. Kodansha Ltd., Tokyo; Academic Press, New York, San Francisco, and London.

Hill, E. C. 1973. Clear cell carcinoma of the cervix and vagina in young women. Am. J. Obstet. Gynecol. 116:470–484.

Hollstein, M., J. McCann, F. A. Angelosanto, and W. W. Nichols. 1979. Short-term tests for carcinogens and mutagens. Mutat. Res. 65:133–226.

Homburger, F. 1978. Negative lifetime carcinogen studies in rats and mice fed 50,000 ppm saccharin. Pp. 359–373 in C. L. Galli, R. Paoletti, and G. Vettorazzi, eds. Chemical Toxicology of Food. Elsevier/North-Holland Biomedical Press, Amsterdam, New York, and Oxford.

Hooper, N. K., B. N. Ames, M. A. Saleh, and J. E. Casida. 1979. Toxaphene, a complex mixture of polychloroterpenes and a major insecticide, is mutagenic. Science 205:591–593.

Hoopingarner, R., A. Samuel, and D. Krause. 1972. Polychlorinated biphenyl interactions with tissue culture cells. Environ. Health Perspect. 1:155–158.

Hoover, R. N., and P. H. Strasser. 1980. Editorial: Saccharin: A bitter aftertaste? N. Engl. J. Med. 302:573–575.

Howard, J. W., and T. Fazio. 1980. Review of polycyclic aromatic hydrocarbons in foods. Analytical methodology and reported findings of polycyclic aromatic hydrocarbons in foods. J. Assoc. Off. Anal. Chem. 63:1077-1104.

Howe, G. R., J. D. Burch, A. B. Miller, B. Morrison, P. Gordon, L. Weldon, L. W. Chambers, G. Fodor, and G. M. Winsor. 1977. Artificial sweeteners and human bladder cancer. Lancet 2:578-581.

Howe, G. R., J. D. Burch, A. B. Miller, G. M. Cook, J. Esteve, G. Morrison, P. Gordon, L. W. Chambers, G. Fodor, and G. M. Winsor. 1980. Tobacco use, occupation, coffee, various nutrients, and bladder cancer. J. Natl. Cancer Inst. 64:701-713.

Huang, C. C. 1973. Effect on growth but not on chromosomes of the mammalian cells after treatment with three organophosphorus insecticides. Proc. Soc. Exp. Biol. Med. 142:36-40.

Huberman, E., H. Bartsch, and L. Sachs. 1975. Mutation induction in Chinese hamster V79 cells by two vinyl chloride metabolites, chloro-ethylene oxide and 2-chloroacetaldehyde. Int. J. Cancer 16:639-644.

Huggins, C., and N. C. Yang. 1962. Induction and extinction of mammary cancer. Science 137:257-262.

Infante, P. F., S. S. Epstein, and W. A. Newton, Jr. 1978. Blood dyscrasias and childhood tumors and exposure to chlordane and heptachlor. Scand. J. Work Environ. Health 4:137-150.

Innes, J. R. M., B. M. Ulland, M. G. Valerio, L. Petrucelli, L. Fishbein, E. R. Hart, A. J. Pallotta, R. R. Bates, H. L. Falk, J. J. Gart, M. Klein, I. Mitchell, and J. Peters. 1969. Bioassay of pesticides and industrial chemicals for tumorigenicity in mice: A preliminary note. J. Natl. Cancer Inst. 42:1101-1114.

International Agency for Research on Cancer. 1974. IARC Monographs on the Evaluation of the Carcinogenic Risk of Chemicals to Man. Volume 5. Some Organochlorine Pesticides. International Agency for Research on Cancer, Lyon, France. 241 pp.

International Agency for Research on Cancer. 1978. Pp. 37-103 in IARC Monographs on the Evaluation of the Carcinogenic Risk of Chemicals to Humans. Volume 18. Polychlorinated Biphenyls and Polybrominated Biphenyls. International Agency for Research on Cancer, Lyon, France.

International Agency for Research on Cancer. 1979. IARC Monographs on the Evaluation of the Carcinogenic Risk of Chemicals to Humans. Volume 20. Some Halogenated Hydrocarbons. International Agency for Research on Cancer, Lyon, France. 609 pp.

International Agency for Reseach on Cancer. 1980. IARC Monographs on the Evaluation of the Carcinogenic Risk of Chemicals to Humans. Volume 22. Some Non-Nutritive Sweetening Agents. International Agency for Research on Cancer, Lyon, France. 208 pp.

Ishidate, M., Jr., and S. Odashima. 1977. Chromosome tests with 134 compounds on Chinese hamster cells in vitro--a screening for chemical carcinogens. Mutat. Res. 48:337-353.

Ishii, H., T. Koshimizu, S. Usami, and T. Fujimoto. 1981. Toxicity of aspartame and its diketopiperazine for Wistar rats by dietary administration for 104 weeks. Toxicology 21:91-94.

Ito, N., H. Nagasaki, M. Arai, S. Makiura, S. Sugihara, and K. Hirao. 1973. Histopathologic studies on liver tumorigenesis induced in mice by technical polychlorinated biphenyls and its promoting effect on liver tumors induced by benzene hexachloride. J. Natl. Cancer Inst. 51:1637-1646.

Ivett, J. L., and R. R. Tice. 1981. Diethylstilbestrol-diphosphate induces chromosomal aberrations but not sister chromatid exchanges in murine bone marrow cells in vivo. Environ. Mutagenesis 3:445-452.

Jager, J. W. 1970. Aldrin, Dieldrin, Endrin and Telodrin. An Epidemiological and Toxicological Study of Long-Term Occupational Exposure. Elsevier, Amsterdam, London, and New York. 234 pp.

Jedlička, V., Z. Heřmanská, I. Smída, and A. Kouba. 1958. Paramyeloblastic leukaemia appearing simultaneously in two blood cousins after simultaneous contact with gammexane (hexachlorcyclohexane). Acta Med. Scand. 161:447-451.

Jelinek, C. 1981. Occurrence and methods of control of chemical contaminants in foods. Environ. Health Perspect. 39:143-151.

Jelinek, C. F., and P. E. Corneliussen. 1976. Levels of PCB's in the U.S. food supply. Pp. 147-154 in National Conference on Polychlorinated Biphenyls, November, 1975. Chicago, Illinois. EPA-560/6-75-004, Office of Toxic Substances, U. S. Environmental Protection Agency, Washington, D. C.

Jukes, T. H. 1974. Estrogens in beefsteaks. J. Am. Med. Assoc. 229:1920-1921.

Jukes, T. H. 1976. Diethylstilbestrol in beef production: What is the risk to consumers? Prev. Med. 5:438-453.

Kay, K. 1977. Polybrominated biphenyls (PPB) environmental contamination in Michigan, 1973-1976. Environ. Res. 13:74-93.

Kennaway, E. L., and N. M. Kennaway. 1947. A further study of the incidence of cancer of the lung and larynx. Br. J. Cancer 1:260-298.

Kessler, I. I. 1970. Cancer mortality among diabetics. J. Natl. Cancer Inst. 44:673-686.

Kessler, I. I., and J. P. Clark. 1978. Saccharin, cyclamate, and human bladder cancer. No evidence of an association. J. Am. Med. Assoc. 240:349-355.

Khera, K. S. 1974. Teratogenicity and dominant lethal studies on hexachlorobenzene in rats. Food Cosmet. Toxicol. 12:471-477.

Kimbrough, R. D., and R. E. Linder. 1974. Induction of adenofibrosis and hepatomas of the liver in BALB/cJ mice by polychorinated biphenyls (Aroclor 1254). J. Natl. Cancer Inst. 53:547-552.

Kimbrough, R. D., R. A. Squire, R. E. Linder, J. D. Strandberg, R. J. Montali, and V. W. Burse. 1975. Induction of liver tumors in Sherman strain female rats by polychlorinated biphenyl Aroclor 1260. J. Natl. Cancer Inst. 55:1453-1459.

Kimbrough, R. D., V. W. Burse, and J. A. Liddle. 1978. Persistent liver lesions in rats after a single oral dose of polybrominated biphenyls (FireMaster FF-1) and concomitant PBB tissue levels. Environ. Health Perspect. 23:265-273.

Kimbrough, R. D., D. F. Groce, M. P. Korver, and V. W. Burse. 1981. Induction of liver tumors in female Sherman strain rats by polybrominated biphenyls. J. Natl. Cancer Inst. 66:535-542.

Kimura, N. T., T. Kanematsu, and T. Baba. 1976. Polychlorinated biphenyl(s) as a promoter in experimental hepatocarcinogenesis in rats. Z. Krebsforsch. Klin. Onkol. 87:257-266.

Klein, M. 1963. Susceptibility of strain B6AF$_1$/J hybrid infant mice to tumorigenesis with 1,2-benzanthracene, deoxycholic acid, and 3-methylcholanthrene. Cancer Res. 23:1701-1707.

Kroes, R., P. W. J. Peters, J. M. Berkvens, H. G. Verschuuren, T. de Vries, and G. J. van Esch. 1977. Long term toxicity and reproduction study (including a teratogenicity study) with cyclamate, saccharin and cyclohexylamine. Toxicology 8:285-300.

Kuratsune, M. 1976. Epidemiologic studies on Yusho. Pp. 9-23 in K. Higuchi, ed. PCB Poisoning and Pollution. Kodansha Ltd., Tokyo; Academic Press, New York, San Francisco, and London.

Kuratsune, M., Y. Masuda, and J. Nagayama. 1976. Some of the recent findings concerning Yusho. Pp. 14-29 in National Conference on Polychlorinated Biphenyls, November 1975. Chicago, Illinois. EPA-560/6-75-004, Office of Toxic Substances, Environmental Protection Agency, Washington, D. C.

Kutz, F. W., and S. C. Strassman. 1976. Residues of polychlorinated biphenyls in the general population of the United States. Pp. 139-143 in National Conference on Polychlorinated Biphenyls, November 1975, Chicago, Illinois. EPA-560/6-75-004, Office of Toxic Substances, Environmental Protection Agency, Washington, D. C.

Larionov, L. T., and N. G. Soboleva. 1938. Gastric tumors experimentally produced in mice by means of benzopyrene and dibenzanthracene. Vestn. Rentgenol. Radiol. 20:276-286.

Laws, E. R., Jr., A. Curley, and F. J. Biros. 1967. Men with intensive occupational exposure to DDT. A clinical and chemical study. Arch. Environ. Health 15:766-775.

Lijinsky, W., and H. W. Taylor. 1976. Carcinogenesis in Sprague-Dawley rats of N-nitroso-N-alkylcarbamate esters. Cancer Lett. 1:275-279.

Lo, M.-T., and E. Sandi. 1978. Polycyclic aromatic hydrocarbons (polynuclears) in foods. Residue Rev. 69:35-86.

Loprieno, N., R. Barale, S. Baroncelli, C. Bauer, G. Bronzetti, A. Cammellini, G. Cercignani, C. Corsi, G. Gervasi, C. Leporini, R. Nieri, A. M. Rossi, G. Stretti, and G. Turchi. 1976. Evaluation of the genetic effects induced by vinyl chloride monomer (VCM) under mammalian metabolic activation: Studies in vitro and in vivo. Mutat. Res. 40:85-95.

Machemer, L., and D. Lorke. 1976. Evaluation of the mutagenic potential of cyclohexylamine on spermatogonia of the Chinese hamster. Mutat. Res. 40:243-250.

Makiura, S., H. Aoe, S. Sugihara, K. Hirao, M. Arai, and N. Ito. 1974. Inhibitory effect of polychlorinated biphenyls on liver tumorigenesis in rats treated with 3'-methyl-4-dimethylaminoazobenzene, N-2-fluorenylacetamide, and diethylnitrosamine. J. Natl. Cancer Inst. 53:1253-1257.

Maltoni, C. 1977. Vinyl chloride carcinogenicity: An experimental model for carcinogenesis studies. Pp. 119-146 in H. H. Hiatt, J. D. Watson, and J. A. Winsten, eds. Origins of Human Cancer, Book A. Incidence of Cancer in Humans. Cold Spring Harbor Laboratory, Cold Spring Harbor, N.Y.

Maltoni, C., G. Lefemine, P. Chieco, and D. Carretti. 1974. Vinyl chloride carcinogenesis: Current results and perspectives. Med. Lav. 65:421-444.

Maltoni, C., A. Ciliberti, L. Gianni, and P. Chieco. 1975. [In Italian.] Gli effetti oncogeni del cloruro di vinile somministrato per via orale mel ratto. Gli Ospedali della Vita 2(6):102-104.

Marshall, T. C., H. W. Dorough, and H. E. Swim. 1976. Screening of pesticides for mutagenic potential using Salmonella typhimurium mutants. J. Agric. Food Chem. 24:560-563.

Martin, C. N., A. C. McDermid, and R. C. Garner. 1978. Testing of known carcinogens and noncarcinogens for their ability to induce unscheduled DNA synthesis in HeLa cells. Cancer Res. 38:2621-2627.

Masuda, Y., K. Mori, T. Hirohata, and M. Kuratsune. 1966. Carcinogenesis in the esophagus. III. Polycyclic aromatic hydrocarbons and phenols in whisky. Gann 57:549-557.

Mazur, R. H. 1976. Aspartame--A sweet surprise. J. Toxicol. Environ. Health 2:243-249.

McCann, J. C. 1977. Short-term tests. Pp. 91-108 in Cancer Testing Technology and Saccharin. Office of Technology Assessment, Congress of the United States, Washington, D. C.

McCann, J., and B. N. Ames. 1976. Detection of carcinogens as mutagens in the Salmonella/microsome test: Assay of 300 chemicals: Discussion. Proc. Natl. Acad. Sci. U.S.A 73:950-954.

McCann, J., E. Choi, E. Yamasaki, and B. N. Ames. 1975. Detection of carcinogens as mutagens in the Salmonella/microsome test: Assay of 300 chemicals. Proc. Natl. Acad. Sci. U.S.A. 72:5135-5139.

McChesney, E. W., F. Coulston, and K.-F. Benitz. 1977. Six-year study of saccharin in rhesus monkeys. Toxicol. Appl. Pharmacol. 41:164. Abstract 79.

Miller, C. T., C. I. Neutel, R. C. Nair, L. D. Marrett, J. M. Last, and W. E. Collins. 1978. Relative importance of risk factors in bladder carcinogenesis. J. Chronic Dis. 31:51-56.

Milvy, P. 1978. Letter to the Editor. Mutat. Res. 57:110-112.

Milvy, P., and M. Wolff. 1977. Mutagenic studies with acrylonitrile.
Mutat. Res. 48:271-278.

Mohn, G. 1973. Comparison of the mutagenic activity of eight organophosphorus insecticides in Escherichia coli. Mutat. Res. 21:196.
Abstract 21.

Mohr, U., U. Green, J. Althoff, and P. Schneider. 1978. Syncarcinogenic
action of saccharin and sodium-cyclamate in the induction of bladder
tumours in MNU-pretreated rats. Pp. 64-69 in B. Guggenheim, ed.
Health and Sugar Substitutes. S. Karger, Basel, Munich, Paris, London
New York, and Sydney.

Mondal, S., D. W. Brankow, and C. Heidelberger. 1978. Enhancement of
oncogenesis in C3H/10T1/2 mouse embryo cell cultures by saccharin.
Science 201:1141-1142.

Monson, R. R., J. M. Peters, and M. N. Johnson. 1974. Proportional
mortality among vinyl-chloride workers. Lancet 2:397-398.

Moreau, P., A. Bailone, and R. Devoret. 1976. Prophage Υ induction in
Escherichia coli K12 envA uvrB: A highly sensitive test for
potential carcinogens. Proc. Natl. Acad. Sci. U.S.A. 73:3700-3704.

Morgan, R. W., and M. G. Jain. 1974. Bladder cancer: Smoking,
beverages and artificial sweeteners. Can. Med. Assoc. J.
111:1067-1070.

Morrison, A. S. 1979. Use of artificial sweeteners by cancer patients.
J. Natl. Cancer Inst. 62:1397-1399.

Morrison, A. S., and J. E. Buring. 1980. Artificial sweeteners and
cancer of the lower urinary tract. N. Engl. J. Med. 302:537-541.

Mussman, H. C. 1975. Drug and chemical residues in domestic animals.
Fed. Proc. Fed. Am. Soc. Exp. Biol. 34:197-201.

Nagao, M., and T. Sugimura. 1978. Mutagenesis: Microbial systems.
Pp. 99-121 in H. V. Gelboin and P. O. P. Ts'o, eds. Polycyclic
Hydrocarbons and Cancer, Volume 2. Molecular and Cell Biology.
Academic Press, New York, San Francisco, and London.

Nagasaki, H., S. Tomii, T. Mega, M. Marugami, and N. Ito. 1971. Letter
to the Editor: Development of hepatomas in mice treated with benzene
hexachloride. Gann 62:431.

Nagasaki, H., S. Tomii, and T. Mega. 1975. [In Japanese; English Title.] Factors on liver tumor in mice induced by benzene hexachloride (BHC) and technical polychlorinated biphenyls (PCBs). Nippon Eiseigaku Zasshi 30:134. Abstract 235.

National Academy of Sciences. 1977. Drinking Water and Health, Volume 1. Safe Drinking Water Committee, National Academy of Sciences, Washington, D. C. 939 pp.

National Academy of Sciences. 1978. Saccharin: Technical Assessment of Risks and Benefits, Part I. Committee for a Study on Saccharin and Food Safety Policy, National Academy of Sciences, Washington, D. C. [250] pp.

National Cancer Institute. 1976. Report on Carcinogenesis Bioassay of Technical Grade Chlordecone (Kepone). Carcinogenesis Program, Division of Cancer Cause and Prevention, National Cancer Institute, Bethesda, Md. [25] pp.

National Cancer Institute. 1977a. Bioassay of Captan for Possible Carcinogenicity. NCI Carcinogenesis Technical Report Series No. 15. DHEW Publication No. (NIH) 77-815. PB-273 475. Carcinogenesis Program, National Cancer Institute, Bethesda, Md. 99 pp.

National Cancer Institute. 1977b. Bioassay of Heptachlor for Possible Carcinogenicity. NCI Carcinogenesis Technical Report Series No. 9, DHEW Publication No. (NIH) 77-809. PB-271 966. Carcinogenesis Program, National Cancer Institute, Bethesda, Md. 111 pp.

National Cancer Institute. 1977c. Bioassay of Lindane for Possible Carcinogenicity. NCI Carcinogenesis Technical Report Series No. 14. DHEW Publication No. (NIH) 77-814. PB-273 480. Carcinogenesis Program, National Cancer Institute, Bethesda, Md. 99 pp.

National Cancer Institute. 1977d. Bioassay of Chlordane for Possible Carcinogenicity. NCI Carcinogenesis Technical Report Series No. 8. DHEW Publication No. (NIH) 77-808. PB 271-977. Carcinogenesis Program, National Cancer Institute, Bethesda, Md. 117 pp.

National Cancer Institute. 1978a. Bioassay of Malathion for Possible Carcinogenicity. NCI Carcinogenesis Technical Report Series No. 24. DHEW Publication No. (NIH) 78-824. Carcinogenesis Testing Program, National Cancer Institute, Bethesda, Md. 102 pp.

National Cancer Institute. 1978b. Bioassays of Aldrin and Dieldrin for Possible Carcinogenicity. NCI Carcinogenesis Technical Report Series No. 21. DHEW Publication No. (NIH) 78-821. Carcinogenesis Testing Program, National Cancer Institute, Bethesda, Md. 184 pp.

National Cancer Institute. 1978c. Bioassay of Dieldrin for Possible
    Carcinogenicity. NCI Carcinogenesis Technical Report Series No. 22.
    DHEW Publication No. (NIH) 78-822. Carcinogenesis Testing Program,
    National Cancer Institute, Bethesda, Md. 50 pp.

National Cancer Institute. 1978d. Bioassays of DDT, TDE and p,p'-DDE
    for Possible Carcinogenicity. NCI Carcinogenesis Technical Report
    Series No. 131. Carcinogenesis Testing Program, National Cancer
    Institute, Bethesda, Md. [230] pp.

National Cancer Institute. 1978e. Bioassay of Pentachloronitrobenzene
    for Possible Carcinogenicity. NCI Carcinogenesis Technical Report
    Series No. 61. Carcinogenesis Testing Program, National Cancer
    Institute, Bethesda, Md. [82] pp.

National Cancer Institue. 1978f. Bioassay of Methoxychlor for Possible
    Carcinogenicity. NCI Carcinogenesis Technical Report Series No. 35.
    DHEW Publication No. (NIH) 78-835. Carcinogenesis Testing Program,
    National Cancer Institute, Bethesda, Md. [86] pp.

National Cancer Institute. 1979a. Bioassay of Butylated Hydroxytoluene
    (BHT) for Possible Carcinogenicity. NCI Carcinogenesis Technical
    Report Series No. 150. NIH Publication No. 79-1706. Carcinogenesis
    Testing Program, National Cancer Institute, Bethesda, Md. 114 pp.

National Cancer Institute. 1979b. Bioassay of Aldicarb for Possible
    Carcinogenicity. NCI Carcinogenesis Technical Report Series No.
    136. NIH Publication No. 179-1391. PB 298-511. Carcinogenesis
    Testing Program, National Cancer Institute, Bethesda, Md. 106 pp.

National Cancer Institute. 1979c. Bioassay of Diazinon for Possible
    Carcinogenicity. NCI Carcinogenesis Technical Report Series No.
    137. NIH Publication No. 79-1392. PB-293 889. Carcinogenesis
    Testing Program, National Cancer Institute, Bethesda, Md. 96 pp.

National Cancer Institute. 1979d. Bioassay of Malathion for Possible
    Carcinogenicity. NCI Carcinogenesis Technical Report Series No.
    192. NIH Publication No. 79-1748. PB-300 301. Carcinogenesis
    Testing Program, National Cancer Institute, Bethesda, Md. 72 pp.

National Cancer Institute. 1979e. Bioassay of Methyl Parathion for
    Possible Carcinogenicity. NCI Carcinogenesis Technical Report Series
    No. 157. DHEW Publication No. (NIH) 79-1713. Carcinogenesis Testing
    Program, National Cancer Institute, Bethesda, Md. 112 pp.

National Cancer Institute. 1979f. Bioassay of Parathion for Possible
    Carcinogenicity. NCI Carcinogenesis Technical Report Series No. 70.
    DHEW Publication No. (NIH) 79-1320. Carcinogenesis Testing Program,
    National Cancer Institute, Bethesda, Md. 104 pp.

National Cancer Institute. 1979g. Bioassay of Toxaphene for Possible Carcinogenicity. NCI Carcinogenesis Technical Report Series No. 37. DHEW Publication No. (NIH) 79-837. Carcinogenesis Testing Program, National Cancer Institute, Bethesda, Md. 104 pp.

National Institute of Hygienic Sciences. 1973. Chronic Toxicity Study of Sodium Saccharin: 21 Months Feeding in Mice. National Institute of Hygienic Sciences, Tokyo.

Neal, J., and R. H. Rigdon. 1967. Gastric tumors in mice fed benzo(a)-pyrene: A quantitative study. Tex. Rep. Biol. Med. 25:553-557.

Nicholson, W. J., E. C. Hammond, H. Seidman, and I. J. Selikoff. 1975. Mortality experience of a cohort of vinyl chloride-polyvinyl chloride workers. Ann. N.Y. Acad. Sci. 246:225-230.

Nishizumi, M. 1976. Enhancement of diethylnitrosamine hepatocarcino-genesis in rats by exposure to polychlorinated biphenyls or phenobarbital. Cancer Lett. 2:11-15.

Norris, J. M. 1977. Status Report on the 2 Year Study Incorporating Acrylonitrile in the Drinking Water of Rats. Health and Environmental Research. The Dow Chemical Company, Midland, Mich. [14] pp.

O'Berg, M. T. 1980. Epidemiologic study of workers exposed to acrylonitrile. J. Occup. Med. 22:245-252.

Ochi, H., and A. Tonomura. 1978. Presence of unscheduled DNA synthesis in cultured human cells after treatment with sodium saccharin. Mutat. Res. 54:224. Abstract 26.

Office of Technology Assessment. 1979. Environmental Contaminants in Food. Office of Technology Assessment, Congress of the United States, Washington, D. C. 229 pp.

Ohshima, H., and H. Bartsch. 1981. Quantitative estimation of endogenous nitrosation in man by monitoring N-nitrosoproline excreted in the urine. Cancer Res. 41:3658-3662.

Ortelee, M. F. 1958. Study of men with prolonged intensive occupational exposure to DDT. Arch. Ind. Health 18:433-440.

Oser, B. L., S. Carson, G. E. Cox, E. E. Vogin, and S. S. Sternberg. 1975. Chronic toxicity study of cyclamate:saccharin (10:1) in rats. Toxicology 4:315-330.

Peirce, W. E. H. 1961. Tumour-promotion by lime oil in the mouse forestomach. Nature 189:497-498.

Peraino, C., R. J. M. Fry, E. Staffeldt, and J. P. Christopher. 1977. Enhancing effects of phenobarbitone and butylated hydroxytoluene on 2-acetylaminofluorene-induced heptatic tumorigenesis in the rat. Food Cosmet. Toxicol. 15:93-96.

Poncelet, F., M. Roberfroid, M. Mercier, and J. Lederer. 1979. Absence of mutagenic activity in Salmonella typhimurium of some impurities found in saccharin. Food Cosmet. Toxicol. 17:229-231.

Pott, P. 1775. Cancer scroti. Pp. 63-68 in Chirurgical Observations. Hawes, Clarke, and Collins, London.

Preston, B. D., J. P. Van Miller, R. W. Moore, and J. R. Allen. 1981. Promoting effects of polychlorinated biphenyls (Aroclor 1254) and polychlorinated dibenzofuran-free Aroclor 1254 on diethylnitrosamine-induced tumorigenesis in the rat. J. Natl. Cancer Inst. 66:509-515.

Purchase, I. F. H., C. R. Richardson, and D. Anderson. 1975. Letter to the Editor: Chromosomal and dominant lethal effects of vinyl chloride. Lancet 2:410-411.

Rao, M. S., and A. B. Qureshi. 1972. Induction of dominant lethals in mice by sodium saccharin. Indian J. Med. Res. 60:599-603.

Rigdon, R. H., and J. Neal. 1969. Relationship of leukemia to lung and stomach tumors in mice fed benzo(a)pyrene. Proc. Soc. Exp. Biol. Med. 130:146-148.

Roe, F. J. C., L. S. Levy, and R. L. Carter. 1970. Feeding studies on sodium cyclamate, saccharin and sucrose for carcinogenic and tumour-promoting activity. Food Cosmet. Toxicol. 8:135-145.

Rösli, M., B. Zimmerli, and B. Marek. 1975. [In German; English Summary.] Ruckstände von Vinylchlorid-Monomer in Speiseölen. Mitt. Geb. Lebensmittelunters. Hyg. 66:507-511.

Rudali, G., E. Coezy, and I. Muranyi-Kovacs. 1969. [In French.] Recherches sur l'action cancérigène du cyclamate de soude chez les souris. C. R. Hebd. Seances Acad. Sci. Ser. D. 269:1910-1912.

Rurainski, R. D., H. J. Theiss, and W. Zimmermann. 1977. [In German.] Über das Vorkommen von natürlichen und synthetischen Östrogenen im Trinkwasser. GWF Gas-Wasserfach:Wasser/Abwasser 118:288-291.

Rustia, M. 1979. Role of hormone imbalance in transplacental carcinogenesis induced in Syrian golden hamsters by sex hormones. Natl. Cancer Inst. Monogr. 51:77-87.

Rustia, M., and P. Shubik. 1976. Transplacental effects of diethyl-stilbestrol on the genital tract of hamster offspring. Cancer Lett. 1:139-146.

Schmähl, D. 1973. [In German; English Summary.] Lack of carcinogenic effects of cyclamate, cyclohexylamine and saccharine in rats. Arzneim. Forsch. 23:1466-1470.

Schwartz, L. 1943. An outbreak of halowax acne ("cable rash") among electricians. J. Am. Med. Assoc. 122:158-161.

Sciorra, L. J., B. N. Kaufmann, and R. Maier. 1974. The effects of butylated hydroxytoluene on the cell cycle and chromosome morphology of phytohaemagglutinin-stimulated leucocyte cultures. Food Cosmet. Toxicol. 12:33-44.

Searle, G. D., and Co. 1972a. An Evaluation of Mutagenic Potential Employing the Host-Mediated Assay in the Rat. P-T No. 1028H72. Final Report. G. D. Searle and Co., Skokie, Ill. 15 pp.

Searle, G. D., and Co. 1972b. An Evaluation of Mutagenic Potential Employing the Host-Mediated Assay in the Rat. P-T No. 1029H72. Final Report. G. D. Searle and Co., Skokie, Ill. 15 pp.

Searle, G. D., and Co. 1973a. A 26-Week Urinary Bladder Tumorigenicity Study in the Mouse by the Intravesical Pellet Implant Technique. P-T No. 10310T72. Final Report. G. D. Searle and Co., Skokie, Ill.

Searle, G. D., and Co. 1973b. Two Year Toxicity Study in the Rat. P-T No. 838H71. Final Report. G. D. Searle and Co., Skokie, Ill. 104 pp.

Searle, G. D., and Co. 1973c. 106-Week Oral Toxicity Study in the Dog. P-T No. 855S270. G. D. Searle and Co., Skokie, Ill.

Searle, G. D., and Co. 1973d. An Evaluation of the Mutagenic Potential in the Rat Employing the Dominant Lethal Assay. P-T No. 1007S72. G. D. Searle and Co., Skokie, Ill. 35 pp.

Searle, G. D., and Co. 1974a. 104-Week Toxicity Study in the Mouse. P-T No. 984H73. Final Report. G. D. Searle and Co., Skokie, Ill. 295 pp.

Searle, G. D., and Co. 1974b. Lifetime Toxicity Study in the Rat. P-T No. 892H72. Final Report. G. D. Searle and Co., Skokie, Ill. 255 pp.

Searle, G. D., and Co. 1974c. An Evaluation of Mutagenic Potential Employing the Host-Mediated Assay in the Mouse. P-T No. 1095S73. G. D. Searle and Co., Skokie, Ill. 23 pp.

Searle, G. D., and Co. 1978a. An Evaluation of Mutagenic Potential Employing the Ames Salmonella/Microsome Assay. Final Report. S.A. No. 13-77. G. D. Searle and Co., Skokie, Ill.

Searle, G. D., and Co. 1978b. An Evaluation of Mutagenic Potential Employing the Ames Salmonella/Microsome Assay. Final Report. S. A. No. 13-78. G. D. Searle and Co., Skokie, Ill.

Searle, G. D., and Co. 1978c. An Evaluation of the Mutagenic Potential Employing the Ames Salmonella/Microsome Assay. Final Report. S.A. 13-85. G. D. Searle and Co., Skokie, Ill.

Simmon, V. F., D. C. Poole, and G. W. Newell. 1976. In vitro mutagenic studies of twenty pesticides. Toxicol. Appl. Pharmacol. 37:109. Abstract 42.

Simmon, V. F., D. C. Poole, E. S. Riccio, D. E. Robinson, A. D. Mitchell, and M. D. Waters. 1979. In vitro mutagenicity and genotoxicity assays of 38 pesticides. Environ. Mutagenesis 1:142-143. Abstract Ca-9.

Simon, D., S. Yen, and P. Cole. 1975. Coffee drinking and cancer of the lower urinary tract. J. Natl. Cancer Inst. 54:587-591.

Simon, G. S., B. R. Kipps, R. G. Tardiff, and J. F. Borzelleca. 1978. Failure of kepone and hexachlorobenzene to induce dominant lethal mutations in the rat. Toxicol. Appl. Pharmacol. 45:330-331. Abstract 260.

Snell, K. C., and H. L. Stewart. 1962. Pulmonary adenomatosis induced in DBA/2 mice by oral administration of dibenz(a,h)anthracene. J. Natl. Cancer Inst. 28:1043-1051.

Soós, K. 1980. The occurrence of carcinogenic polycyclic hydrocarbons in foodstuffs in Hungary. Arch. Toxicol. Suppl. 4:446-448.

Subcommittee on the Health Effects of Polychlorinated Biphenyls and Polybrominated Biphenyls. 1978. Final report of the Subcommittee on the Health Effects of Polychlorinated Biphenyls and Polybrominated Biphenyls of the DHEW Committee to Coordinate Toxicology and Related Programs. Environ. Health Perspect. 24:129-239.

Suess, M. J. 1976. The environmental load and cycle of polycyclic aromatic hydrocarbons. Sci. Total Environ. 6:239-250.

Tabershaw, I. R., and W. R. Gaffey. 1974. Mortality study of workers in the manufacture of vinyl chloride and its polymers. J. Occup. Med. 16:509-518.

Tardiff, R. G., G. P. Carlson, and V. Simmon. 1976. Halogenated organics in tap water: A toxicological evaluation. Pp. 213-227 in R. L. Jolley, ed. The Environmental Impact of Water Chlorination. CONF-751096, UC-11,41,48. Oak Ridge National Laboratory, Oak Ridge, Tenn.

Taylor, J. M., and L. Friedman. 1974. Combined chronic feeding and three-generation reproduction study of sodium saccharin in the rat. Toxicol. Appl. Pharmacol. 29:154. Abstract 200.

Terracini, B., M. C. Testa, J. R. Cabral, and N. Day. 1973. The effects of long-term feeding of DDT to BALB/c mice. Int. J. Cancer 11:747-764.

Thiess, A. M., and I. Fleig. 1978. Analysis of chromosomes of workers exposed to acrylonitrile. Arch. Toxicol. 41:149-152.

Thorpe, E., and A. I. T. Walker. 1973. The toxicology of dieldrin (HEOD). II. Comparative long-term oral toxicity studies in mice with dieldrin, DDT, phenobarbitone, β-BHC and γ-BHC. Food Cosmet. Toxicol. 11:433-442.

Tisdel, M. O., P. O. Nees, D. L. Harris, and P. H. Derse. 1974. Long-term feeding of saccharin in rats. Pp. 145-158 in G. E. Inglett, ed. Symposium: Sweeteners. AVI Publishing Company, Westport, Conn.

Tokumitsu, T. 1971. Some aspects of cytogenetic effects of sodium cyclamate on human leucocytes in vitro. Proc. Jpn. Acad. 47:635-639.

Tong, C., M. F. Laspia, S. Telang, and G. M. Williams. 1981. The use of adult rat liver cultures in the detection of the genotoxicity of various polycyclic aromatic hydrocarbons. Environ. Mutagenesis 3:477-487.

Trosko, J. E., B. Dawson, L. P. Yotti, and C. C. Chang. 1980. Saccharin may act as a tumour promoter by inhibiting metabolic cooperation between cells. Nature 285:109-110.

Trosko, J. E., L. P. Yotti, S. Warren, G. Tsushimoto, and C. C. Chang. 1982. Inhibition of cell-cell communication by tumor promoters. Pp. 565-585 in E. Hecker, W. Kunz, S. Marx, N. E. Fusenig, and H. W. Phielmann, eds. Carcinogenesis: A Comprehensive Survey. Volume 7, Carcinogenesis and Biological Effects of Tumor Promoters. Raven Press, New York.

U.S. Consumer Product Safey Commission. 1974. Self-pressurized household substances containing vinyl chloride monomer; classification as banned hazardous substance. Fed. Regist. 39:30112-30114.

U.S. Department of Agriculture. 1977. Assessment of Toxaphene in Agriculture. USDA/State Assessment Team on Toxaphene, September 9, 1977. Coordinated by the Office of Environmental Quality Activities, U.S. Department of Agriculture, Washington, D. C. 633 pp.

U.S. Department of Agriculture. 1978. Situation and Outlook. Sugar and Sweetener Report 3(5):1-70.

U.S. Department of Health, Education, and Welfare. 1969. Report of the Secretary's Commission on Pesticides and Their Relationship to Environmental Health, Parts I and II. U.S. Department of Health, Education, and Welfare, Washington, D. C. 677 pp.

U.S. Department of Health, Education, and Welfare. 1973a. Histopathologic Evaluation of Tissues from Rats Following Continuous Dietary Intake of Sodium Saccharin and Calcium Cyclamate for a Maximum Period of Two Years. Final Report, December 21, 1973. Project P-169-170. Division of Pathology, Food and Drug Administration, U. S. Department of Health, Education, and Welfare, Washington, D. C.

U.S. Department of Health, Education, and Welfare. 1973b. Subacute and Chronic Toxicity and Carcinogenicity of Various Dose Levels of Sodium Saccharin. Final Report. Project P-169-170. Divison of Pathology, Food and Drug Administration, U.S. Department of Health, Education, and Welfare, Washington, D.C.

U.S. Environmental Protection Agency. 1975a. Preliminary Assessment of Suspected Carcinogens in Drinking Water. Report to Congress. EPA-560/4-75-005. PB-25096. Office of Toxic Substances, U.S. Environmental Protection Agency, Washington, D. C.

U.S. Environmental Protection Agency. 1975b. Draft Report. Aspects of Pesticidal Uses of Carbaryl (Sevin) on Man and the Environment. Office of Pesticide Programs, U.S. Environmental Protection Agency, Washington, D. C.

U.S. Environmental Protection Agency. 1975c. Scientific and Technical Assessment Report on Particulate Polycyclic Organic Matter (PPOM), EPA-600/6-75-001. March 1975. Office of Research and Development, U.S. Environmental Protection Agency, Washington, D. C. [95] pp.

U.S. Environmental Protection Agency. 1979. Polychlorinated biphenyls (PCBs). Manufacturing, processing, distribution in commerce, and use prohibitions. Fed. Regist. 44:31514-31568.

U.S. Environmental Protection Agency. 1980. Summary of Reported Incidents Involving Toxaphene. Pesticide Incident Monitoring

System Report No. 316. Hazard Evaluation Division, Office of Pesticide Programs, U.S. Environmental Protection Agency, Washington, D. C.

U. S. Food and Drug Administration. 1970. Revocations regarding cyclamate-containing products intended for drug use. Fed. Regist. 35:13644–13645.

U. S. Food and Drug Administration. 1977a. Polychlorinated biphenyls (PCB's). Unavoidable contaminants in food and food packaging materials; Reduction of temporary tolerances. Fed. Regist. 42:17487–17494.

U. S. Food and Drug Administration. 1977b. Butylated hydroxytoluene. Use restrictions. Fed. Regist. 42:27603–27609.

U. S. Food and Drug Administration. 1979. Diethylstilbestrol; Withdrawal of approval of new animal drug applications; Commissioner's decision. Fed. Regist. 44:54852–54900.

U. S. Food and Drug Administration. 1980a. Aspartame: Decision of the Public Board of Inquiry, Department of Health and Human Services. Docket No. 75F-0355. 51 pp.

U. S. Food and Drug Administration. 1980b. FDA Compliance Program Report of Findings, FY 77 Total Diet Studies – Adult (7320.73). Food and Drug Administration, U.S. Department of Health, Education, and Welfare, Washington, D. C.

U. S. Food and Drug Administration. 1981. Aspartame; Commisioner's Final Decision. Fed. Regist. 46:38283–38308.

Urabe, H. 1974. [In Japanese; English Summary.] Foreward. Fukuoka Igaku Zasshi 65:1–4.

Venitt, S., C. T. Bushell, and M. Osborne. 1977. Mutagenicity of acrylonitrile (cyanoethylene) in *Escherichia coli*. Mutat. Res. 45:283–288.

Verburgt, F. G., and E. Vogel. 1977. Vinyl chloride mutagenesis in *Drosophila melanogaster*. Mutat. Res. 48:327–336.

Versteeg, J. P. J., and K. W. Jager. 1973. Long-term occupational exposure to the insecticides aldrin, dieldrin, endrin, and telodrin. Br. J. Ind. Med. 30:201–202.

Voitalovich, E. A., P. P. Deekoon, L. U. Deemarsky, and L. M. Shabad. 1957. [In Russian; English Summary.] Comparative study of malignant tumor frequency in Tookoom District of the Latvian SSR. Vopr. Onkol. 3:351-357.

Wang, H. H., and S. Grufferman. 1981. Aplastic anemia and occupational pesticide exposure: A case-control study. J. Occup. Med. 23:364-366.

Wang, H. H., and B. MacMahon. 1979. Mortality of workers employed in the manufacture of chlordane and heptachlor. J. Occup. Med. 21:745-748.

Waxweiler, R. J., W. Stringer, J. K. Wagoner, J. Jones, H. Falk, and C. Carter. 1976. Neoplastic risk among workers exposed to vinyl chloride. Ann. N. Y. Acad. Sci. 271:40-48.

Weil, C. S., and C. P. Carpenter. 1965. Results of a Three-Generation Reproductive Study on Rats Fed Sevin in Their Diets. Report 28-53. Mellon Institute, Carnegie-Mellon University, Pittsburgh, Penn. 18 pp.

Weil, C. S., and C. P. Carpenter. 1974. Aldicarb. Inclusion in the Diet of Rats for Three Generations and a Dominant Lethal Mutagenesis Test. Special Report 37-90. Carnegie-Mellon Institute of Research, Carnegie-Mellon University, Pittsburgh, Penn. 46 pp.

Wertz, G. F., and G. Ficsor. 1978. Cytogenetic and teratogenic test of polybrominated biphenyls in rodents. Environ. Health Perspect. 23:129-132.

West, I. 1967. Lindane and hematologic reactions. Arch. Environ. Health 15:97-101.

Wiegand, R. G. 1978. Practical considerations for synthetic sweeteners: Past, present and future--Cyclamates. Pp. 263-267 in J. H. Shaw and G. G. Roussos, eds. Sweeteners and Dental Caries. Information Retrieval, Inc., Arlington, Va.

Williams, D. T. 1976a. Gas-liquid chromatographic headspace method for vinyl chloride in vinegars and alcoholic beverages. J. Assoc. Off. Anal. Chem. 59:30-31.

Williams, D. T. 1976b. Confirmation of vinyl chloride in foods by conversion to 1-chloro-1,2-dibromoethane. J. Assoc. Off. Anal. Chem. 59:32-34.

Williams, D. T., and W. F. Miles. 1975. Gas-liquid chromatographic determination of vinyl chloride in alcoholic beverages, vegetable oils, and vinegars. J. Assoc. Off. Anal. Chem. 58:272-275.

Witschi, H. P. 1981. Enhancement of tumor formation in mouse lung by dietary butylated hydroxytoluene. Toxicology 21:95-104.

Witschi, H., D. Williamson, and S. Lock. 1977. Enhancement of urethan tumorigenesis in mouse lung by butylated hydroxytoluene. J. Natl. Cancer Inst. 58:301-305.

Witschi, H. P., P. J. Hakkinen, and J. P. Kehrer. 1981. Modification of lung tumor development in A/J mice. Toxicology 21:37-45.

Wolff, S., and B. Rodin. 1978. Saccharin-induced sister chromatid exchanges in Chinese hamster and human cells. Science 200:543-545.

World Health Organization. 1958. Procedures for the Testing of Intentional Food Additives to Establish Their Safety for Use. Second Report of the Joint FAO/WHO Expert Committee on Food Additives. W.H.O. Tech. Rep. Ser. 144:1-19.

World Health Organization. 1973. Safe Use of Pesticides. W.H.O. Tech. Rep. Ser. 513:1-54.

Wynder, E. L., and S. D. Stellman. 1980. Artificial sweetener use and bladder cancer: A case-control study. Science 207:1214-1216.

Wynder, E. L., K. Mabuchi, N. Maruchi, and J. G. Fortner. 1973. Epidemiology of cancer of the pancreas. J. Natl. Cancer Inst. 50:645-667.

Wyndham, C., J. Devenish, and S. Safe. 1976. The in vitro metabolism, macromolecular binding and bacterial mutagenicity of 4-chlorobiphenyl, a model PCB substrate. Res. Commun. Chem. Pathol. Pharmacol. 15:563-570.

Yoshida, S., M. Masubuchi, and K. Hiraga. 1978. Induced chromosome aberrations by artificial sweeteners in CHO-K1 cells. Mutat. Res. 54:262. Abstract 45.

15 Inhibitors of Carcinogenesis

In recent years, a number of foods and constituents of foods have been studied for their inhibitory effects on carcinogenesis. Results from both epidemiological and experimental studies have indicated that some of the substances studied do have inhibitory effects, but the mechanisms are not yet clear.

This chapter contains a review of the most conclusive data pertaining to the inhibitory effects of nonnutritive constituents of the diet.

EPIDEMIOLOGICAL STUDIES

Epidemiological studies have produced data suggesting that certain substances in foods may protect against the development of cancer. A substantial number of these studies have demonstrated an inverse relationship between consumption of vegetables and risk of cancer, especially cancer of the gastrointestinal tract. Vegetables contain nutritive constituents with inhibitory capacities (as discussed in Section A and Chapter 9) as well as nonnutritive inhibitors, which are described in this chapter. The epidemiological data are not sufficient to permit a definition of the individual roles played by each of the several putative inhibitors that may be present in the same food. Nevertheless, the data are of considerable interest even though the mechanism of inhibition is unclear.

In one study of stomach cancer, Graham et al. (1972) found that consumption of raw vegetables, including cole slaw and red cabbage, was higher among controls than among cases. In a study of Hawaiian Japanese, Haenszel et al. (1972) reported lower risk of stomach cancer for consumers of several Western vegetables, many of which are eaten raw. In a corresponding study in Japan, the same investigators reported a lower risk of stomach cancer for consumers of lettuce and celery (Haenszel et al., 1976). In case-control studies conducted in Norway and in the United States (Minnesota), Bjelke (1978) also demonstrated an inverse relationship between incidence of stomach cancer and the indices for consumption of vegetables, especially among younger patients and women. He also reported preliminary findings from a prospective cohort study, showing a reduced risk of stomach cancer for consumers of large amounts of vegetables in Norway, but not in the United States. In Japan, Hirayama (1977) found that the risk for stomach cancer was lower for nonsmokers who ate green and yellow vegetables than for nonsmokers who did not eat these vegetables.

Much of the epidemiological evidence pertains to cancer of the large bowel. Modan et al. (1975) compared cases of colon and rectal cancer with both hospital and neighborhood controls and found an inverse association between colon cancer (but not for rectal cancer) and the frequent consumption of fiber-containing foods, including cabbage. Other inverse associations between consumption of fiber-containing foods and colon cancer (see Chapter 8) could also reflect different intakes of cruciferous vegetables. Graham et al. (1978) reported that a decreased risk for colon cancer was associated with frequent ingestion of raw vegetables, especially cabbage, brussels sprouts, and broccoli, in a case-control study conducted in New York State. Similar but less impressive findings were obtained for rectal cancer.

Haenszel et al. (1980) found an inverse association for cabbage consumption in a case-control study of colorectal cancer in Japan, but not in Hawaii (Haenszel et al., 1973). In the previously cited, ongoing cohort study in Minnesota and Norway, Bjelke (1978) noted that the risk for colorectal cancer is associated inversely with an index of vegetable consumption in Minnesota, but not in Norway. This result paralleled his earlier finding that the intake of vegetables, particularly cabbage, by colorectal cancer cases was less than for controls in Minnesota.

EXPERIMENTAL STUDIES

As discussed in Chapters 8, 9, and 10, certain vitamins, minerals, and fiber have been found to inhibit some forms of carcinogenesis. During the past decade, studies have shown that foods also contain nonnutritive organic compounds that are also inhibitors of carcinogenesis. These compounds fall into a category frequently referred to as "secondary plant constituents." Among these constituents are phenols, indoles, aromatic isothiocyanates, flavones, protease inhibitors, and the plant sterol β-sitosterol, which are discussed below along with related studies of the effects of individual foods.

Effects of Selected Chemicals

The administration of selected chemicals in this category has been shown to inhibit both initiation and promotion of chemically induced neoplasia in virtually all organs of laboratory animals. As will become apparent in subsequent discussions, much remains to be learned about these numerous and virtually omnipresent dietary constituents, including their possible adverse as well as beneficial effects.

The mechanisms by which these compounds prevent neoplasia is incompletely understood. Some inhibitors, so-called "blocking agents," exert their effects when administered before and during exposure to carcinogens. Others act during the promotion phase of carcinogenesis, and still others inhibit only when given following exposures to inhibitors and promoters from other external sources. Finally, some inhibitors are effective at more than one point during the process of carcinogenesis. Of the inhibitors identified thus far, the largest number falls into the category of blocking agents, appearing to act by preventing carcinogens or their metabolites from reaching or reacting with critical target sites. In many instances, they alter the activity of enzyme systems that metabolize carcinogenic agents (Wattenberg, 1981a).

A second general form of inhibition is particularly relevant to promotion. The inhibitor is assumed either to suppress free radical formation resulting from exposure to tumor promoters or to trap these radicals. Protease inhibitors and phenolic antioxidants have been postulated to inhibit neoplasia in this manner.

The fact that a compound inhibits chemically induced carcinogenesis in laboratory animals should not be interpreted as indicating that an increased intake of the substance is desirable for humans. Knowledge of possible adverse effects of these compounds is incomplete (see discussion at the end of this chapter).

Phenols. Two categories of phenolic inhibitors of carcinogenesis are found in food. One is synthetic and the other occurs naturally. The synthetic antioxidant, butylated hydroxyanisole (BHA) is a widely used food additive and has been extensively studied for its capacity to inhibit carcinogen-induced neoplasia (Wattenberg, 1978). Table 15-1 lists experiments in which BHA has been shown to have inhibitory effects. In these studies, BHA was administered before and/or during exposure to the carcinogen. BHA has also been shown to inhibit host-mediated mutagenesis resulting from exposure to hycanthone, metrifonate, praziquantel, and metronidazole (Batzinger et al., 1978). Slaga (1981) reported that BHA inhibited tumor promotion in the mouse skin when administered after the carcinogen.

Studies of the mechanism by which BHA inhibits chemically induced carcinogenesis have shown that this phenolic compound produces a co-ordinated enzyme response that may be interpreted as causing a greater rate of detoxification (Wattenberg, 1981a). Mice that have been fed BHA for 1 to 2 weeks in carcinogen inhibition experiments show marked increases in both glutathione S-transferase activity and tissue glutathione levels (Benson et al., 1978, 1979). Glutathione S-transferase is an important enzyme for detoxifying chemical carcinogens (Benson et al., 1978; Jakoby, 1978; Wattenberg, 1981a). The activity of uridine diphosphate (UDP)-glucuronyl transferase, which is another important conjugating enzyme in the detoxification systems, is also increased (Cha and Bueding, 1979). The feeding of BHA has also been reported to increase epoxide hydrolase activity (Cha et al., 1978) and to alter the microsomal monooxygenase system (Lam et al., 1980; Speier et al., 1978).

TABLE 15-1

Inhibition of Carcinogen-Induced Neoplasia by BHA[a]

Carcinogen Inhibited	Species	Site of Neoplasm
Benzo[a]pyrene	Mouse	Lung
Benzo[a]pyrene	Mouse	Forestomach
Benzo[a]pyrene-7-8-dihydrodiol	Mouse	Forestomach, lung, and lymphoid tissue
7,12-Dimethylbenz[a]anthracene	Mouse	Lung
7,12-Dimethylbenz[a]anthracene	Mouse	Forestomach
7,12-Dimethylbenz[a]anthracene	Mouse	Skin
7,12-Dimethylbenz[a]anthracene	Rat	Breast
7-Hydroxymethyl-12-methyl-benz[a]anthracene	Mouse	Lung
Dibenz[a,h]anthracene	Mouse	Lung
Nitrosodiethylamine	Mouse	Lung
4-Nitroquinoline-N-oxide	Mouse	Lung
Uracil mustard	Mouse	Lung
Urethan	Mouse	Lung
Methylazoxymethanol acetate	Mouse	Large intestine
trans-5-Amino-3-[2-(5-nitro-2-furyl)vinyl]-1,2,4-oxadiazole	Mouse	Forestomach, lung, and lymphoid tissue

---

[a]From Wattenberg, 1979a.

15-4

The amount of BHA consumed in the average U.S. diet is estimated to be several milligrams per day at most. This level, when corrected for body weight, is far less than that given to laboratory animals in experimental studies. However, exposure to carcinogens is almost certainly orders of magnitude lower in the human population than in experimental studies in animals. No conclusion can be drawn at this time as to whether inhibitory effects of BHA occur at the low concentrations of carcinogens to which humans are generally exposed.

Recent studies have shown that several naturally occurring phenolic compounds inhibit carcinogenesis in mice (Wattenberg et al., 1981a). The phenols studied thus far are cinnamic acid derivatives that are common constituents of plants. They include o-hydroxycinnamic acid, p-hydroxycinnamic acid, 3,4-dihydroxycinnamic acid (caffeic acid), and 4-hydroxy-3-methoxycinnamic acid (ferulic acid). Limited data on these derivatives indicate that their inhibition of benzo[a]-pyrene-induced neoplasia in the mouse is considerably weaker than that of BHA (Wattenberg et al., 1981a). There are many other phenols in plants, including plants consumed by humans, but their inhibitory activity is unknown.

Indoles. Indole-3-acetonitrile, 3,3'-diindolylmethane, and indole-3-carbinol are found in edible cruciferous vegetables such as brussels sprouts, cabbage, cauliflower, and broccoli. Indole-3-acetonitrile is the most abundant of the three. These indoles have been studied for their effects on neoplasia induced by benzo[a]pyrene (BaP) and 7,12-dimethylbenz[a]anthracene (DMBA) in rodents (Wattenberg and Loub, 1978). When added to the diet of mice before and during administration of BaP, all three indoles inhibited BaP-induced neoplasia of the forestomach and pulmonary adenoma formation. In other experiments, indole-3-carbinol and 3,3'-diindolylmethane inhibited DMBA-induced mammary tumor formation in female Sprague-Dawley rats. Indole-3-acetonitrile was inactive in the rat (Wattenberg and Loub, 1978). The original rationale for testing the three indoles stemmed from their ability to alter microsomal monooxygenase oxidase activity. All three compounds increased the activity of this enzyme system (Loub et al., 1975; Pantuck et al., 1976) -- indole-3-carbinol and 3,3'-diindolylmethane more strongly than indole-3-acetonitrile. The three of them also increased glutathione S-transferase activity. There have been no studies in which these compounds were administered after the carcinogen.

Aromatic Isothiocyanates. Benzyl isothiocyanates and phenethyl isothiocyanate are also constituents of cruciferous plants. These aromatic isothiocyanates have been shown to inhibit neoplasia induced by polycyclic aromatic hydrocarbons (PAH's) when they were administered during the initiation phase under several different experimental conditions. These results were obtained when the aromatic isothiocyanate was fed both before and during administration of the PAH's

(Wattenberg, 1977, 1979b). Little is known about their mechanism of inhibition other than the fact that benzyl isothiocyanate is a potent inducer of glutathione S-transferase activity. In further studies, mammary tumor formation resulting from exposure to DMBA was inhibited by the administration of benzyl isothiocyanate subsequent to the carcinogen. It has also been demonstrated that this compound inhibited 1,2-dimethylhydrazine-induced neoplasia of the large intestine when the exposures were begun 1 week after administration of the carcinogen (Wattenberg, 1981b). The mechanism of these inhibitory effects is not known.

Flavones. The study of flavones (found in fruits and vegetables) as possible inhibitors was undertaken as a result of data showing that several inducers of increased microsomal mixed function oxidase activity inhibit chemically induced carcinogenesis.

Inhibition of BaP-induced carcinogenesis has been studied with three flavones: two synthetic compounds -- β-naphthoflavone (5,6-benzoflavone) and quercetin pentamethyl ether -- and one naturally occurring compound -- rutin (3,3',4',5,7-pentahydroxyflavone-3-rutinoside). Quercetin pentamethyl ether is sometimes substituted for tangeretin, a naturally occurring pentamethoxy flavone found in citrus fruits. All three flavones induce aryl hydrocarbon hydroxylase (AHH) activity: β-naphthoflavone is the most potent inducer, quercetin pentamethyl ether is a moderate inducer, and rutin has the weakest inducing capacity. When added to the diet of A/HeJ mice subsequently challenged with orally administered BaP, β-naphthoflavone caused almost total inhibition of pulmonary adenoma formation, and quercetin pentamethyl ether reduced the number of these neoplasms by one-half. The number of adenomas was the same in animals fed rutin and the control diet. Thus, the inhibitory effects of BaP-induced neoplasia paralleled the potency of the three flavones in inducing increased AHH activity (Wattenberg and Leong, 1968, 1970). Recently, β-naphthoflavone has been shown to induce activity of conjugating enzymes, including glutathione S-transferase.

The mutagenic flavones have multiple hydroxyl groups. Flavones exerting protective effects do not have free polar groups; they either contain methoxy substituents or are unsubstituted (MacGregor and Jurd, 1978). The mutagenic and carcinogenic effects of flavones are discussed in Chapter 13.

Protease Inhibitors. Protease inhibitors are widely distributed in plants, and are particularly abundant in seeds. Soybeans, a major source of protein in many vegetarian diets, and lima beans contain a variety of these compounds.

Protease inhibitors have in common the ability to inhibit protease enzymes as well as tumor promotion (Troll, 1981). Inhibition of this type has been demonstrated using the two-stage model to study skin carcinogenesis in the mouse. In addition, a reduced incidence of breast cancer has been observed in irradiated rats fed a diet rich in protease inhibitors after exposure to the radiation (Troll, 1981). Protease inhibitors have also been shown to block promotion in in vitro systems. The transformation of C3H10T1/2 cells by x-rays followed by incubation with 12-o-tetradecanoylphorbol-13-acetate (TPA) is blocked if protease inhibitors are present after exposure to the radiation (Kennedy and Little, 1981). Troll (1980) suggested that protease inhibitors prevent formation of free radicals by tumor promoters. Since BHA and some related antioxidants inhibit promotion, there may be common mechanisms among inhibitors that would lead to synergistic effects.

β-Sitosterol. β-Sitosterol is a common plant sterol that is present in many different vegetables and vegetable oils. Its protective effects have been studied in an experimental system with N-nitroso-methylurea—a direct-acting carcinogen. β-Sitosterol reduced the incidence of large bowel cancer from 54% to 33% when fed in the diet through the entire course of the experiment or only during the promotion phase of carcinogenesis (Cohen and Raicht, 1981; Raicht et al., 1980). Other plant sterols of similar structure have not been studied for potential inhibitory effects.

Effects of Individual Foods on Carcinogen-Metabolizing Enzyme Systems

Studies in Animals. Several enzyme systems involved in metabolizing carcinogens are highly responsive to compounds entering the body from the environment. For example, animals fed purified diets and kept in filtered air show almost no monooxygenase oxidase activity for PAH's and azo dyes in the small bowel and lungs (Wattenberg, 1970, 1972).

One source of naturally occurring inducers of increased microsomal monooxygenase activity is vegetables. In laboratory animals, cruciferous vegetables such as brussels sprouts, cabbage, cauliflower, and broccoli have a moderately potent inducing effect on monooxygenase oxidase activity. Other vegetables such as alfalfa, spinach, and celery have some inducing activity, but it is weak (Wattenberg, 1972).

More recently, studies have been conducted to examine the effects of individual foods on glutathione S-transferase, which is a major detoxification system that catalyzes the binding of a vast variety of electrophiles to the sulfhydryl group of glutathione (Chasseaud, 1979; Jakoby, 1978). Since the reactive ultimate carcinogenic forms of chemicals are electrophiles, the glutathione S-transferase system takes on considerable importance as a mechanism for carcinogen detoxification. Enhancement of the activity of this system, as measured in vitro, has been shown to be associated with decreased response of tissues to chemical carcinogens (Sparnins and Wattenberg, 1981).

The activity of glutathione S-transferase is much greater in tissues of animals fed normal rather than purified diets. Diets containing large quantities of cruciferous vegetables induce increased glutathione S-transferase activity (Sparnins, 1980). The extent to which green coffee beans induce such activity is quite remarkable. In mice fed a diet containing green coffee beans, glutathione S-transferase activity was enhanced sixfold in the liver and sevenfold in the small bowel (Sparnins et al., 1981). Considerably less inducing activity has been found in roasted coffee beans, commercial instant coffee, and instant decaffeinated coffee, indicating that some destruction of the inducing compounds has occurred during processing. Two potent inducers of glutathione S-transferase activity have been isolated from green coffee beans. These compounds are kahweol palmitate and cafestol palmitate (Lam et al., 1982).

Studies in Humans. Diets containing large amounts of cabbage and brussels sprouts were fed to healthy volunteers between 21 and 32 years of age. The effects of this diet on the metabolism of antipyrine and phenacetin were studied. These compounds, like many carcinogens, are initially metabolized by the microsomal monooxygenase system and their oxidative metabolites subsequently conjugated. The results indicated that subjects eating diets rich in vegetables metabolized both drugs more rapidly than did subjects on a control diet (Pantuck et al., 1979).

Possible Adverse Effects of Inhibitors

Several of the inhibitors discussed above, e.g., indole-3-carbinol and 3,3'-diindolylmethane, are moderate or strong inducers of microsomal monooxygenase activity. Compounds with this characteristic are potentially hazardous (Wattenberg, 1979a). For example, the microsomal monooxygenase enzyme system produces two different categories of carcinogen metabolites: detoxification products and activated species. In the metabolism of aromatic amines, ring hydroxylation results in detoxification, whereas hydroxylation of the nitrogen leads to the formation of a proximate carcinogen. Thus, administration of compounds that increase monooxygenase activity can result in competing reactions, and the net effect is uncertain.

A second possible adverse effect of compounds that induce microsomal monooxygenase activity is that they may act as tumor promoters. An additional consideration is that the microsomal monooxygenase system metabolizes some physiological compounds such as steroid hormones. This alteration of activity might cause adverse effects by changing the levels of these compounds or their metabolites.

Two compounds have been shown experimentally to have dual effects, i.e., they can inhibit carcinogenesis and they also can cause or enhance neoplasia. One such compound is butylated hydroxytoluene (BHT). This compound can inhibit carcinogenesis under certain conditions. It is also a tumor promoter, as discussed in Chapter 14. The second compound is coumarin, which can inhibit carcinogenesis, but when fed to rats for 18 months, it produces bile duct carcinomas. Thus, a particular compound may have diverse effects. When this occurs, its overall impact is difficult to predict.

SUMMARY

Epidemiological Studies

Epidemiological evidence from several case-control studies suggests that certain vegetables, especially cruciferous vegetables, have a possible protective effect against cancer at several sites. The responsible constituent or constituents cannot be identified on the basis of present information.

Experimental Studies

Food contains many compounds that have been shown to inhibit carcinogenesis in laboratory animals. Because there are so many of these compounds and because their nature is so diverse, they are likely to be present in the diet of most humans.

The mechanisms of inhibition are incompletely understood. Some inhibitors modify the activity of enzyme systems that have the capacity to detoxify carcinogenic agents. Others may act by suppressing formation of free radicals or by trapping free radicals arising during the process of carcinogenesis.

A number of compounds inhibiting chemically induced carcinogenesis in laboratory animals are present in cruciferous vegetables. These compounds include aromatic isothiocyanates, indoles, and phenols.

CONCLUSION

The committee concluded that there is sufficient epidemiological evidence to suggest that consumption of certain vegetables, especially carotene-rich (i.e., dark green and deep yellow) vegetables and cruciferous vegetables (e.g., cabbage, broccoli, cauliflower, and brussels sprouts), is associated with a reduction in the incidence of cancer at several sites in humans. A number of nonnutritive and nutritive compounds that are present in these vegetables also inhibit carcinogenesis in laboratory animals. Investigators have not yet established which, if any, of these compounds may be responsible for the protective effect observed in epidemiological studies.

The fact that a compound has been shown to inhibit carcinogen-induced neoplasia in laboratory animals should not be interpreted as indicating that it is desirable for humans. These compounds may have adverse effects. Information on this subject is incomplete.

REFERENCES

Batzinger, R. P., S.-Y. L. Ou, and E. Bueding. 1978. Antimutagenic
    effects of 2(3)-tert-butyl-4-hydroxyanisole and of antimicrobial
    agents. Cancer Res. 38:4478-4485.

Benson, A. M., R. P. Batzinger, S.-Y. L. Ou, E. Bueding, Y.-N. Cha,
    and P. Talalay. 1978. Elevation of hepatic glutathione S-
    transferase activities and protection against mutagenic metab-
    olites of benzo(a)pyrene by dietary antioxidants. Cancer Res.
    38:4486-4495.

Benson, S. M., Y.-N. Cha, E. Bueding, H. S. Heine, and P. Talalay.
    1979. Elevation of extrahepatic glutathione S-transferase and
    epoxide hydratase activities by 2(3)-tert-butyl-4-hydroxyanisole.
    Cancer Res. 39:2971-2977.

Bjelke, E. 1978. Dietary factors and the epidemiology of cancer of
    the stomach and large bowel. Aktuel. Ernaehrungsmed. Klin. Prax.
    Suppl. 2:10-17.

Cha, Y.-N., and E. Bueding. 1979. Effect of 2(3)-tert-butyl-4-
    hydroxyanisole administration on the activities of several hepatic
    microsomal and cytoplasmic enzymes in mice. Biochem. Pharmacol.
    28:1917-1921.

Cha, Y.-N., F. Martz, and E. Bueding. 1978. Enhancement of liver
    microsome epoxide hydratase activity in rodents by treatment with
    2(3)-tert-butyl-4-hydroxyanisole. Cancer Res. 38:4496-4498.

Chasseaud, L. F. 1979. The role of glutathione and glutathione
    S-transferases in the metabolism of chemical carcinogens and other
    electrophilic agents. Adv. Cancer Res. 29:175-274.

Cohen, B. I., and R. F. Raicht. 1981. Plant sterols: Protective
    role in chemical carcinogenesis. Pp. 189-201 in M. S. Zedeck and
    M. Lipkin, eds. Inhibition of Tumor Induction and Development.
    Plenum Press, New York and London.

Graham, S., W. Schotz, and P. Martino. 1972. Alimentary factors in
    the epidemiology of gastric cancer. Cancer 30:927-938.

Graham, S., H. Dayal, M. Swanson, A. Mittelman, and G. Wilkinson.
    1978. Diet in the epidemiology of cancer of the colon and rectum.
    J. Natl. Cancer Inst. 51:709-714.

Haenszel, W., M. Kurihara, M. Segi, and R. K. C. Lee. 1972. Stomach cancer among Japanese in Hawaii. J. Natl. Cancer Inst. 49:969-988.

Haenszel, W., J. W. Berg, M. Segi, M. Kurihara, and F. B. Locke. 1973. Large-bowel cancer in Hawaiian Japanese. J. Natl. Cancer Inst. 51:1765-1779.

Haenszel, W., M. Kurihara, F. B. Locke, K. Shimuzu, and M. Segi. 1976. Stomach cancer in Japan. J. Natl. Cancer Inst. 56:265-274.

Haenszel, W., F. B. Locke, and M. Segi. 1980. A case-control study of large bowel cancer in Japan. J. Natl. Cancer Inst. 64:17-22.

Hirayama, T. 1977. Changing patterns of cancer in Japan with special reference to the decrease in stomach cancer mortality. Pp. 55-75 in H. H. Hiatt, J. D. Watson, and J. A. Winsten, eds. Origins of Human Cancer, Book A: Incidence of Cancer in Humans. Cold Spring Harbor Laboratory, Cold Spring Harbor, N.Y.

Jakoby, W. B. 1978. The glutathione S-transferases: A group of multifunctional detoxification proteins. Adv. Enzymol. Relat. Areas Mol. Biol. 46:383-414.

Kennedy, A. R., and J. B. Little. 1981. Effects of protease inhibitors on radiation transformation in vitro. Cancer Res. 41:2103-2108.

Lam, L. K. T., A. V. Fladmoe, J. B. Hochalter, and L. W. Wattenberg. 1980. Short time interval effects of butylated hydroxyanisole on the metabolism of benzo(a)pyrene. Cancer Res. 40:2824-2828.

Lam, L. K. T., V. L. Sparnins, and L. Wattenberg. 1982. Isolation and identification of kahweol palmitate and cafestol palmitate as active constituents of green coffee beans that enhance glutathione S-transferase activity in the mouse. Cancer Res. 42:1193-1198.

Loub, W. D., L. W. Wattenberg, and D. W. Davis. 1975. Aryl hydrocarbon hydroxylase induction in rat tissues by naturally occurring indoles of cruciferous plants. J. Natl. Cancer Inst. 54:985-988.

MacGregor, J. T., and L. Jurd. 1978. Mutagenicity of plant flavonoids: Structural requirements for mutagenic activity in Salmonella typhimurium. Mutat. Res. 54:297-309.

MacLennan, R., J. Da Costa, N. E. Day, C. H. Law, Y. K. Ng, and K. Shanmugaratnam. 1977. Risk factors for lung cancer in Singapore Chinese, a population with high female incidence rates. Int. J. Cancer 20:854-860.

Modan, B., V. Barrell, F. Lubin, M. Modan, R. A. Greenberg, and S. Graham. 1975. Low-fiber intake as an etiologic factor in cancer of the colon. J. Natl. Cancer Inst. 55:15-18.

Pantuck, E. J., K.-C. Hsiao, W. D. Loub, L. W. Wattenberg, R. Kuntzman, and A. H. Conney. 1976. Stimulatory effect of vegetables on intestinal drug metabolism in the rat. J. Pharmacol. Exp. Ther. 198:278-283.

Pantuck, E. J., C. B. Pantuck, W. A. Garland, B. H. Min, L. W. Wattenberg, K. E. Anderson, A. Kappas, and A. H. Conney. 1979. Stimulatory effect of Brussels sprouts and cabbage on human drug metabolism. Clin. Pharmacol. Ther. 25:88-95.

Raicht, R. F., B. I. Cohen, E. P. Fazzini, A. N. Sarwal, and M. Takahashi. 1980. Protective effect of plant sterols against chemically induced colon tumors in rats. Cancer Res. 40:403-405.

Slaga, T. 1981. Food additives and contaminants as modifying factors in cancer induction. Prog. Cancer Res. Ther. 17:279-290.

Sparnins, V. L. 1980. Effects of dietary constituents on glutathione-S-transferase (G-S-T) activity. Proc. Am. Assoc. Cancer Res. Am. Soc. Clin. Oncol. 21:80. Abstract 319.

Sparnins, V. L., and L. W. Wattenberg. 1981. Enhancement of glutathione S-transferase activity of the mouse forestomach by inhibitors of benzo[a]pyrene-induced neoplasia of forestomach. J. Natl. Cancer Inst. 66:769-771.

Sparnins, V. L., L. K. T. Lam, and L. W. Wattenberg. 1981. Effects of coffee on glutathione S-transferase (G S T) activity and 7,12-dimethylbenz(a)anthracene (DMBA)-induced neoplasia. Proc. Am. Assoc. Cancer Res. Am. Soc. Clin. Oncol. 22:114. Abstract 453.

Speier, J. L., L. K. T. Lam, and L. W. Wattenberg. 1978. Effects of administration to mice of butylated hydroxyanisole by oral intubation on benzo[a]pyrene-induced pulmonary adenoma formation and metabolism of benzo[a]pyrene. J. Natl. Cancer Inst. 60:605-609.

Troll, W. 1981. Blocking of tumor promotion by protease inhibitors. Pp. 549-555 in J. H. Burchenal and H. F. Oettgen, eds. Cancer: Achievements, Challenges and Prospects for the 1980's, Volume 1. Grune and Stratton, New York, London, Toronto, Sydney, and San Francisco.

Wattenberg, L. W. 1970. The role of the portal of entry in inhibition of tumorigenesis. Prog. Exp. Tumor Res. 14:89-104.

Wattenberg, L. W. 1972. Enzymatic reactions and carcinogenesis. Pp. 241-254 in Environment and Cancer. Williams and Wilkins Company, Baltimore, Md.

Wattenberg, L. W. 1977. Inhibition of carcinogenic effects of polycyclic hydrocarbons by benzyl isothiocyanate and related compounds. J. Natl. Cancer Inst. 58:395-398.

Wattenberg, L. W. 1978. Inhibitors of chemical carcinogenesis. Adv. Cancer Res. 26:197-226.

Wattenberg, L. W. 1979a. Inhibitors of chemical carcinogens. Pp. 241-263 in P. Emmelot and E. Kriek, eds. Environmental Carcino-genesis. Elsevier/North-Holland Biomedical Press, Amsterdam.

Wattenberg, L. W. 1979b. Naturally occurring inhibitors of chemical carcinogenesis. Pp. 315-329 in E. C. Miller, J. A. Miller, I. Hirono, T. Sugimura, and S. Takayama, eds. Naturally Occurring Carcinogens-Mutagens and Modulators of Carcinogenesis. Japan Scientific Societies Press, Tokyo; University Park Press, Baltimore, Md.

Wattenberg, L. W. 1981a. Inhibitors of chemical carcinogens. Pp. 517-539 in J. H. Burchenal and H. F. Oettgen, eds. Cancer: Achieve-ments, Challenges, and Prospects for the 1980's, Volume 1. Grune and Stratton, New York, London, Toronto, Sydney, and San Francisco.

Wattenberg, L. W. 1981b. Inhibition of carcinogen-induced neoplasia by sodium cyanate, tert-butyl isocyanate and benzyl isothiocyanate administered subsequent to carcinogen exposure. Cancer Res. 41:2991-2994.

Wattenberg, L. W., and J. L. Leong. 1968. Inhibition of the carcino-genic action of 7,12-dimethylbenz(a)anthracene by beta-naphthofla-vone. Proc. Soc. Exp. Biol. Med. 128:940-943.

Wattenberg, L. W., and J. L. Leong. 1970. Inhibition of the carcino-genic action of benzo(a)pyrene by flavones. Cancer Res. 30:1922-1925.

Wattenberg, L. W., and W. D. Loub. 1978. Inhibition of polycyclic hydrocarbon-induced neoplasia by naturally occurring indoles. Cancer Res. 38:1410-1413.

Wattenberg, L. W., J. B. Coccia, and L. K. T. Lam. 1980. Inhibitory effects of phenolic compounds on benzo(a)pyrene-induced neoplasia. Cancer Res. 40:2820-2823.

Section C Patterns of Diet and Cancer

In Sections A and B the committee reviewed the evidence concerning the role of specific nutrients and nonnutritive dietary components. This section provides a more comprehensive assessment of the overall contribution of diet to cancer.

Chapter 16 contains an overview of the evidence relating diet to cancer in light of the trends in cancer incidence and mortality and the influence of other environmental factors on these trends. In Chapter 17, the epidemiological evidence is reassembled by each cancer site to provide a perspective on the contribution of all dietary factors to the occurrence of cancer at specific sites.

The committee recognized at the start that the current state of knowledge is insufficient to permit a precise quantification of the effect of the diet on the incidence of cancer. Therefore, in Chapter 18, the committee has presented merely a framework for assessing risk, with particular emphasis on the different elements that need to be considered when assessing the risks posed by initiators and modifiers that may be present in the diet. Attempts made by other investigators to determine the quantitative contribution of diet to the overall risk of cancer are also discussed.

C-1

16 Cancer Incidence and Mortality

A number of authors (e.g., Doll, 1967, 1977; Higginson, 1969; Higginson and Muir, 1979; Wynder and Gori, 1977) have pointed to the large differences in cancer incidence and mortality that exist between countries and the likelihood that these differences are largely due to environmental factors. Here the term environment is used in its widest sense, encompassing all factors external to humans, as distinct from differences that are attributable to man's genetic makeup. Higginson (1969) calculated the proportion of cancers that were theoretically preventable and suggested that approximately 90% of all cancers in humans are influenced by exogenous factors. This observation has stimulated attempts to distinguish between occupation and way of life (Fox and Adelstein, 1978) and to identify those components linked to lifestyle (Higginson and Muir, 1979; Miller, 1981)--specifically, to examine diet as a component of lifestyle (Miller et al., 1980; Wynder and Gori, 1977).

This chapter reviews those aspects of descriptive epidemiology that indicate the importance of dietary factors in explaining differences in cancer incidence and mortality among various population groups. In general, incidence data are used when available, since they more directly relate to etiology, being uninfluenced by changes in survival due to advances in the management and treatment of cancer. In the absence of incidence data, mortality data have been used. As pointed out by Doll and Peto (1981), mortality data have certain advantages as well. Their interpretation is less often complicated by changes in diagnostic practices or cancer registration.

The diet is generally associated with cancers of the gastrointestinal tract (i.e., esophagus, stomach, colon, rectum, pancreas, and liver) and cancers of some sex-hormone-responsive sites (i.e., breast, prostate, endometrium, and ovary). There is also evidence that diet is associated to some degree with cancers of the respiratory system and bladder. Incidence data for 1973-1977, as compiled by the National Cancer Institute Surveillance, Epidemiology, and End Results (NCI-SEER) Program (Young et al., 1981), indicate that cancer of the stomach, colon, breast, bladder, and prostate comprise ∿39% of the cancers in males and ∿43% of cancers in females. Thus, these presumably diet-sensitive sites account for approximately 40% of the cancers in both sexes (Young et al., 1981). If we add the incidence of lung cancer in males, which may be influenced by diet as well as by smoking, the total for cancer in males reaches 60%.

GEOGRAPHICAL DIFFERENCES RELATED TO ETHNICITY

In the United States, incidence data for whites and blacks have been compared. Table 16-1 provides such comparisons for gastrointestinal

372

TABLE 16-1

Cumulative Incidence Rate (Age 0-74) per 100 Persons for
Malignant Neoplasms in All Areas of the United States
(Excluding Puerto Rico), 1973-1977[a]

Site	Whites		Blacks	
	Males	Females	Males	Females
Esophagus	0.5	0.2	1.7	0.4
Stomach	1.1	0.4	2.1	0.9
Colon	3.1	2.7	3.2	2.7
Rectum and rectosigmoid	1.8	1.0	1.4	1.0
Liver	0.2	0.1	0.5	0.2
Gallbladder	0.1	0.1	0.1	0.1
Pancreas	1.1	0.7	1.7	1.1
Lung	7.7	2.3	11.5	2.4
Breast	0.1	8.2	0.1	7.0
Corpus uteri		3.1		1.4
Ovary		1.4		0.9
Prostate	5.2		9.6	
Bladder	2.4	0.6	1.2	0.5
Kidney	0.9	0.4	0.8	0.4

[a]Data from Young et al., 1981.

16-2

cancers and for some other sites (Young et al., 1981). The measure used
(i.e., cumulative incidence to age 74) is an approximation of the lifetime risk of developing cancer of that site in the absence of death from
other causes (Day, 1976). Rates are higher for blacks of both sexes for
cancers of the esophagus, stomach, liver, and pancreas, and there is a
substantial excess of prostate cancer in black males. However, the incidence of bladder cancer is lower in blacks.

A number of cancer registries provide incidence data for different
racial groups (Waterhouse et al., 1976). For example, the age-adjusted
rates for stomach and large bowel cancer among Chinese living in the San
Francisco Bay area are similar to those for whites, whereas rates for
prostate and bladder cancer are lower. In Hawaii, the rates for stomach
cancer are higher for Hawaiians and Japanese of both sexes and for
Chinese and Filipino females than the corresponding rates for Caucasians
(Table 16-2) (Young et al., 1981).

The differences in the rates of cancer among racial and ethnic
groups do not necessarily have a ready interpretation. Some, such as
the similarity of rates among the various ethnic groups (Henderson et
al., in press) suggest the possibility of a genetic contribution to
cancer at some sites. However, other explanations should also be
considered. Most of the differences would indicate that cultural and,
thus, environmental factors are involved in the etiology of cancers at
the various sites. Among these, dietary factors are likely to be of
critical importance.

CHANGES SUBSEQUENT TO MIGRATION

The hypothesis that differences in cancer incidence and mortality
among racial or ethnic groups are due largely to cultural rather than
genetic factors receives considerable support from data on groups that
have migrated (Haenszel, 1961; Kmet, 1970). In general, the incidence of
cancer in migrant groups is similar to that of the country of origin or
is intermediate between that of the country of origin and the host country. After one or more generations, it becomes the same as that of the
host country. These trends have been well documented for gastric, colon,
and breast cancer in Japanese who migrated to Hawaii and to the western
continental United States and Canada (Buell, 1973; Kolonel et al., 1980);
Eastern Europeans who migrated to the United States and Canada (Kmet,
1970); Icelanders who migrated to Manitoba, Canada (Choi et al., 1971);
and Southern Europeans who migrated to Australia (McMichael et al., 1980).
The changes seem to be most rapid for colon cancer and somewhat less
rapid for stomach cancer. They are slowest for breast cancer, requiring
more than one, or possibly two, generations for a full effect to be manifested. These different rates of change may reflect differences in the
stage of life during which factors exert an effect, or they may reflect
the differences in the action of carcinogenic initiators or promoting
agents.

TABLE 16-2

Average Annual Age-Adjusted Incidence (per 100,000) in
Different Ethnic Groups in Hawaii, 1973-1977[a]

Site	Sex	Race Hawaiian	Caucasian	Chinese	Filipino	Japanese
Stomach	M	51.4	15.6	14.6	13.3	47.3
	F	23.9	7.0	9.4	7.3	19.9
Colon	M	20.2	33.8	39.3	24.3	36.5
	F	17.5	24.4	28.2	13.2	24.4
Rectum and	M	15.9	17.6	20.6	16.5	28.2
rectosigmoid	F	10.9	10.2	11.0	10.0	11.0
Liver	M	12.6	2.9	10.3	13.3	7.5
	F	9.7	1.9	3.6	2.1	2.8
Gallbladder	M	2.3	--	3.3	2.4	1.4
	F	1.5	0.9	2.2	1.0	2.2
Pancreas	M	12.9	11.4	11.5	8.6	11.7
	F	9.2	8.7	7.6	1.8	6.1
Breast	F	104.3	99.9	64.1	29.2	51.3
Corpus uteri	F	40.4	41.5	33.4	17.3	22.4
Ovary	F	11.8	10.7	8.1	5.4	8.0
Prostate	M	66.3	86.7	40.0	46.9	54.1
Kidney and	M	5.8	13.5	2.9	4.7	6.1
pelvis	F	5.5	3.0	4.6	3.8	2.5
Bladder	M	6.8	31.3	9.9	10.8	13.7
	F	8.3	5.2	1.5	5.6	4.8

[a]Data from Young et al., 1981.

When interpreting the effects of migration, it is important to recognize that migrants are not necessarily representative of the population from which they were derived. They may have led more active lives or have a socioeconomic background that is not typical for the general population in their country of origin, or they may have come from a specific region with atypical characteristics. Furthermore, migrant groups may retain some cultural habits, possibly including different dietary practices, while in their host country, even after several generations. MacDonald (1966) compared the diet of 65 Japanese men, age 50 or more who had migrated to Canada 35 to 55 years before, with 65 non-Japanese control subjects. The Japanese ate more fish and rice than did the control group and ingested less beef, potatoes, bread, milk, and cereals other than rice. Fruit and vegetable consumption was similar in the two groups. Hence, there may be differences in cancer incidence among groups from different countries for some time after they migrated. In the United States, breast cancer in postmenopausal women has been linked to German ethnicity (Blot et al., 1977b). Mortality from colon and rectal cancer is elevated in counties in the United States where there are large populations with Irish, German, or Czechoslovakian descent (Blot et al., 1976). Mortality from renal cancer is also elevated in counties where a large percentage of the population is of German, Scandinavian, or, especially, Russian descent (Blot and Fraumeni, 1979).

Where differences have been explored in detail, the findings support the operation of environmental factors, as distinct from those of genetic origin, even when "genetic isolates" are considered (Gaudette et al., 1978; Martin et al., 1980).

CHANGING TIME TRENDS IN INCIDENCE AND MORTALITY

For various reasons, cancer incidence and mortality in the United States are reported neither completely nor accurately. Generally speaking, although reporting of incidence has improved during the past 25 years, reporting is probably more accurate and complete for mortality. There have also been recent improvements in the reporting of categories of cancer. Therefore, long-term trends must be interpreted cautiously, and even recent trends are the subject of controversy.

Because of population growth and changes in its age distribution, the annual number of cancer cases is steadily increasing in the United States. For 1981, approximately 400,000 cancer deaths are projected, and about 800,000 new cases expected to occur. Cancer is the second most frequent cause of death (about 20% of total deaths). Against a background of drastic environmental modification and rapid technological change, some have suggested that a vast cancer "epidemic" may have begun. However, since more people are living longer and cancer rates are higher among older people, adjustment for age corrects the impression that cancer rates are being driven upward dramatically by an increasing environmental threat. In fact, examination of recent age-adjusted rates indicates that there has been little change overall, although there are some increases and decreases in cancer incidence at certain sites.

Apart from the smoking-associated cancers, stomach cancer, and cervical cancer, the incidence of and mortality from cancer at nearly all sites have remained remarkably stable for the last 30 to 40 years (Devesa and Silverman, 1978; Miller, 1980). There has been a slight increase in the rates of nonrespiratory cancers for white males age 75 or more (but, if anything, a decrease at ages 55-59 and 40-44). For other age groups, the rates have been stable. In females, there has been an increase in the 74-84 age group, but decreases in the age groups 85 or more, 70-74, and 40-54, and a relative stability for other age groups. The data indicate that rates for the youngest age groups (especially for women) appear to be falling. This is a critical observation because the youngest age groups would have been expected to show the effect first if the environment were becoming increasingly carcinogenic.

There has been an increased incidence of breast cancer, especially in postmenopausal women, but there has been little or no change in mortality from cancer at this site (Barclay et al., 1975; Cutler et al., 1971; Fabia et al., 1977; Grace et al., 1977). This finding is probably due to a combination of factors. For example, improved cancer registration has provided a more accurate reflection of cancer incidence. Furthermore, increased awareness by the general population and physicians and intensified pathological examination of resected tissue have led to early detection and, thus, slightly more successful treatment.

In Iceland, the age-specific curves for breast cancer have shifted from higher rates for premenopausal women (similar to the pattern in Japan in this century) to higher rates for postmenopausal women (similar to the pattern in North American women) (Bjarnason et al., 1974). However, an analysis of the data by birth cohort demonstrated that the shapes of the age-specific curves were the same and that the incidence at each age increased in successive birth cohorts. This suggests that the incidence of breast cancer may have increased because more recent birth cohorts were exposed to environmental factors that increase the risk of breast cancer.

The incidence of endometrial cancer increased remarkably during the 1970's, then fell sharply beginning in 1976, especially on the west coast of the United States. There now seems to be little doubt that these changes are due to the excessive use and then partial withdrawal of conjugated estrogens at the time of menopause (Jick et al., 1980). Despite the dramatic changes in incidence, mortality has remained stable.

Both incidence of and mortality from stomach cancer have declined steadily in Western countries during the past 30 to 40 years (Devesa and Silverman, 1978; Miller, 1980). More recently, they have started to decline in Japan (Hirayama, 1977).

These trends and stabilities are reflected in international incidence data, apart from minor fluctuations due to changing registration practices (Stukonis, 1978).

Recently, controversy has arisen over whether the general incidence of cancer has been increasing significantly over the past several dec- ades, in particular during the past 5 years. Resolution of this contro- versy is complicated by the inadequacies in the data and by the different trends for specific cancer sites. If lung and skin cancer are excluded (the former because most of it is attributed to cigarette smoking, the latter because it is easily curable and poorly reported), the remaining aggregated cancer incidence appears to be roughly stable up to 1971. Differences of interpretation have arisen from the comparison of SEER data (collected after 1973) with the earlier data because they represent different population samples and different methods of data collection.

Thus, Pollack and Horm (1980) suggested that cancer incidence is rising in the United States, even for cancers not associated with smoking. Their report was based on data from the third National Cancer Survey (1959-1971) and the SEER Program for 1973-1976. Although the authors took pains to exclude methodological reasons for the increase and to regard it as real, it still seems possible that most of the ob- served increases are artifactual, caused by more efficient registration following the change from the earlier methods of a one-time survey to those of a permanent registration system. The matter should be resolved in the next few years as SEER data continue to accumulate.

INTERSITE CORRELATIONS OF INCIDENCE

Burkitt (1971) pointed out that similar frequencies for different diseases might imply common etiological factors. Using data from the third National Cancer Survey (Cutler and Young, 1975), Winkelstein et al. (1977) studied the geographic variation in the occurrence of cancers at sites common to both sexes and at five sex-specific sites. They found strong correlations among the incidence rates for cancer at three gastro- intestinal sites, i.e., cancers of the colon and rectum were directly cor- related with each other, and inversely correlated with stomach cancer. In addition, there was a strong direct correlation between colorectal cancer and bladder cancer in both men and women. There was also a strong direct correlation among cancer of the breast, corpus uteri, and ovary in women. These two groups of interrelated sites were also correlated with one another.

Berg (1975) pointed out that international incidence rates for the hormone-dependent cancers (i.e., breast, corpus uteri, and ovarian can- cers in females and testis and prostate cancers in males) were closely

correlated with the rates for large bowel cancer. Table 16-3 shows the
extent to which the the cancer incidence rates for certain sites are
intercorrelated. The lowest correlation between males and females was
found for esophageal cancer; the highest, for colon cancer. Significant
direct correlations within the same sex occur for colon and rectal cancer
and for both sites combined with pancreatic cancer. There are significant
inverse correlations for colon and stomach cancer. In men, esophageal
cancer is directly correlated with liver cancer; in women, liver cancer
is inversely correlated with colon and rectal cancer. Colon and, to a
lesser extent, rectal and pancreatic cancers are directly correlated with
breast, endometrial, and ovarian cancers in women.

ASSOCIATIONS WITH SOCIOECONOMIC STATUS

Using data for 1950 to 1969, Blot et al. (1977a) analyzed mortality
in the United States by county. This study has provided a number of
opportunities to evaluate mortality rates by socioeconomic status, which
may reflect differences in diet. Thus, mortality from colon and rectal
cancer has been associated with higher income and education levels (Blot
et al., 1976); mortality from breast cancer in postmenopausal women has
been linked to higher socioeconomic status (Blot et al., 1977a); and
mortality from renal cancer has been directly correlated in both sexes
with higher socioeconomic status (Blot and Fraumeni, 1979).

In the United Kingdom, the Registar General's Decennial Supplement
for England and Wales (Registrar General's Office for England and Wales,
1978) and a report by Fox and Adelstein (1978) have shed further light on
the relative importance of socioeconomic status and occupational factors.
Standardization for social class has shown that nearly all significantly
high standardized mortality ratios for occupational groups are reduced to
nonsignificance after social class is considered. Fox and Adelstein
(1978) have calculated that occupation accounts for approximately 12% of
the variation in cancer mortality between social class groups, and that
lifestyle accounts for 88%. The corresponding proportions for all causes
of death are 18% and 82%, respectively.

Teppo et al. (1980), using data from the Finnish Cancer Registry,
reported an association between social class and cancer at a number of
sites. They found inverse correlations between social class and cancer
of the lip and stomach in males and direct correlations between social
class and colon cancer in both sexes and breast and lung cancer in
females. After examining the incidence of breast cancer by province and
selected municipalities in Finland, Hakama et al. (1979) reported an
association with taxable income. They concluded that factors reflected
by the standard of living and fertility might act independently.

TABLE 16-3

Correlation of Worldwide Incidence of Various Cancers
for Males and Females[a]

Females	Males Esophagus	Stomach	Colon	Rectum	Liver	Gallbladder	Pancreas
Esophagus	0.38[b]	0.05	-0.03	-0.19	0.80	-0.22	0.20
Stomach	0.11	0.94[b]	-0.40	-0.24	0.04	0.20	-0.17
Colon	0.12	-0.40	0.95[b]	0.85	-0.15	-0.24	0.60
Rectum	-0.08	-0.18	0.67	0.76[b]	-0.22	0.14	0.41
Liver	0.05	0.06	-0.33	-0.39	0.89[b]	-0.14	0.05
Gallbladder	-0.28	0.13	-0.27	-0.01	-0.08	0.74[b]	-0.07
Pancreas	-0.14	-0.23	0.54	0.44	-0.23	0.17	0.77[b]
Breast	-0.17	-0.46	0.84	0.72	-0.39	-0.15	0.63
Cervix uteri	0.06	0.09	-0.12	-0.14	0.20	0.14	0.13
Endometrium	-0.29	-0.28	0.69	0.45	-0.15	-0.16	0.49
Ovary	-0.25	-0.40	0.63	0.51	-0.26	0.04	0.60

[a]Data derived from Waterhouse et al., 1976.
[b]Correlation between same site in males and females. All coefficients above and to the right refer to males; all below and to the left to females. A coefficient >0.22 is significant at $p<0.05$; >0.31 at $p<0.01$; and >0.43 at $p<0.001$.

Urban-rural differences in cancer incidence and mortality have long been recognized as indicators of the effect of socioeconomic status and lifestyle. However, only the Norwegian Cancer Registry routinely reports its data in this form, since reports are grouped according to the official administrative boundaries (Waterhouse et al., 1976). In urban areas, there is a marked excess of esophageal and liver cancer in males and of lung cancer in both sexes and a moderate excess of colon and pancreatic cancer in males, breast cancer in females, and bladder and other urinary tract cancers in both sexes. In rural areas, there is a marked excess of lip cancer in males.

RELIGIOUS PRACTICES AND CANCER INCIDENCE AND MORTALITY

Religious groups whose lifestyles and dietary habits differ from those of the general population have been a fruitful source for assessing the possible effect of dietary variables.

Phillips and colleagues have studied Seventh-Day Adventists (SDA's), a religious group with approximately 600,000 members in North America (Phillips, 1975; Phillips et al., 1980b). SDA's abstain from smoking and drinking, and approximately 50% of them follow a lacto-ovovegetarian diet. In earlier studies, Phillips (1975) suggested that the lacto-ovovegetarian diet may protect against colon cancer; the evidence for breast cancer was less clear. These studies compared cancer mortality among California SDA's with mortality data for the general California population. In more recent analyses, Phillips et al. (1980a,b) used as a non-SDA control group Californians who enrolled in a concurrent prospective study conducted among the general population by the American Cancer Society. This study showed that the risk of dying from colorectal cancer and cancers related to smoking is clearly lower among SDA's than among non-SDA's of comparable age, sex, and socioeconomic status. The risk of dying from breast cancer was also reduced, but not significantly. This may be clarified in further analyses that take into account important risk factors for breast cancer. But since a number of SDA's are adult converts, their risk of breast cancer may have been at least partially determined by exposures in early (adolescent or young adult) life, before they adopted SDA practices. However, the SDA age-specific mortality curve for breast cancer is consistent with those of other low--risk populations, in which postmenopausal women have been observed to have a lower risk for cancer at this site (Phillips et al., 1980b).

The Mormons comprise another religious group whose lifestyle differs markedly from that of the general U.S. population. For at least 80 years, these members of the Church of Jesus Christ of Latter-Day Saints have proscribed the use of alcohol, tobacco, coffee, and tea in all forms to help ensure good health (Lyon et al., 1980). In addition, they recommend a well-balanced diet, especially the use of grains, fruits, and vegetables, and moderate consumption of meat (Enstrom, 1980). In a study based on data from the Utah Cancer Registry, Lyon et al. (1976) reported that the incidence of cancers associated with cigarette smoking; breast, uterine, cervical, and ovarian cancer in females; and stomach cancer in males was much lower in Mormons than in non-Mormons. Colon cancer was also significantly lower in females, but not in males. In an update of these analyses (Lyon et al., 1980), the same reductions were observed, but for colon and rectal cancer they had become significant for both sexes. In states adjacent to Utah (Idaho and Wyoming), mortality from smoking-associated cancers and from cancers of the rectum and breast is almost identical to that of Utah (Rawson, 1980). Thus, there may be some general environmental variable peculiar to this entire area affecting cancer incidence and mortality.

In India, cancer incidence differs among religious groups, especially between the Parsi and Hindu communities of Bombay (Jussawalla, 1976). In the Parsi community, the rates of colon, rectal, and breast cancer are substantially greater than those in the Hindu population, although they are not as high as those in Western countries.

There are many differences other than dietary factors between religious groups and the general population. Although attempts have been made to control for the nondietary differences (e.g., Phillips et al., 1980b), studies of groups will probably never be as effective as direct evaluations of the effect of dietary factors and other variables in individuals. Nevertheless, these studies of subgroups of the population have value because they indicate which hypotheses should be evaluated more directly by other means.

CORRELATIONS OF INCIDENCE AND MORTALITY WITH DIETARY AND OTHER VARIABLES

In several studies, dietary and other variables have been found to be strongly correlated with geographical differences in the incidence of and mortality from cancer at a number of sites (Armstrong and Doll, 1975; Carroll, 1975; Knox, 1977). Armstrong and Doll (1975) correlated incidence rates for cancer at 27 sites in 23 countries and mortality rates for cancer at 14 sites in 32 countries with a wide range of dietary and other variables. They reported strong correlations between dietary variables and cancer at several sites, especially meat and fat intake with cancers of the colorectum, breast, corpus uteri, and ovary. Direct correlations with dietary variables were also found for cancer of the small intestine (sugar), pancreas (eggs, animal protein, and fat), and ovary and bladder (fats and oils); inverse associations were reported for gastric cancer (meat, animal protein, and fat) and cervical cancer (total protein and fruit). Many of the dietary variables were strongly intercorrelated, especially fat and protein of animal origin, and were also correlated with gross national product. Carroll (1975) observed a strong correlation between per capita intake of dietary fat and age-adjusted mortality from breast cancer. The correlation was strongest for total fat, almost as strong for animal fat, but almost completely absent for vegetable fat. Knox (1977) suggested that associations between alcohol intake and cancer of the mouth and larynx, between total fat intake and cancer of the large intestine and breast, and between beer intake and cancer of the rectum were causal. In Japan, Hirayama (1977) found that the intakes of fat and pork were associated with mortality from breast cancer in 12 different prefectures. After having reviewed data for cancer and fat intake, Enig et al. (1979) retracted their original suggestion that cancer was correlated with the intake of total fat and vegetable fat, but not with animal fat.

One disadvantage of this type of study, especially in relation to breast and gastric cancer, is that current dietary factors are usually correlated with current information on incidence and mortality, whereas a more appropriate time relationship might be established by taking dietary information recorded some 20 or 30 years ago and correlating it with current incidence or mortality rates (Miller et al., 1980).

By conducting personal interviews with 4,137 subjects to determine their usual weekly food consumption, Kolonel et al. (1981) determined the average daily consumption of several components of fat in the diets of the five main ethnic groups in Hawaii. The intake of total fat correlated with the ethnic-specific incidence rates of breast cancer in Hawaii, but not with colon or prostate cancer incidence. There was no correlation between cholesterol consumption and incidence of colon cancer. One possible difficulty with this study is that many of the means of dietary intake for the different ethnic groups were rather close. Furthermore, current diet as measured in this study may not be relevant to current incidence, especially for sites where incidence is changing.

Evidence associating fiber intake with certain cancer sites has also been contradictory. Drasar and Irving (1973) were unable to find any association of breast and colon cancer incidence with per capita fiber intake using data from 37 countries, although they demonstrated a high correlation with fat and animal protein intake. However, the International Agency for Research on Cancer Intestinal Microecology Group (1977) found that differences in dietary fiber in Scandinavian populations appeared to correlate well with incidence of and mortality from colon cancer.

Dietary correlation studies have produced evidence for groups, rather than for individuals. Although the variation in the intake of nutrients is great internationally, it is not necessarily extensive for groups within countries. The variation of incidence and mortality within countries may also be low. Furthermore, the dietary information is generally derived from food disappearance data (i.e., per capita intake), and not necessarily from individual food consumption data. Hence, lack of correlation, either nationally or internationally, does not suffice to disprove a hypothesis. Conversely, one should not rely too heavily on observed correlations in case they are confounded by some factor that could not be studied or has not yet been identified (Stavraky, 1976).

16-12

ASSOCIATIONS WITH OTHER DISEASES

Burkitt (1971) noted an association between a number of chronic diseases and "affluence." He suggested that such "diseases of affluence"
might have a common etiology and that dietary fiber may play a role in
protecting against such illnesses as cancer of the colon and other sites,
coronary heart disease, diverticulitis, etc. There has been a recent
decline in mortality from ischemic heart disease in the United States,
Australia, and Canada, but not in the United Kingdom (Dwyer and Hetzel,
1980). This decline has been associated by some investigators with increased consumption of polyunsaturated fats and reduced cigarette smoking. We may therefore question why there has not been any indication of
a reduction in cancers associated with dietary components, especially
fat. Since the amount of vegetable fat in the U.S. diet has been increasing (Page and Friend, 1978), one possible explanation could be that
such fat has an adverse influence on colorectal and breast cancer incidence (Enig et al., 1978). An alternative explanation might be that the
substitution of polyunsaturated fats for saturated fats may help to reduce cardiovascular diseases, but for this substitution to have an effect
on fat-associated cancers, a concurrent reduction in total fat consumption may also be necessary (Miller et al., 1980). It is also possible
that any effect of fat on cancer incidence would take longer to appear
than its effect on cardiovascular disease; however, in view of the rapid
changes in colorectal cancer rates after migration, this appears to be an
unlikely explanation for cancer at this site. Finally, dietary changes
may not have had any influence on changes in cardiovascular disease.

SUMMARY

The incidence of cancers differs greatly among countries and to a
limited extent within countries. Studies of migrants (e.g., Japanese who
migrated to the United States) suggest environmental causes for these
differences. In affluent countries, stomach cancer rates have fallen,
rates for intestinal and breast cancer are stable, and pancreatic cancer
rates, which have increased, are now descreasing for males. The incidence of cancer of the colon, rectum, breast, corpus uteri, ovary, and
prostate are directly correlated with each other, but cancer of the colon
or rectum is inversely correlated with stomach cancer. Mortality from
colorectal and breast cancer is directly associated with socioeconomic
status, and stomach cancer is inversely associated. In males, incidence
of cancer of the esophagus, liver, colon, pancreas, and lung is higher in
urban areas. Seventh-Day Adventists and Mormons have a low risk for
colon and breast cancer. Internationally, the intake of fat has been
directly correlated with cancer of the breast, colon, rectum, pancreas,
corpus uteri, and ovary.

REFERENCES

Armstrong, B., and R. Doll. 1975. Environmental factors and cancer incidence and mortality in different countries, with special reference to dietary practices. Int. J. Cancer 15:617-631.

Barclay, T. H. C., M. M. Black, B. F. Hankey, and S. J. Cutler. 1975. The increasing incidence of breast cancer in Saskatchewan. Pp. 282-288 in P. Bucalossi, U. Veronesi, and N. Cascinelli, eds. Proceedings of the XI International Cancer Congress, Volume 3. Excerpta Medica, Amsterdam.

Berg, J. W. 1975. Can nutrition explain the pattern of international epidemiology of hormone-dependent cancers? Cancer Res. 35:3345-3350.

Bjarnason, O., N. Day, G. Snaedal, and H. Tulinius. 1974. The effect of year of birth on the breast cancer age-incidence curve in Iceland. Int. J. Cancer 13:689-696.

Blot, W. J., and J. F. Fraumeni, Jr. 1979. Geographic patterns of renal cancer in the United States. J. Natl. Cancer Inst. 63: 363-366.

Blot, W. J., J. F. Fraumeni, Jr., B. J. Stone, and F. W. McKay. 1976. Geographic patterns of large bowel cancer in the United States. J. Natl. Cancer Inst. 57:1225-1231.

Blot, W. J., T. J. Mason, R. Hoover, and J. F. Fraumeni, Jr. 1977a. Cancer by county: Etiologic implications. Pp. 21-30 in H. H. Hiatt, J. D. Watson, and J. A. Winsten, eds. Origins of Human Cancer. Book A, Incidence of Cancer in Humans. Cold Spring Harbor Laboratory, Cold Spring Harbor, N.Y.

Blot, W. J., J. F. Fraumeni, Jr., and B. J. Stone. 1977b. Geographic patterns of breast cancer in the United States. J. Natl. Cancer Inst. 59:1407-1411.

Buell, P. 1973. Changing incidence of breast cancer in Japanese-American women. J. Natl. Cancer Inst. 51:1479-1483.

Burkitt, D. P. 1971. Guest editorial: Some neglected leads to cancer causation. J. Natl. Cancer Inst. 47:913-919.

Carroll, K. K. 1975. Experimental evidence of dietary factors and hormone-dependent cancers. Cancer Res. 35:3374-3383.

Choi, N. W., D. W. Entwistle, W. Michaluk, and N. Nelson. 1971. Gastric cancer in Icelanders in Manitoba. Isr. J. Med. Sci. 7:1500-1508.

Cutler, S. J., and J. L. Young, Jr., eds. 1975. Third National Cancer Survey: Incidence data. Nat. Cancer Inst. Monogr. 41:1-454.

Cutler, S. J., B. Christine, and T. H. C. Barclay. 1971. Increasing incidence and decreasing mortality rates for breast cancer. Cancer 28:1376-1380.

Day, N. E. 1976. A new measure of age standardized incidence, the cumulative rate. Pp. 443-445 in J. Waterhouse, C. Muir, P. Correa, and J. Powell, eds. Cancer Incidence in Five Continents, Volume III. IARC Scientific Publications No. 15. International Agency for Research on Cancer, Lyon, France.

Devesa, S. S., and D. T. Silverman. 1978. Cancer incidence and mortality trends in the United States: 1935-74. J. Natl. Cancer Inst. 60:545-571.

Doll, R. 1967. Prevention of Cancer. Pointers from Epidemiology. The Nuffield Provincial Hospitals Trust, London. 143 pp.

Doll, R. 1977. Strategy for detection of cancer hazards to man. Nature 265:589-596.

Doll, R., and R. Peto. 1981. The causes of cancer: Quantitative estimates of avoidable risks of cancer in the United States today. J. Natl. Cancer Inst. 66:1191-1308.

Drasar, B. S., and D. Irving. 1973. Environmental factors and cancer of the colon and breast. Br. J. Cancer 27:167-172.

Dwyer, T., and B. S. Hetzel. 1980. A comparison of trends of coronary heart disease mortality in Australia, USA and England and Wales with reference to three major risk factors--hypertension, cigarette smoking and diet. Int. J. Epidemiol. 9:65-71.

Enig, M. G., R. J. Munn, and M. Keeney. 1978. Dietary fat and cancer trends--a critique. Fed. Proc. Fed. Am. Soc. Exp. Biol. 37:2215-2220.

Enig, M. G., R. J. Munn, and M. Keeney. 1979. Response to letters. Fed. Proc. Fed. Am. Soc. Exp. Biol. 38:2437-2439.

Enstrom, J. E. 1980. Health and dietary practices and cancer mortality among California Mormons. Pp. 69-90 in J. Cairns, J. L. Lyon, and M. Skolnick, eds. Cancer Incidence in Defined Populations. Banbury Report 4. Cold Spring Harbor Laboratory, Cold Spring Harbor, N. Y.

Fabia, J., P.-M. Bernard, and G. Hill. 1977. Recent time-trends of age-specific death rates for breast cancer: Quebec and other provinces, 1965 through 1974. Can. Med. Assoc. J. 116:1135-1138.

Fox, A. J., and A. M. Adelstein. 1978. Occupational mortality: Work or way of life. J. Epidemiol. Community Health 32:73-78.

Gaudette, L. A., T. M. Holmes, L. M. Laing, K. Morgan, and M. G. A. Grace. 1978. Cancer incidence in a religious isolate of Alberta, Canada, 1953-74. J. Natl. Cancer Inst. 60:1233-1238.

Grace, M., L. A. Gaudette, and P. E. Burns. 1977. The increasing incidence of breast cancer in Alberta, 1953-1973. Cancer 40:358-363.

Haenszel, W. 1961. Cancer mortality among the foreign-born in the United States. J. Natl. Cancer Inst. 26:37-132.

Hakama, M., I. Soini, E. Kuosma, M. Lehtonen, and A. Aromaa. 1979. Breast cancer incidence: Geographical correlations in Finland. Int. J. Epidemiol. 8:33-40.

Henderson, B., L. Kolonel, and F. Foster. In press. Cancer in the Polynesians. Natl. Cancer Inst. Mongr. Series.

Higginson, J. 1969. Present trends in cancer epidemiology. Pp. 40-75 in J. F. Morgan, ed. Proceedings of the Eighth Canadian Cancer Research Conference. Pergamon Press, Oxford, London, Edinburgh, New York, Toronto, Paris, and Frankfurt.

Higginson, J., and C. S. Muir. 1979. Guest editorial: Environmental carcinogenesis: Misconceptions and limitations to cancer control. J. Natl. Cancer Inst. 63:1291-1298.

Hirayama, T. 1977. Changing patterns of cancer in Japan with special reference to the decrease in stomach cancer mortality. Pp. 55-75 in H. H. Hiatt, J. D. Watson, and J. A. Winsten, eds. Origins of Human Cancer. Book A, Incidence of Cancer in Humans. Cold Spring Harbor Laboratory, Cold Spring Harbor, N. Y.

International Agency for Research on Cancer Intestinal Microecology Group. 1977. Dietary fibre, transit-time, faecal bacteria, steroids, and colon cancer in two Scandinavian populations. Lancet 2:207-211.

Jick, H., A. M. Walker, and K. J. Rothman. 1980. The epidemic of endometrial cancer: A commentary. Am. J. Public Health 70:264-267.

Jussawalla, D. J. 1976. The problem of cancer in India: An epidemiological assessment. Gann Monogr. Cancer Res. 18:265-273.

Kmet, J. 1970. The role of migrant population in studies of selected cancer sites: A review. J. Chronic Dis. 23:305-324.

Knox, E. G. 1977. Foods and diseases. Br. J. Prev. Soc. Med. 31:71-80.

Kolonel, L. N., M. W. Hinds, and J. H. Hankin. 1980. Cancer patterns among migrant and native-born Japanese in Hawaii in relation to smoking, drinking and dietary habits. Pp. 327-340 in H. V. Gelboin, B. MacMahon, T. Matsushima, T. Sugimura, S. Takayama, and H. Takebe, eds. Genetic and Environmental Factors in Experimental and Human Cancer. Japan Scientific Societies Press, Tokyo.

Kolonel, L. N., J. H. Hankin, A. M. Nomura, and S. Y. Chu. 1981. Dietary fat intake and cancer incidence among five ethnic groups in Hawaii. Cancer Res. 41:3727-3728.

Lyon, J. L., M. R. Klauber, J. W. Gardner, and C. R. Smart. 1976. Cancer incidence in Mormons and non-Mormons in Utah, 1966-1970. N. Engl. J. Med. 294:129-133.

Lyon, J. L., J. W. Gardner, and D. W. West. 1980. Cancer risk and life-style: Cancer among Mormons from 1967-1975. Pp. 3-27 in J. Cairns, J. L. Lyon, and M. Skolnick, eds. Cancer Incidence in Defined Populations. Banbury Report 4. Cold Spring Harbor Laboratory, Cold Spring Harbor, N.Y.

MacDonald, W. C. 1966. Gastric cancer among the Japanese of British Columbia: Dietary studies. Pp. 451-459 in R. W. Bigg, C. P. Leblond, R. L. Noble, R. J. Rossiter, R. M. Taylor, and A. C. Wallace, eds. Proceedings of the Sixth Canadian Cancer Research Conference. Pergamon Press, London, Edinburgh, New York, Toronto, Paris, and Frankfurt.

Martin, A. O., J. K. Dunn, and B. Smalley. 1980. Use of a genealogically linked data base in the analysis of cancer in a human isolate. Pp. 235-251 in J. Cairns, J. L. Lyon, and M. Skolnick, eds. Cancer Incidence in Defined Populations. Banbury Report 4. Cold Spring Harbor Laboratory, Cold Spring Harbor, N.Y.

McMichael, A. J., M. G. McCall, J. M. Hartshorne, and T. L. Woodings. 1980. Patterns of gastro-intestinal cancer in European migrants to Australia: The role of dietary change. Int. J. Cancer 25:431-437.

Miller, A. B. 1980. The epidemiology of malignant disease. A basis for public policy. Health Community Informatics 6:283-294.

Miller, A. B. 1981. Epidemiology of gastrointestinal cancer. Compr. Therapy 7:53-58.

Miller, A. B., G. B. Gori, S. Graham, T. Hirayama, M. Kunze, B. S. Reddy, and J. H. Weisburger. 1980. Nutrition and cancer. Prev. Med. 9:189-196.

Page, L., and B. Friend. 1978. The changing United States diet. BioScience 28:192-197.

Phillips, R. L. 1975. Role of life-style and dietary habits in risk of cancer among Seventh-Day Adventists. Cancer Res. 35:3513-3522.

Phillips, R. L., J. W. Kuzma, and T. M. Lotz. 1980a. Cancer mortality among comparable members versus nonmembers of the Seventh-Day Adventist Church. Pp. 93-102 in J. Cairns, J. L. Lyon, and M. Skolnick, eds. Cancer Incidence in Defined Populations. Banbury Report 4. Cold Spring Harbor Laboratory, Cold Spring Harbor, N.Y.

Phillips, R. L., J. W. Kuzma, W. L. Beeson, and T. Lotz. 1980b. Influence of selection versus lifestyle on risk of fatal cancer and cardiovascular disease among Seventh-Day Adventists. Am. J. Epidemiol. 112:296-314.

Pollack, E. S., and J. W. Horm. 1980. Trends in cancer incidence and mortality in the United States, 1969-1976. J. Natl. Cancer Inst. 64:1091-1103.

Rawson, R. W. 1980. The total environment in the epidemiology of neoplastic disease: The obvious "ain't necessarily so." Pp. 109-119 in J. Cairns, J. L. Lyon, and M. Skolnick, eds. Cancer Incidence in Defined Populations. Banbury Report 4. Cold Spring Harbor Laboratory, Cold Spring Harbor, N.Y.

Registrar General's Office for England and Wales. 1978. Occupational Mortality: The Registrar General's Decennial Supplement for England and Wales, 1970-72, XVIII. Series D S 1. HMSO No. [0 11 6906448]. Her Majesty's Stationery Office, London.

Stavraky, K. M. 1976. The role of ecologic analysis in studies of the etiology of disease: A discussion with reference to large bowel cancer. J. Chronic Dis. 29:435-444.

Stukonis, M. K. 1978. Cancer Incidence Cumulative Rates--International Comparison Based on Data from "Cancer Incidence in Five Contients".

IARC Technical Report No. 78/002. International Agency for Research on Cancer, Lyon, France. 54 pp.

Teppo, L., E. Pukkala, M. Hakama, T. Hakulinen, A. Herva, and E. Saxén. 1980. Way of life and cancer incidence in Finland. A municipality-based ecological analysis. Scand. J. Soc. Med. Suppl. 19:1-84.

Waterhouse, J., C. Muir, P. Correa, and J. Powell, eds. 1976. Cancer Incidence in Five Continents, Volume III. IARC Scientific Publications No. 15. International Agency for Research on Cancer, Lyon, France. 584 pp.

Winkelstein, W., Jr., S. T. Sacks, V. L. Ernster, and S. Selvin. 1977. Correlations of incidence rates for selected cancers in the nine areas of the Third National Cancer Survey. Am. J. Epidemiol. 105:407-419.

Wynder, E. L., and G. B. Gori. 1977. Contribution of the environment to cancer incidence: An epidemiologic exercise. J. Natl. Cancer Inst. 58:825-832.

Young, J. L., Jr., C. L. Percy, and A. J. Asire, eds. 1981. Surveillance, epidemiology, and end results: Incidence and mortality data, 1973-1977. Natl. Cancer Inst. Monogr. 57:1-1081.

17 The Relationship of Diet to Cancer at Specific Sites

To present more clearly what is known about the relationship between diet and cancer at specific sites, the committee has reassembled the epidemiological literature and summarized it by site: esophagus, stomach, colon and rectum, liver, pancreas, gallbladder, lung, urinary bladder, kidneys, breast, endometrium, ovary, and prostate. Since most of these data have already been discussed in earlier chapters on specific dietary constituents, the information contained in the following pages has been greatly condensed. The organization of this chapter reflects the design of most epidemiological studies, which generally examine cancer at specific sites.

ESOPHAGEAL CANCER

The incidence of esophageal cancer varies widely among different regions of the world. A belt of particularly high risk runs from the Middle East (notably the Caspian littoral of Iran) through central Asia to China. Other regions of high risk are the eastern and southern areas of Africa, and France has unusually high rates, especially in Normandy and Brittany.

Correlational analyses have shown direct associations of alcohol drinking with incidence of and mortality from esophageal cancer in some parts of the world. These studies were based on both estimated per capita intakes and dietary interview data in special population groups in Western countries (Breslow and Enstrom, 1974; Hinds et al., 1980; Kolonel et al., 1980; Lyon et al., 1980a,b; Schoenberg et al., 1971). Chilvers et al. (1979) found a consistent relationship between mortality from esophageal cancer and total ethanol intake in England and Wales. Other investigators reported high correlations of esophageal cancer mortality with death rates from cirrhosis and alcoholism (Lipworth and Rice, 1979; Tuyns et al., 1979).

The results from a number of case-control studies have confirmed the association with alcohol. Various investigators have demonstrated a dose-response relationship after controlling for cigarette smoking (Keller, 1980; Martínez, 1969; Pottern et al., 1981; Tuyns et al., 1979; Williams and Horm, 1977; Wynder and Bross, 1961; Wynder and Stellman, 1977). Schmidt and Popham (1981) found a significantly increased risk for esophageal cancer in a retrospective cohort study of male alcoholics. Smoking and alcohol appear to act synergistically to increase the risk for esophageal cancer as they do for cancers of the oral cavity and larynx (Rothman and Keller, 1972; Tuyns et al., 1977).

17-1

There has been no consistency in the type of alcoholic beverage most strongly associated with the risk of esophageal cancer. Some investigators found no specificity at all (Breslow and Enstrom, 1974; Williams and Horm, 1977); some found a stronger association with hard liquor than with beer or wine (Pottern et al., 1981; Wynder and Bross, 1961); and some reported a stronger association with beer (Hinds et al., 1980; Mettlin et al., 1980).

Alcohol consumption cannot explain the pattern of esophageal cancer in Africa and Asia (Bradshaw and Schonland, 1974; Burrell, 1962; Collis et al., 1971; Gatei et al., 1978; Higginson and Oettle, 1960; Joint Iran-International Agency for Research on Cancer Study Group, 1977; Yang, 1980). Correlation studies have indicated that the intakes of pulses (e.g., lentils), green vegetables, fresh fruit, animal and fish protein, and the estimated intakes of vitamin A, vitamin C, and riboflavin, are lower in high risk regions of the Caspian littoral in Iran (Hormozdiari et al., 1975; Joint Iran-International Agency for Research on Cancer Study Group, 1977). Similar studies in China have implicated low intakes of trace elements (particularly molybdenum), animal products, fat, fruits, vegetables, calcium, and riboflavin; high intakes of pickles, pickled vegetables, and moldy foods containing N-nitroso compounds (possibly produced by the fungal contaminants); and consumption of foods at very high temperatures (Coordinating Group for Research on Etiology of Esophageal Cancer in North China, 1975; Yang, 1980). In Japan, Segi (1975) found a direct association between mortality from esophageal cancer and the intake of tea-cooked rice gruel. On the other hand, Stocks (1970) and Howell (1974) found no associations between international per capita food and beverage intakes and corresponding mortality rates for esophageal cancer.

In view of the findings that nitrosamines and fungi contaminate some foods in China, it is notable that Marasas et al. (1979) found higher contamination levels of Fusarium mycotoxins in samples of corn (a dietary staple) from a high risk area for esophageal cancer in the African Republic of Transkei, compared with levels in a low risk area. However, these mycotoxins, unlike aflatoxin, have not been shown to be carcinogenic. Furthermore, results of the studies in Iran indicated that there were no differences in aflatoxin (or nitrosamine) levels in foods in regions of high and low risk for esophageal cancer.

A case-control study in Iran confirmed the inverse relationship between esophageal cancer and consumption of fresh fruit and cooked vegetables (Cook-Mozaffari, 1979; Cook-Mozaffari et al., 1979). The authors concluded that the disease might be caused by opium use in combination with diets low in fresh fruit and vegetables. In a case-control study of white males in the United States, Mettlin et al. (1980) also found a statistically significant inverse relationship, including a dose-response gradient, between risk of esophageal cancer and frequency of consumption of fruits and vegetables. Similar inverse associations were found for indices of vitamin A and C intake, especially for vitamin C intake. In a case-control study among Chinese in Singapore, de Jong et al. (1974)

found that a significant decrease in risk for esophageal cancer among males was associated with consumption of bread, potatoes, and bananas. They also found a direct association with consumption of very hot beverages. Ziegler et al. (1981) examined the role of nutrition in the etiology of esophageal cancer among blacks in the United States. They found that nutrition in general was poorer among cases than controls, but they identified no specific nutrient deficiency as responsible for the effect, which appeared to be independent of ethanol consumption.

Warwick and Harington (1973) reported that large quantities of grain, especially wheat and maize, are commonly consumed in most areas with high risk for esophageal cancer. This observation was recently extended by van Rensburg (1981), who examined esophageal cancer incidence and relative frequencies with which dietary staples were consumed in several populations, primarily in Africa and Asia. The low-risk populations consumed millet, cassava, yams, or peanuts; the high-risk populations consumed primarily wheat or corn, which provide diets relatively deficient in zinc, magnesium, nicotinic acid, and possibly riboflavin. He suggested that such nutritional deficiencies, which may also occur in abusers of alcohol, might increase susceptibility of the esophageal epithelium to neoplastic transformation. Thus, it is possible that a common mechanism is involved in the causation of esophageal cancer throughout the world.

In summary, a number of dietary factors appear to be associated with the risk of esophageal cancer. An increased risk in some parts of the world is associated with alcohol drinking, especially in combination with cigarette smoke, high intakes of pickles and moldy foods possibly containing mycotoxins or N-nitroso compounds, trace mineral deficiencies, and consumption of very hot beverages. Frequent consumption of fresh fruits and vegetables appears to be associated with a lower risk for esophageal cancer.

STOMACH CANCER

There is a high incidence rate of stomach cancer in Japan, in other parts of Asia, and in South America; but in North America and Europe, the incidence is low and is decreasing (Stukonis, 1978; Waterhouse et al., 1976). In Japan, gastric cancer has been associated with chronic gastritis (Imai et al., 1971) and with the consumption of spiced and pickled foods (Haenszel et al., 1976).

Surveys have shown that there is substantial variation in incidence among different areas of Colombia (Cuello et al., 1976). These variations have been correlated with different levels of nitrate in the diet and drinking water (Correa et al., 1976; Tannenbaum et al., 1979). Broitman et al. (1981) studied iron-deficient patients in Medellin, Colombia, who exhibited lesions that were precursors to gastric cancer. They found that hypochlorhydria and achlorhydria associated with iron deficiency permitted bacterial colonization of the stomach. Reduction of dietary nitrate to nitrite, and subsequent endogenous synthesis of N-nitroso compounds from nitrite, could thus be mediated by the gastric flora. Ruddell et al. (1978) suggested a similar mechanism to explain the increased risk for gastric cancer in patients with pernicious anemia.

An association between gastric cancer and high concentrations of nitrate in drinking water was suggested by Hill et al. (1973), who observed that mortality rates for stomach cancer were higher in Worksop, England, where the water supply contained higher concentrations of nitrate, than in nine control towns. However, Davies (1980) pointed out that Worksop was a coal-mining town, and that stomach cancer has been associated with coal-mining regions in Great Britain. Adjustment for coal mining and socioeconomic status abolished the excess mortality from stomach cancer in males in Worksop and reduced it markedly in females.

In Chile, exposure of the general population to high concentrations of nitrate in drinking water or in food appeared to be associated with high rates of stomach cancer (Armijo and Coulsen, 1975; Zaldívar, 1977). However, although nitrate levels were significantly higher in the urine of schoolchildren from two areas of central Chile with high mortality from stomach cancer than they were in the urine of schoolchildren from a northern, low risk area, levels of nitrate were also significantly higher in vegetables obtained from the low risk area (Armijo et al., 1981).

Dungal (1966) observed that large quantities of smoked foods (e.g., mutton and trout) were consumed in high incidence areas of Iceland and that there was a lower incidence of stomach cancer in sailors than in farmers in Iceland. He noted that sailors often stock food obtained at foreign ports; thus, their diet contains a higher proportion of fresh food. Choi et al. (1971) showed that the mortality from gastric cancer among Icelanders in Manitoba was twice as high as that among people born in Manitoba. A dietary survey showed that the people born in Iceland had consumed high levels of smoked and pickled foods.

Hakama and Saxén (1967) analyzed age- and sex-adjusted mortality rates for stomach cancer in 16 countries. They found a strong correlation (r = 0.75) with the per capita intake of cereals used for flour during 1934-1938.

In the United States, counties with high mortality from stomach cancer tend to be concentrated in Minnesota, Wisconsin, and the upper peninsula of Michigan (Mason et al., 1975). Kriebel and Jowett (1979) pointed out that although high rates in migrants from Northern Europe may explain part of this increased mortality, the rates are disproportionately high. They suggested that native-born Americans have shared the increased risk of the migrants, possibly by adopting the "high-risk" diet of the foreign-born residents.

Over several generations, there has been a gradual decline in the incidence of stomach cancer in Japanese migrants to the United States (Kolonel et al., 1980), suggesting that the risk factors for this cancer exert their effect early in life.

Data from several countries indicate that there is a strong correlation between mortality from gastric cancer and cerebrovascular disease. Joossens and Geboers (1981) suggested that both diseases are related to salt intake. However, the use of salt to preserve food is often accompanied by the use of nitrate for the same purpose (Weisburger et al., 1980). Furthermore, Okamura and Matsuhisa (1965) found no correlation between the salt content of salted fish and the death rate from gastric cancer in Japan.

In a number of case-control studies, investigators have attempted to define more specifically the role of diet and other factors in the etiology of gastric cancer. Acheson and Doll (1964) and Wynder et al. (1963) found no association with dietary factors. In another study, however, Meinsma (1964) observed that cases had eaten more bacon and less citrus fruits (and, thus, less ascorbic acid) than had the controls. Higginson (1966) found that cases had also consumed fried foods more frequently, especially bacon drippings and animal fats used for cooking. Hirayama (1967) reported that the daily consumption of milk was less frequent and the daily use of salted foods was more frequent among cases. Graham et al. (1972) observed that a low risk of gastric cancer was associated with the consumption of raw lettuce, tomatoes, carrots, coleslaw, and red cabbage and that there was a dose-response relationship for these food items.

Haenszel et al. (1972) studied Japanese living in Hawaii. Migrants (Issei) continued to display an increased risk in Hawaii, but the Nisei offspring, who adhered to Western-style diets, did not. There were elevated risks for both Issei and Nisei users of pickled vegetables and dried/salted fish. Low risks were associated with the consumption of several Western vegetables, many of which are eaten raw. Using a similar protocol, Haenszel et al. (1976) showed that farmers in Japan, representing the lower socioeconomic class, had the highest risk for gastric cancer. A lower risk was found for those whose diet included more frequent use of lettuce and celery. Modan et al. (1974) reported that starches were consumed more frequently by gastric cancer patients than by controls.

Bjelke (1978) found an inverse relationship between stomach cancer and consumption of vegetables and vitamin C, especially in younger patients and among women. He also reported preliminary findings from a prospective study, showing a reduced risk for those with a high consumption of vegetables in Norway, but not in Minnesota. The Norwegian study also suggested that frequent use of salted fish may be associated with a high risk of stomach cancer.

In a large cohort study conducted in Japan, Hirayama (1977) reported that a protective effect against gastric cancer was associated with the consumption of two glasses of milk daily and that there was an increased risk in cigarette smokers. Nonsmokers who ate green or yellow vegetables also had a lower risk of stomach cancer.

Weisburger and Raineri (1975) suggested that "gastric cancer in humans may result from the in vivo nitrosation in the stomach of as yet unknown substrates, with the production of alkylnitrosamides." They postulated that exposure to reducing agents such as ascorbic acid may interfere with the endogenous production of N-nitroso compounds by the reaction of dietary nitrite with amines or amides (Weisburger et al., 1980). Such a mechanism could explain the protective effect of green or yellow vegetables, raw lettuce, and other vitamin-C-containing vegetables.

In summary, studies in migrants to the United States suggest that gastric cancer is related in part to dietary factors that exert their influence early in life. The factors increasing risk may include frequent consumption of smoked food (which in some parts of the world leads to increased exposure to polycyclic aromatic hydrocarbons) and frequent ingestion of salt-pickled foods or foods containing nitrate and nitrite (which may result in subsequent in vivo production of nitrosamines) and other carcinogens produced in food by preservation treatments and cooking. Protective factors may include consumption of milk, raw green or yellow vegetables, especially lettuce, and other foods containing vitamin C.

COLON AND RECTAL CANCER

Haenszel (1961) reported that the rates of colon and rectal cancer in migrants from Italy, Norway, Poland, and the Soviet Union more closely resembled those in the host country (the United States) than those in their country of origin, in contrast to the findings for stomach cancer.

Haenszel and Dawson (1965) observed that mortality for cancer of the colon and rectum was higher in urban regions in the United States. Urban-born people who migrate to rural areas acquire the lower mortality of the rural areas; the reverse occurs for those who migrate from rural to urban areas. Mortality is higher in the North than in the South for long-term residents of these regions.

De Jong et al. (1972) found that in areas of high and intermediate risk there is a decreasing incidence from the ascending colon to the descending colon and a sharp increase at the sigmoid colon. Rectal cancer rates are generally higher than those for the sigmoid. In low incidence areas, there may be a low rate for sigmoid cancers.

Berg and Howell (1974) reviewed international mortality from cancer of the bowel from 1952 to 1953 and from 1966 to 1967. The highest death rates were reported in Scotland, but these rates were falling, as were those for England and Wales. The rates for whites in the United States appeared to be stable, but those for the Federal Republic of Germany, Italy, and Japan were rising. The investigators interpreted differences between colon and rectal cancer rates as indicating that, although much of rectal cancer is caused by the same factors that cause colon cancer, there is a second set of factors that affect rectal cancers alone.

Lee (1976) found that death rates from large bowel cancer in Japan have risen rapidly since World War II and that colon cancer has increased at a greater rate than rectal cancer. In Japan, each successive birth cohort had an increased rate of colon cancer, whereas those in the United States did not.

Haenszel et al. (1975) investigated the incidence of large-bowel cancer in Cali, Colombia in relation to place of residence, by census tract. They found that the upper socioeconomic classes were at higher risk. Lynch et al. (1975) also reported a greater frequency of colon cancer in patients living in census tracts with higher average incomes. Similarly, Teppo et al. (1980) found a higher incidence of colon cancer in higher socioeconomic areas of Finland.

Studies of the international incidence of and mortality from large bowel cancer in relation to dietary variables strongly support an association of colon cancer and, to a lesser extent, rectal cancer with total dietary fat (Armstrong and Doll, 1975; Wynder, 1975). Irving and Drasar (1973) failed to find a correlation between cancer of the colon and the per capita intake of various fiber-containing foods. In studies of mortality rates for colon cancer, Berg and Howell (1974) and Howell (1975) reported that the highest correlations were found for per capita meat intake, and that the highest was for beef. However, Enstrom (1975) pointed out that the trends in per capita beef and fat intake in the United States do not correlate with trends in incidence of and mortality from colorectal cancer.

Jansson et al. (1978) correlated the selenium concentration in water samples from the eastern part of the United States with the incidence of colorectal cancer. They found a strong, direct relationship between the selenium content of water and colorectal cancer and observed that the mean mortality rate increased with increasing levels of selenium in the drinking water. Other studies, however, have shown an inverse correlation between the intake of selenium and colon cancer (Schrauzer et al., 1977a,b; also see the section on selenium in Chapter 10).

Lui et al. (1979) evaluated food disappearance data for 1954-1965 and data on mortality from colon cancer for 1967-1973 from 20 industrialized countries. They found that the per capita intakes of total fat, saturated fat, monounsaturated fat, and cholesterol were directly correlated and that fiber intake was inversely correlated with mortality from colon cancer. The correlation of dietary cholesterol with colon cancer was highly significant and remained so when they controlled for fat or fiber. However, the correlations of fat or of fiber with colon cancer mortality were no longer significant when they controlled for cholesterol.

Bingham et al. (1979) related the average intake of foods, nutrients, and dietary fiber in Great Britain to the regional pattern of death from colon and rectal cancer. They found that intakes of the pentosan fraction of total dietary fiber and of vegetables other than potatoes were inversely correlated with death rates for colon cancer.

The possible importance of dietary cholesterol (and/or dietary fat) is supported by the correlations of mortality from colon cancer with mortality from coronary heart disease in different countries (Rose et al., 1974), correlations with large-bowel cancer among different social classes in Cali, Colombia (Haenszel et al., 1975), and for cancer of the colon and rectum together and individually within 34 health-planning subdivisions in the Commonwealth of Massachusetts (Lipworth and Rice, 1979). Stemmermann et al. (1979) noted the high rate of colon cancer among Japanese who migrated to Hawaii and observed that myocardial infarction, severe atherosclerosis, diverticulosis, and polyposis of the colon also occurred more frequently in this population, compared to Japanese living in Japan.

In studies of cancer incidence in Seventh-Day Adventists, Phillips and colleagues reported that a lacto-ovovegetarian diet had a protective effect against colon cancer (Phillips, 1975; Phillips et al., 1980a,b). The findings among Mormons in Utah (Lyon and Sorenson, 1978; Lyon et al., 1976, 1980a,b) and in California (Enstrom, 1980) confirmed that this group had a lower incidence of colon cancer than the U.S. average, but were less clear with respect to the impact of dietary factors. In a preliminary dietary survey, Lyon and Sorenson (1978) found little difference in meat, fat, and fiber intake by the population of Utah and by the general U.S. population.

Malhotra (1977) suggested that the virtual absence of colon cancer among Punjabis from northern India is due to their diet, which is rich in roughage, cellulose, vegetable fiber, and short-chain fatty acids contained in fermented milk products.

MacLennan et al. (1978) evaluated the diets consumed by adult men from Kuopio, Finland and compared them with the diets consumed by a similar sample from Copenhagen, Denmark, where the incidence of colon cancer is 4 times higher. They found that the high incidence group consumed more refined wheat breads, meats (especially pork), and beer, but less potatoes and milk than did the low incidence group in Finland. The estimated consumption of fat was similar, but the consumption of fiber was higher in the low incidence group.

Reddy et al. (1978) studied the dietary patterns and fecal constituents of a high risk group in New York and the low risk group in rural Kuopio. The average daily intake of dietary fat and protein was the same in the two groups, but a greater proportion of fat came from dairy products in Kuopio and from meat in New York. The daily stool output and fecal fiber excretion were also greater in Kuopio, where there was a high dietary intake of cereal products rich in fiber.

These investigators found more mutagenic activity in the stools from New York subjects who were not Seventh-Day Adventists than in the stools obtained from subjects in Kuopio, who had a similar fat but a higher fiber intake (Reddy et al., 1980). However, they found no mutagenic activity in the stools from vegetarian Seventh-Day Adventist volunteers from New York, who had a lower average fat intake than the other two groups, but an intermediate level of fiber intake.

A number of case-control studies have been conducted to examine the relationship between diet and cancer of the large bowel. Wynder and Shigematsu (1967) could not identify environmental factors that differed significantly between cases and controls. A study of Japanese patients with bowel cancer and hospital controls in Hawaii indicated that there was a higher risk for persons who regularly ate Western-style meals (Haenszel et al., 1973). Control for beef produced the largest downward displacement in estimated risks for other dietary variables. In Japan, a study conducted with similar methodology did not replicate these findings (Haenszel et al., 1980); however, reduced risk was associated with consumption of cabbage.

Modan et al. (1975) found that fiber-containing foods were consumed less frequently by cases of colon cancer than by controls, but there were no differences for cases with rectal cancer. They also observed no differences in consumption of fat-containing foods by either cancer group or the controls.

Parallel studies in Norway and Minnesota indicated that there was a slightly lower consumption of cereal products, milk, and coffee by colorectal cancer cases, compared to controls, and several vegetables were eaten less frequently by the cases (Bjelke, 1978). The cases also had lower indices for consumption of vitamin A and crude fiber, both of which are associated with vegetable intake. In the United States, Phillips (1975) found that consumption of beef, lamb, and fish, and the heavy use of dairy products other than milk and other high-fat foods, were directly associated with the risk of colon cancer, and that there was a slight inverse association with the consumption of milk, vegetable protein products, and green leafy vegetables.

Dales et al. (1979) reported that foods with at least 0.5% fiber content were consumed less frequently by colon cancer cases than by the controls, and that there was a consistent dose-response relationship. Cases tended to have eaten foods with at least 5% saturated fat more often than controls. Significantly more cases than controls reported a high saturated fat, low fiber food consumption pattern.

Graham et al. (1978) reported that a decreased risk of colon cancer was associated with frequent ingestion of vegetables, especially cabbage, brussels sprouts, and broccoli. Decreased risk of rectal cancer was associated only with frequent ingestion of raw vegetables and cabbage.

However, Martinez et al. (1979) reported that cases had consumed significantly higher quantities of meats, cereals, total fats, total residue,
and fiber.

Jain et al. (1980) observed that an increased risk of both colon and
rectal cancer was associated with elevated consumption of calories, total
fat, total protein, saturated fat, oleic acid, and cholesterol, but that
there was no association with consumption of crude fiber, vitamin C, and
linoleic acid. The highest risk was found for saturated fat consumption,
and there was evidence of a dose-response relationship.

The only cohort studies that have yet provided data on dietary variables are the ongoing parallel studies in Norway and Minnesota (Bjelke,
1978). These studies indicate that there is a reduced risk of colorectal
cancer in the Minnesota subjects who have a high index of vegetable consumption. No such effect has been observed in Norway, but the number of
cases in that country is small.

Most information on the association between colon cancer and cholesterol levels has been derived from epidemiological studies and intervention trials to determine risk for cardiovascular disease. The findings
have been conflicting, and it is not certain whether reported increases
in risk of cancer (especially colon cancer) at low serum cholesterol
levels reflect a causal association (Feinleib, 1981; Lilienfeld, 1981).

Rectal cancer has been associated with intake of beer in some studies (Breslow and Enstrom 1974; Dean et al., 1979; Enstrom, 1977; Stocks,
1957), but not in all studies (Jensen, 1979; Schmidt and Popham, 1981).
McMichael et al. (1979) suggested that there is a better correlation between trends in mortality from rectal cancer and changes in beer intake
than has been found for saturated fat.

Wynder and Shigematsu (1967) showed that the proportion of beer
drinkers among male colorectal cancer patients was significantly higher
than in one control group, but not in a second control group. In a
prospective study conducted by Bjelke (1973), there was a dose-response
relationship between the risk of colorectal cancer and the frequency of
beer and liquor consumption. The gradient was steeper for beer consumption. Conversely, case-control studies of intestinal cancer in Finland,
Kansas, and Norway (Bjelke, 1971, 1973; Higginson, 1966; Pernu, 1960)
indicated that there was no significant relationship with beer drinking.
Vitale et al. (1981) reported a correlation coefficient of 0.78 between
alcohol consumed as beer and colon cancer in 20 countries. There were
poor correlations for colon cancer and the intake of total ethanol,
distilled spirits, or wine.

In summary, three hypotheses appear to be supported by data of various strengths obtained from epidemiological studies of both colon and

and rectal cancer: (1) a causal association with total, and perhaps saturated, fat; (2) a protective effect of dietary fiber; and (3) a protective effect of cruciferous vegetables. The diverse results concerning the importance of fat and fiber may be partly due to differences in the degrees of precision in the dietary methodology used in the various studies. The possible role of alcohol in the induction of rectal cancer requires further study.

LIVER CANCER

Primary liver cancer is relatively uncommon in the United States and most Western countries, but it is a major form of cancer in sub-Saharan Africa and Southeast Asia. Several different dietary agents have been reported as possible hepatic carcinogens, including alcohol, aflatoxin, safrole, pyrrolizidine alkaloids, and cycasin (Anthony, 1977).

Oettlé (1965) suggested that the geographic distribution of liver cancer in Africa could be explained by differing levels of exposure to aflatoxin in the diet. In a number of studies, aflatoxin contamination of foodstuffs has been correlated with liver cancer incidence and mortality by geographic area or for different population groups in Africa (Alpert et al., 1971; Keen and Martin, 1971; Peers and Linsell, 1973; Peers et al., 1976; van Rensburg et al., 1974). Similar correlations have been found in Thailand, China, and Taiwan, which also have high rates of liver cancer (Armstrong, 1980; Shank et al., 1972a,b; Tung and Ling, 1968; Wogan, 1975). There is a strong correlation between the estimated levels of aflatoxin ingestion and liver cancer rates in these various studies, and no populations with documented high levels of aflatoxin ingestion have low rates of liver cancer (Linsell and Peers, 1977).

Numerous reports (e.g., Chien et al., 1981) have also documented a high correlation between primary liver cancer and exposure to hepatitis B viral infection, which has a worldwide distribution similar to that of aflatoxin. Many investigators believe that although primary liver cancer could be initiated by aflatoxin, there is a higher probability that liver cancer develops in individuals exposed to the hepatitis B virus.

In Guam and Okinawa, which have high rates of liver cancer, the ingestion of cycasin (a toxic substance contained in cycad nuts) has been proposed as an etiologic factor. However, in a descriptive study conducted in the Miyako Islands of Okinawa, investigators found no correlation between mortality from hepatoma and the ingestion of cycad nuts (Hirono et al., 1970).

Alcohol is the main dietary factor that has been suggested as an etiologic agent for liver cancer in Western, low-risk countries, although Armstrong and Doll (1975) reported a weak correlation between liver cancer incidence (but not mortality) and per capita intake of potatoes in more than 20 countries. Interest in alcohol as a causal factor for primary liver cancer was generated by reports of hepatomas occurring at increased rates in cirrhotic patients with histories of heavy alcohol use and by other reports of high rates of alcoholic cirrhosis in hepatoma patients (Lee, 1966; Purtilo and Gottlieb, 1973). However, the cirrhosis usually associated with liver cancer is the macronodular form, which is characteristically associated with hepatitis B viral infection (Anthony, 1977). Furthermore, ethanol itself has not been shown to be carcinogenic in animals (Vitale and Gottlieb, 1975).

Most descriptive epidemiological data do not support the association between alcohol intake and risk of liver cancer. Esophageal cancer has been linked to alcohol consumption; however, the incidence rates for esophageal cancer in various countries have been significantly correlated with liver cancer in men, but not in women (Miller, 1981). Despite differences in alcohol consumption between Mormons and non-Mormons in Utah and between Issei and Nisei Japanese in Hawaii, both groups in Utah and both in Hawaii have similar incidence rates for liver cancer (Kolonel et al., 1980; Lyon et al., 1976, 1980a,b). There is also no significant correlation between ethnic patterns of liver cancer incidence in Hawaii and alcohol consumption (Hinds et al., 1980).

There have been few analytical studies of the relationship between alcohol and liver cancer. In a proportional mortality analysis, Monson and Lyon (1975) found no increase in deaths from liver cancer among alcoholics admitted to mental hospitals in Massachusetts. Conversely, Hakulinen et al. (1974) found that liver cancer cases in two alcohol abuser populations in Finland exceeded the number expected, based on data in the Finnish Cancer Registry. In a retrospective cohort study of male alcoholics in Ontario, Canada, Schmidt and Popham (1981) observed that liver cancer deaths were 2 times higher than expected, based on the general population of Ontario, but the numbers were small and the difference was not statistically significant.

In summary, high intake of foods contaminated with aflatoxin is associated with liver cancer in high incidence areas of the world, i.e., Asia and Africa. Chronic infection with hepatitis B virus, which has the same geographic distribution as aflatoxin contamination, has been proposed as a primary etiologic factor in liver cancer. The evidence that excessive alcohol consumption may indirectly contribute to the development of some types of liver cancer is extremely tenuous.

PANCREATIC CANCER

The per capita intake of several foods has been associated with pancreatic cancer incidence and mortality in a number of international studies. Analyses of mortality data have produced direct associations with intake of fats and oils, sugar, animal protein, eggs, milk, and coffee (Armstrong and Doll, 1975; Lea, 1967; Stocks, 1970; Wynder et al.,

1973). From incidence data, there was a direct correlation only with per capita intake of eggs (Armstrong and Doll, 1975). In a correlation analysis by county in the United States, Blot et al. (1978) found that there was a direct association with alcohol intake. In contrast, Hinds et al. (1980) reported that pancreatic cancer incidence in five ethnic groups in Hawaii correlated directly with beer consumption, after controlling for cigarette smoking and consumption of other types of alcoholic beverages. This finding was in agreement with the observation of Kolonel et al. (1980) that pancreatic cancer incidence rates are the same for migrant and native-born Japanese groups in Hawaii, which have similar rates for beer consumption but not for total alcohol consumption. Lyon et al. (1980a,b) observed that non-Mormons in Utah have higher incidence rates of pancreatic cancer than do Mormons, who drink less alcohol, tea, and coffee.

Reports of several case-control studies have indicated an association between diet and pancreatic cancer. Based on data obtained from relatives of cases and controls, who responded to a mailed questionnaire, Burch and Ansari (1968) found a direct association between pancreatic cancer and chronic alcoholism. Using a similar design, Ishii et al. (1968) found direct associations with alcohol and meat consumption (men only) and an inverse association with vegetable intake. Lin and Kessler (1981) reported that the consumption of wine by female cases was greater than that of controls, a finding not observed in the males. In contrast, Wynder et al. (1973) and MacMahon et al. (1981) found no association between pancreatic cancer and alcohol consumption. Wynder et al. (1973) did find a direct association with early-onset diabetes in women, and MacMahon et al. (1981) reported a direct association with coffee consumption and a dose-response gradient for women only. Lin and Kessler (1981) also noted a greater consumption of decaffeinated coffee by cases than by controls.

Two cohort studies have reproduced the association of pancreatic cancer with diabetes in women, which was observed in the case-control study of Wynder et al. (1973) and in the correlational analyses of Blot et al. (1978). After studying a cohort of diabetics for 29 years, Kessler (1970) found excess deaths from pancreatic cancer, despite fewer overall cancer deaths than expected. Armstrong et al. (1976b) also followed a cohort of diabetics and found a slight increase in mortality from pancreatic cancer (although not statistically significant) and an overall decrease in mortality from all cancers. Hirayama (1977) reported a relative risk of 2.5 for daily meat consumption and pancreatic cancer in a cohort study conducted in Japan, thereby reproducing a similar finding in the case-control study of Ishii et al. (1968).

In summary, there is limited evidence that certain dietary factors (e.g., the intake of alcohol, coffee, and meat) are associated with an elevated risk for cancer of the pancreas.

GALLBLADDER CANCER

There is a high incidence of gallbladder cancer in Latin America, Japan, and Southeast Asia for both sexes--but it is higher for females than for males (Waterhouse et al., 1976). Cancer at this site is relatively uncommon among blacks and whites in the United States, but occurs more frequently among North American Indians and Mexican-American females. It has also been associated with gallstones, obesity, and type IV hyperlipoproteinemia (Fraumeni, 1975a). Among the dietary risk factors that have been postulated are both high calorie and high fat diets. However, the uniformly poor correlation of gallbladder cancer with other cancers associated with high fat diets appears to militate against high fat diets as a causal factor. No case-control study of dietary factors and cancer of this site has been reported.

The evidence for a dietary etiology of this cancer is therefore indirect and rather weak at this time, other than an association with obesity and, therefore, possibly an excess of calories.

LUNG CANCER

Lung cancer is the most prevalent cancer in men in most technically advanced countries, and it is rapidly approaching this level in women (Miller, 1980; Waterhouse et al., 1976). The most important causal factor is cigarette smoking (Surgeon General, 1979). Occupational exposures contribute substantially to the incidence in males (Fraumeni, 1975b). In women, cigarette smoking probably accounts for more than one-half of the cases (Surgeon General, 1980).

Bjelke (1975) conducted a prospective study of 8,278 Norwegian men who responded to a mailed questionnaire designed to determine the association between vitamin A intake and lung cancer. As a result of observations made during a 5-year follow-up of this group, Bjelke was one of the first to suggest a relationship between vitamin A intake and cancer at this site. He found that the relative risk for lung cancer was 2.5 times higher for current and former smokers in the low vitamin A intake group than for those in the high intake group.

Subsequently, a number of other investigators studied this association. Basu et al. (1976) and Sakula (1976) found that levels of vitamin A in the plasma of bronchial carcinoma patients were lower than those in the serum of controls. MacLennan et al. (1977) studied the relationship between consumption of dark green, leafy vegetables rich in vitamin A precursors and the risk of lung cancer in Chinese female cases and controls in Singapore. They found a relative risk of 2.2 for low indices of vegetable intake. Smith and Jick (1978) assessed the frequency with which preparations containing vitamin A were used by newly diagnosed lung cancer patients and patients with nonmalignant conditions. They found an inverse association among men, but not among women. Mettlin et al. (1979)

found a dose-response relationship for lung cancer up to risk ratios
of 2.4 for heavy smoking men with a low index of vitamin A consumption.
Shekelle et al. (1981) studied a prospective cohort of 1,954 men in
Chicago. After 19 years of followup, they found a significant inverse
association between lung cancer incidence and the intake of carotene,
after adjustment for cigarette smoking. In contrast, lung cancer was
not significantly associated with the intake of preformed vitamin A.

In summary, there is evidence that low dietary levels of foods containing vitamin A and/or vitamin A precursors (e.g., β-carotene) are
associated with increased risk of lung cancer, especially among heavy
smokers. Because the indices of vitamin A intake in these studies were
derived from foods that also contain other natural inhibitors of carcinogenesis, it is also possible that dietary constituents other than preformed vitamin A or carotene are the relevant risk-reducing factors.

BLADDER CANCER

Most of the epidemiological literature on the association between
diet and bladder cancer pertains to coffee and nonnutritive sweeteners.
In both correlation and case-control studies, direct associations have
been found between coffee consumption and bladder cancer (C. T. Miller et
al., 1978; Simon et al., 1975; Wynder and Goldsmith, 1977); however, in
most of the case-control studies, investigators failed to find a dose-
response gradient. In other epidemiological studies, no association at
all was found between coffee consumption and bladder cancer. These
studies are reviewed in Chapter 12.

There are similarly conflicting findings in the epidemiological
literature on nonnutritive sweetener use and bladder cancer. Both correlational data and observations in studies of diabetics have failed to
implicate nonnutritive sweetener use in the etiology of bladder cancer
(Armstrong et al., 1976b; Kessler, 1970). In some case-control studies,
investigators found an association; in others, they did not. With the
exception of a study by Howe et al. (1977), direct associations were
observed only in very select, low-risk subgroups, e.g., nonsmoking women
without occupational exposure to bladder carcinogens (Hoover and Strasser,
1980). These studies are discussed in detail in Chapter 14.

The epidemiological literature pertaining to the association of other
dietary exposures and bladder cancer is much more limited. In an analysis
based on international data, Armstrong and Doll (1975) found a direct
association of bladder cancer mortality, but not incidence, with per
capita intake of fats and oils, particularly in women. In another cor-

relation study, based on data by state in the United States, there was a direct association between beer intake and bladder cancer mortality in men (Breslow and Enstrom, 1974).

In a report of a case-control study, Mettlin and Graham (1979) observed that there was an inverse association between bladder cancer and an index of "vitamin A" intake as well as with consumption of carrots and milk. In another case-control study, Howe et al. (1980) found a direct association between bladder cancer and consumption of coffee and no association with consumption of tea, alcohol, soft drinks, fiddlehead greens (related to bracken fern, which is a bladder carcinogen in cattle), or meats preserved with nitrite (such as hams and sausages). Nitrosamines (presumably formed from precursors of dietary origin) have been found in the urine of patients with urinary tract infections (Hicks et al., 1977; Radomski et al., 1978).

In summary, bladder cancer has frequently been associated with coffee consumption, although the relationship does not appear to be causal. The use of nonnutritive sweeteners (primarily saccharin) does not appear to be a significant risk factor, except perhaps in some very select low risk groups. A possible inverse association with an index of "vitamin A" intake has been reported in one study.

RENAL CANCER

The epidemiological data on dietary factors related to renal cancer are meager. International incidence and mortality data have shown correlations of renal cancer with per capita intake of coffee, milk, meat, total fat, and animal protein (Armstrong and Doll, 1975; Shennan, 1973). In a correlation study of ethnic-specific incidence rates for renal cancer with corresponding intakes of alcohol based on representative interview data, Hinds et al. (1980) found a direct association for beer consumption, but not for the consumption of wine or hard liquor. A similar direct correlation for beer intake and renal cancer was reported by Breslow and Enstrom (1974), who compared mortality data and per capita alcohol intake by state in the United States.

These associations have not been reproduced in case-control studies of renal cancer. In a case-control study by Wynder et al. (1974), there were no differences for coffee drinking or alcohol consumption; however, they did report that the relative weight of female (but not male) cases 2 years before the onset of illness was greater than that of the controls. Armstrong et al. (1976a) also found no direct associations with the frequency of intake of coffee, tea, alcohol, chocolate, or the major food sources of animal protein. Kolonel (1976) observed a direct association between renal cancer and combined exposure to cadmium from three sources: diet, cigarette smoking, and occupational setting.

BREAST CANCER

Breast cancer is the commonest cause of death from cancer among women in North America. In the United States, it is the cause of more deaths than any other cause among women between the ages of 40 and 44. It is known that cancer at this site is associated with hormonal activity, but diet has also been suspected as a major cause (MacMahon et al., 1973).

Several types of studies have provided evidence supporting the importance of dietary factors in breast cancer: descriptive epidemiological studies, correlation studies, evaluations of nutrition-mediated risk factors, and case-control studies. Additional evidence for an association has been provided in reports of studies in laboratory animals, which are discussed in Chapter 5.

The evidence from descriptive epidemiological studies suggests that cultural factors or lifestyle, especially diet, are influential in the etiology of breast cancer. For example, the incidence of breast cancer among premenopausal Japanese-American women living in California is now almost as high as that for Caucasian women (Dunn, 1977); whereas the incidence of cancer among them was similar to that in Japan when they first migrated. Moolgavkar et al. (1980) have shown that changes in cancer incidence for certain populations can be related to changes in lifestyle of successive birth cohorts.

The second type of evidence has been provided by studies correlating breast cancer incidence and mortality with per capita intake of total fat and other nutrients in different countries (Armstrong and Doll, 1975; Carroll, 1975; Drasar and Irving, 1973; Hems, 1978; Knox, 1977), including Japan (Hirayama, 1977) and the United States (Enig et al., 1978; Kolonel et al., 1981). Gaskill et al. (1979) found a direct correlation between breast cancer mortality and intake of milk, table fats, beef, calories, protein, and fat, and an inverse correlation with intake of eggs. Milk and egg intake remained significantly associated (directly and inversely, respectively) with breast cancer when the investigators controlled for age at first marriage.

The third type of evidence is derived from evaluating certain, probably nutrition-mediated, factors that affect the risk of breast cancer. These factors include weight, height, body mass (which is dependent on height and weight) (de Waard 1975; de Waard and Baanders-van Halewijn, 1974; de Waard et al., 1977), and age at menarche (MacMahon et al., 1973; Miller, 1978). Women who experienced menarche at an early age, especially before the age of 12, were at higher risk. Evidence that body weight and food intake are related to early onset of estrus in rats (Frisch et al., 1975) supports the hypothesis that the rat's body must contain a minimum amount of fat for estrus to occur. This also appears

to be essential for menarche in women (Frisch and McArthur, 1974); however, not all studies of these factors have confirmed these findings
(Miller, 1981), perhaps reflecting the overriding importance of other
variables more directly related to nutrition.

Gray et al. (1979) evaluated the effect of per capita intake of
total fat and animal protein on international incidence and mortality
rates for breast cancer, while controlling for height, weight, and age
at menarche. They found that a significant effect of the dietary variables persisted after controlling for the other factors.

Case-control or cohort studies should provide the most conclusive
evidence. Thus far, no cohort studies have been reported. Of the three
case-control studies that have been reported, one involved 77 breast
cancer cases and 77 controls (Phillips, 1975). In this study, five
categories of foods were associated with breast cancer: fried foods,
fried potatoes, hard fat used for frying, dairy products (except milk),
and white bread. The relative risks ranged from 1.6 to 2.6.

In the case-control study of 400 cases and 400 neighborhood controls
reported by A. B. Miller et al. (1978), the mean nutrient consumption
was estimated from dietary histories for six nutrients. In the premenopausal group, the strongest association was found for total fat consumption. There were weaker associations for saturated fat and cholesterol. When the effect of each nutrient was controlled for the effect
of the others, the association for total fat consumption became stronger,
whereas the association for saturated fat and cholesterol diminished.
In the postmenopausal group, the only consistent finding was an association for total fat consumption. The risk ratios were low (1.6 for total
fat in premenopausal women and 1.5 for postmenopausal women), and there
was no evidence of a dose-response relationship.

In the third case-control study, which involved 577 cases and 826
controls, Lubin et al. (1981) found that relative risk increased significantly with more frequent consumption of beef and other red meat, pork,
and sweet desserts. Analysis of computed mean daily nutrient intake
supported a link between breast cancer and consumption of animal fat and
protein.

Nomura et al. (1978) compared the diet of Japanese men whose wives
had developed breast cancer with the diets of other Japanese men who had
participated in the Japan-Hawaii Cancer Study. They assumed that the
diets of the husbands and wives were similar. Their results indicated
that the husbands of the cases consumed more beef or other meat, butter/
margarine/cheese, corn, and wieners, and that they ate less Japanese
foods than did the control group.

In summary, information derived from a number of different types of
studies support the association of diet, especially high fat diets, with

breast cancer. The association is weak, if examined for individuals rather than for populations. One explanation for this may be that the effect of diet takes place early in life and is indirect, possibly influencing cancer risk by its effects on hormones (Miller and Bulbrook, 1980).

ENDOMETRIAL CANCER

Endometrial (uterine) cancer has been correlated with other cancers that are associated with dietary factors (e.g., cancers of the breast, ovary, colon, and rectum) (Miller, 1981) and has been associated with higher socioeconomic status. In correlation studies, it has been associated primarily with high per capita intake of total fat (Armstrong and Doll, 1975).

Two indirect indicators of the effect of nutrition have been evaluated in case-control studies. In two such studies, an association was found with obesity (Elwood et al., 1977; Wynder et al., 1966), although the excess risk appeared to be restricted to the most obese group. In one of these studies, Elwood et al. (1977) observed no association with height. Thus far, there have been no case-control studies directly comparing the effects of diet on cases of endometrial cancer and controls.

In summary, the evidence for an association between endometrial cancer and diet is indirect. It is derived mainly from the similarity between the occurrence of this disease and cancer of the breast and colon. The recent dramatic increases in the incidence of endometrial cancer have been clearly related to the use of exogenous estrogens at the time of menopause (Jick et al., 1980); they do not appear to be related to any factor in the diet.

OVARIAN CANCER

The evidence associating dietary factors, especially high fat diets, and ovarian cancer is largely indirect. It includes both international and national correlations between incidence of and mortality from ovarian cancer and other diet-associated cancers, especially cancers of the breast and colon (Miller, 1981), and the correlation of dietary variables, especially per capita intake of total fat, with incidence of and mortality from ovarian cancer (Armstrong and Doll, 1975; Lingeman, 1974).

In one case-control study, Annegers et al. (1979) observed that obesity is not a risk factor for ovarian cancer, and in another, Hildreth et al. (1981) found no effect of height or weight. No case-control studies evaluating dietary variables directly have yet been reported. There is, however, a greater than expected risk of second primary cancers of the corpus uteri, colon, and breast in patients with ovarian cancer (Reimer et al., 1978). This supports the hypothesis that there are common etiological factors for these sites.

PROSTATE CANCER

Several investigators have correlated dietary intake data with incidence of and mortality from prostate cancer. Stocks (1970) reported a direct correlation of prostate cancer mortality with per capita coffee intake in 20 countries. In a similar analysis, Armstrong and Doll (1975) found a significant direct correlation of prostate cancer mortality, but not incidence, with the per capita intake of total fat and the intake of fats and oils. They noted a high intercorrelation of coffee and fat consumption in their data, which they believed could explain the association with coffee drinking reported by Stocks. Howell (1974) found a high direct correlation between mortality from prostate cancer in 41 countries and per capita intake of fats, milk, and meats (especially beef), and an inverse correlation with intake of rice. Blair and Fraumeni (1978) observed that U.S. counties with the highest prostate cancer mortality among whites were those with greater per capita intake of high fat foods (e.g., beef products, milk products, fats and oils, pork, and eggs). A correlational analysis based on dietary data obtained from individual interviews in Hawaii indicated that there was a significant association between incidence of prostate cancer in five ethnic groups and the consumption of animal fat and protein (Kolonel et al., 1981). Furthermore, it has been observed that both prostate cancer incidence and fat intake are higher among Japanese in Hawaii than in Japan (Kato et al., 1973; Waterhouse et al., 1976).

These observations are further supported by international incidence and mortality data indicating that there are significant correlations of prostate cancer with cancers of other sites associated with diet, including cancer of the breast, corpus uteri, and colon (Berg, 1975; Howell, 1974; Wynder et al., 1971). However, there are important exceptions. For example, the Mormons in Utah have high prostate but low breast cancer incidence rates, and the native Hawaiians have low prostate but high breast cancer incidence rates (Kolonel, 1980; Lyon et al., 1976).

There have been few case-control studies of prostate cancer and diet. Rotkin (1977), in an interim report, observed that high fat foods (including beef, pork, eggs, cheeses, milk, creams, and butter/margarine) were consumed more frequently by cases than by matched hospital controls. Schuman et al. (1982) reproduced this finding in a study conducted in Minnesota. They also reported that the consumption of foods rich in vitamin A (e.g., liver) or its precursors (e.g., carrots) were lower for cases than for controls. Kolonel and Winkelstein (1977) found no difference between cases and controls in exposure to cadmium from dietary sources. This lack of association is interesting in light of reports indicating that there are direct associations between prostate cancer and exposure to cadmium in occupational groups (Adams et al., 1969; Kipling and Waterhouse, 1967; Lemen et al., 1976; Potts, 1965), and the knowledge that diet is the main source of exposure to cadmium for the general population (Friberg et al., 1974).

After a 10-year follow-up of a cohort of 122,261 Japanese men aged 40 years and older, Hirayama (1979) found an inverse association between daily intake of green or yellow vegetables and mortality from prostate cancer. Hirayama (1977) also reported that prostate cancer occurred at a lower rate among vegetarian men in this cohort.

In summary, the incidence of prostate cancer is correlated with other cancers associated with diet, e.g., breast cancer. There is good evidence that an increased risk of prostate cancer is associated with certain dietary factors, especially the intake of high fat and high protein foods, which usually occur together in the diet. There is some evidence that foods rich in vitamin A or its precursors and vegetarian diets are associated with a lower risk.

REFERENCES

Acheson, E. D., and R. Doll. 1964. Dietary factors in carcinoma of the stomach: A study of 100 cases and 200 controls. Gut 5:126-131.

Adams, R. G., J. F. Harrison, and P. Scott. 1969. The development of cadmium-induced proteinuria, impaired renal function, and osteomalacia in alkaline battery workers. Q. J. Med. 38:425-443.

Alpert, M. E., M. S. R. Hutt, G. N. Wogan, and C. S. Davidson. 1971. Association between aflatoxin content of food and hepatoma frequency in Uganda. Cancer 28:253-260.

Annegers, J. F., H. Strom, D. G. Decker, M. B. Dockerty, and W. M. O'Fallon. 1979. Ovarian cancer. Incidence and case-control study. Cancer 43:723-729.

Anthony, P. P. 1977. Cancer of the liver: Pathogenesis and recent aetiological factors. Trans. R. Soc. Trop. Med. Hyg. 71:466-470.

Armijo, R., and A. H. Coulsen. 1975. Epidemiology of stomach cancer in Chile--The role of nitrogen fertilizers. Int. J. Epidemiol. 4:301-309.

Armijo, R., A. Gonzalez, M. Orellana, A. H. Coulson, J. W. Sayre, and R. Detels. 1981. Epidemiology of gastric cancer in Chile: II. Nitrate exposures and stomach cancer frequency. Int. J. Epidemiol. 10:57-62.

Armstrong, B. 1980. The epidemiology of cancer in the Peoples Republic of China. Int. J. Epidemiol. 9:305-315.

Armstrong, B., and R. Doll. 1975. Environmental factors and cancer incidence and mortality in different countries, with special reference to dietary practices. Int. J. Cancer 15:617-631.

Armstrong, B., A. Garrod, and R. Doll. 1976a. A retrospective study of renal cancer with special reference to coffee and animal protein consumption. Br. J. Cancer 33:127-136.

Armstrong, B., A. J. Lea, A. M. Adelstein, J. W. Donovan, G. C. White, and S. Ruttle. 1976b. Cancer mortality and saccharin consumption in diabetics. Br. J. Prev. Soc. Med. 30:151-157.

Basu, T. K., D. Donaldson, M. Jenner, D. C. Williams, and A. Sakula. 1976. Plasma vitamin A in patients with bronchial carcinoma. Br. J. Cancer 33:119-121.

Berg, J. W.   1975.   Can nutrition explain the pattern of international epidemiology of hormone-dependent cancers?   Cancer Res. 35:3345-3350.

Berg, J. W., and M. A. Howell.   1974.   The geographic pathology of bowel cancer.   Cancer 34:807-814.

Bingham, S., D. R. R. Williams, T. J. Cole, and W. P. T. James.   1979. Dietary fibre and regional large-bowel cancer mortality in Britain. Br. J. Cancer 40:456-463.

Bjelke, E.   1971.   Case-control study of cancer of the stomach, colon, and rectum.   Pp. 320-334 in R. L. Clark, R. C. Cumley, J. E. McCay, and M. M. Copeland, eds.   Oncology 1970.   Volume 5: A. Environmental Causes.   B.   Epidemiology and Demography.   C.   Cancer Education.   Yearbook Medical Publishers, Chicago.

Bjelke, E.   1973.   Epidemiologic studies of cancer of the stomach, colon, and rectum; with special emphasis on the role of diet, Volumes I-IV.   Ph.D. Thesis, University of Minnesota.   1746 pp.

Bjelke, E.   1975.   Dietary vitamin A and human lung cancer.   Int. J. Cancer 15:561-565.

Bjelke, E.   1978.   Dietary factors and the epidemiology of cancer of the stomach and large bowel.   Aktuel. Ernaehrungsmed. Klin. Prax. Suppl. 2:10-17.

Blair, A., and J. F. Fraumeni, Jr.   1978.   Geographic patterns of prostate cancer in the United States.   J. Natl. Cancer Inst. 61:1379-1384.

Blot, W. J., J. F. Fraumeni, Jr., and B. J. Stone.   1978.   Geographic correlates of pancreas cancer in the United States.   Cancer 42: 373-380.

Bradshaw, E., and M. Schonland.   1974.   Smoking, drinking and oesophageal cancer in African males of Johannesburg, South Africa.   Br. J. Cancer 30:157-163.

Breslow, N. E., and J. E. Enstrom.   1974.   Geographic correlations between cancer mortality rates and alcohol-tobacco consumption in the United States.   J. Natl. Cancer Inst. 53:631-639.

Broitman, S. A., H. Velez, and J. J. Vitale.   1981.   A possible role of iron deficiency in gastric cancer in Colombia.   Adv. Exp. Med. Biol. 135:155-181.

Burch, G. E., and A. Ansari. 1968. Chronic alcoholism and carcinoma of the pancreas: A correlative hypothesis. Arch. Intern. Med. 122:273-275.

Burrell, R. J. W. 1962. Esophageal cancer among Bantu in the Transkei. J. Natl. Cancer Inst. 28:495-514.

Carroll, K. K. 1975. Experimental evidence of dietary factors and hormone-dependent cancers. Cancer Res. 35:3374-3383.

Carroll, K. K., and G. J. Hopkins. 1979. Dietary polyunsaturated fat versus saturated fat in relation to mammary carcinogenesis. Lipids 14:155-158.

Chien, M.-C., M. J. Tong, K.-J. Lo, J.-K. Lee, D. R. Milich, G. N. Vyas, and B. L. Murphy. 1981. Hepatitis B viral markers in patients with primary hepatocellular carcinoma in Taiwan. J. Natl. Cancer Inst. 66:475-479.

Chilvers, C., P. Fraser, and V. Beral. 1979. Alcohol and oesophageal cancer: An assessment of the evidence from routinely collected data. J. Epidemiol. Community Health 33:127-133.

Choi, N. W., D. W. Entwistle, W. Michaluk, and N. Nelson. 1971. Gastric cancer in Icelanders in Manitoba. Isr. J. Med. Sci. 7:1500-1508.

Collis, C. H., P. J. Cook, J. K. Foreman, and J. F. Palframan. 1971. A search for nitrosamines in East African spirit samples from areas of varying oesophageal cancer frequency. Gut 12:1015-1018.

Cook-Mozaffari, P. 1979. The epidemiology of cancer of the oesophagus. Nutr. Cancer 1(2):51-60.

Cook-Mozaffari, P. J., F. Azordegan, W. E. Day, A. Ressicaud, C. Sabai, and B. Aramesh. 1979. Oesophageal cancer studies in the Caspian littoral of Iran: Results of a case-control study. Br. J. Cancer 39:293-309.

Coordinating Group for Research on Etiology of Esophageal Cancer in North China. 1975. The epidemiology and etiology of esophageal cancer in North China. A preliminary report. Chin. Med. J. (Peking, Engl. Ed.) 1:167-183.

Correa, P., C. Cuello, E. Duque, L. C. Burbano, F. T. Garcia, O. Bolanos, C. Brown, and W. Haenszel. 1976. Gastric cancer in Colombia. III. Natural history of precursor lesions. J. Natl. Cancer Inst. 57:1027-1035.

Cuello, C., P. Correa, W. Haenszel, G. Gordillo, C. Brown, M. Archer, and S. Tannenbaum. 1976. Gastric cancer in Colombia. I. Cancer risk and suspect environmental agents. J. Natl. Cancer Inst. 57:1015-1020.

Dales, L. G., G. D. Friedman, H. K. Ury, S. Grossman, and S. R. Williams. 1979. A case-control study of relationships of diet and other traits to colorectal cancer in American blacks. Am. J. Epidemiol. 109:132-144.

Davies, J. M. 1980. Stomach cancer mortality in Worksop and other Nottinghamshire mining towns. Br. J. Cancer 41:438-445.

Dean, G., R. MacLennan, H. McLoughlin, and E. Shelley. 1979. Causes of death of blue-collar workers at a Dublin brewery, 1954-1973. Br. J. Cancer 40:581-589.

de Jong, U. W., N. E. Day, C. S. Muir, T. H. C. Barclay, G. Bras, F. H. Foster, D. J. Jussawalla, M. Kurihara, G. Linden, I. Martinez, P. M. Payne, E. Pedersen, N. Ringertz, and T. Shanmugaratnam. 1972. The distribution of cancer within the large bowel. Int. J. Cancer 10:463-477.

de Jong, U. W., N. Breslow, J. G. E. Hong, M. Sridharan, and K. Shanmugaratnam. 1974. Aetiological factors in oesophageal cancer in Singapore Chinese. Int. J. Cancer 13:291-303.

de Waard, F. 1975. Breast cancer incidence and nutritional status with particular reference to body weight and height. Cancer Res. 35:3351-3356.

de Waard, F., and E. A. Baanders-van Halewijn. 1974. A prospective study in general practice on breast-cancer risk in postmenopausal women. Int. J. Cancer 14:153-160.

de Waard, F., J. P. Cornelis, K. Aoki, and M. Yoshida. 1977. Breast cancer incidence according to weight and height in two cities of the Netherlands and in Aichi prefecture, Japan. Cancer 40:1269-1275.

Drasar, D. B., and D. Irving. 1973. Environmental factors and cancer of the colon and breast. Br. J. Cancer 27:167-172.

Dungal, N. 1966. Stomach cancer in Iceland. Pp. 441-450 in R. W. Begg, C. P. Leblond, R. L. Noble, R. J. Rossiter, R. M. Taylor, and A. C. Wallace, eds. Proceedings of the Sixth Canadian Cancer Conference. Pergamon Press, Oxford, London, Edinburgh, New York, Toronto, Paris, and Frankfurt.

Dunn, J. E., Jr. 1977. Breast cancer among American Japanese in the San Francisco Bay area. Natl. Cancer Inst. Monogr. 47:157-160.

Elwood, J. M., P. Cole, K. J. Rothman, and S. D. Kaplan. 1977. Epidemiology of endometrial cancer. J. Natl. Cancer Inst. 59:1055-1060.

Enig, M. G., R. J. Munn, and M. Keeney. 1978. Dietary fat and cancer trends--a critique. Fed. Proc. Fed. Am. Soc. Exp. Biol. 37:2215-2220.

Enstrom, J. E. 1975. Colorectal cancer and consumption of beef and fat. Br. J. Cancer 32:432-439.

Enstrom, J. E. 1977. Colorectal cancer and beer drinking. Br. J. Cancer 35:674-683.

Enstrom, J. E. 1980. Health and dietary practices and cancer mortality among California Mormons. Pp. 69-90 in J. Cairns, J. L. Lyon, and M. Skolnick, eds. Cancer Incidence in Defined Populations. Banbury Report 4. Cold Spring Harbor Laboratory, Cold Spring Harbor, N.Y.

Feinleib, M. 1981. On a possible inverse relationship between serum cholesterol and cancer mortality. Am. J. Epidemiol. 114:5-10.

Fraumeni, J. F., Jr. 1975a. Cancers of the pancreas and biliary tract: epidemiological considerations. Cancer Res. 35:3437-3446.

Fraumeni, J. F., Jr. 1975b. Respiratory carcinogenesis: An epidemiologic appraisal. J. Natl. Cancer Inst. 55:1039-1046.

Friberg, L., M. Piscator, G. F. Nordberg, and T. Kjellström. 1974. Cadmium in the Environment, Second edition. CRC Press, Cleveland, Ohio. 248 pp.

Frisch, R. E., and J. W. McArthur. 1974. Menstrual cycles: Fatness as a determinant of minimum weight for height necessary for their maintenance or onset. Science 185:949-951.

Frisch, R. E., D. M. Hegsted, and K. Yoshinaga. 1975. Body weight and food intake at early estrus of rats on a high-fat diet. Proc. Natl. Acad. Sci. U.S.A. 72:4172-4176.

Gaskill, S. P., W. L. McGuire, C. K. Osborne, and M. P. Stern. 1979. Breast cancer mortality and diet in the United States. Cancer Res. 39:3628-3637.

Gatei, D. G., P. A. Odhiambo, D. A. O. Orinda, F. J. Muruka, and A. Wasunna. 1978. Retrospective study of carcinoma of the esophagus in Kenya. Cancer Res. 38:303-307.

Graham, S., W. Schotz, and P. Martino. 1972. Alimentary factors in the epidemiology of gastric cancer. Cancer 30:927-938.

Graham, S., H. Dayal, M. Swanson, A. Mittelman, and G. Wilkinson. 1978. Diet in the epidemiology of cancer of the colon and rectum. J. Natl. Cancer Inst. 61:709-714.

Gray, G. E., M. C. Pike, and B. E. Henderson. 1979. Breast-cancer incidence and mortality rates in different countries in relation to known risk factors and dietary practices. Br. J. Cancer 39:1-7.

Haenszel, W. 1961. Cancer mortality among the foreign-born in the United States. J. Natl. Cancer Inst. 26:37-132.

Haenszel, W., and E. A. Dawson. 1965. A note on mortality from cancer of the colon and rectum in the United States. Cancer 18:265-272.

Haenszel, W., M. Kurihara, M. Segi, and R. K. C. Lee. 1972. Stomach cancer among Japanese in Hawaii. J. Natl. Cancer Inst. 49:969-988.

Haenszel, W., J. W. Berg, M. Segi, M. Kurihara, and F. B. Locke. 1973. Large-bowel cancer in Hawaiian Japanese. J. Natl. Cancer Inst. 51:1765-1779.

Haenszel, W., P. Correa, and C. Cuello. 1975. Social class differences among patients with large-bowel cancer in Cali, Colombia. J. Natl. Cancer Inst. 54:1031-1035.

Haenszel, W., M. Kurihara, F. B. Locke, K. Shimuzu, and M. Segi. 1976. Stomach cancer in Japan. J. Natl. Cancer Inst. 56:265-274.

Haenszel, W., F. B. Locke, and M. Segi. 1980. A case-control study of large bowel cancer in Japan. J. Natl. Cancer Inst. 64:17-22.

Hakama, M., and E. A. Saxén. 1967. Cereal consumption and gastric cancer. Int. J. Cancer 2:265-268.

Hakulinen, T., L. Lehtimäki, M. Lehtonen, and L. Teppo. 1974. Cancer morbidity among two male cohorts with increased alcohol consumption in Finland. J. Natl. Cancer Inst. 52:1711-1714.

Hems, G. 1978. The contributions of diet and childbearing to breast-cancer rates. Br. J. Cancer 37:974-982.

Hicks, R. M., C. L. Walter, I. Elsebai, A.-B. El Aasser, M. El Merzabani, and T. A. Gough. 1977. Demonstration of nitrosamines in human urine: Preliminary observations on a possible etiology for bladder cancer in association with chronic urinary tract infections. Proc. R. Soc. Med. 70:413-417.

Higginson, J. 1966. Etiological factors in gastrointestinal cancer in man. J. Natl. Cancer Inst. 37:527-545.

Higginson, J., and A. G. Oettlé. 1960. Cancer incidence in the Bantu and "Cape Colored" races of South Africa: Report of a cancer survey in the Transvaal (1953-55). J. Natl. Cancer Inst. 24:589-671.

Hildreth, N. G., J. L. Kelsey, V. A. LiVolsi, D. B. Fischer, T. R. Holford, E. D. Mostow, P. E. Schwartz, and C. White. 1981. An epidemiologic study of epithelial carcinoma of the ovary. Am. J. Epidemiol. 114:398-405.

Hill, M. J., G. M. Hawksworth, and G. Tattersall. 1973. Bacteria, nitrosamines and cancer of the stomach. Br. J. Cancer 28:562-567.

Hinds, M. W., L. N. Kolonel, J. Lee, and T. Hirohata. 1980. Associations between cancer incidence and alcohol/cigarette consumption among five ethnic groups in Hawaii. Br. J. Cancer 41:929-940.

Hirayama, T. 1967. The epidemiology of cancer of the stomach in Japan with special reference to the role of diet. Pp. 37-48 in R. J. C. Harris, ed. Proceedings of the 9th International Cancer Congress. UICC Monograph Series Volume 10. Springer-Verlag, Berlin, Heidelberg, and New York.

Hirayama, T. 1977. Changing patterns of cancer in Japan with special reference to the decrease in stomach cancer mortality. Pp. 55-75 in H. H. Hiatt, J. D. Watson, and J. A. Winsten, eds. Origins of Human Cancer. Book A, Incidence of Cancer in Humans. Cold Spring Harbor Laboratory, Cold Spring Harbor, N.Y.

Hirayama, T. 1979. Epidemiology of prostate cancer with special reference to the role of diet. Natl. Cancer Inst. Monogr. 53:149-154.

Hirono, I., H. Kachi, and T. Kato. 1970. A survey of acute toxicity of cycads and mortality rate from cancer in the Miyako Islands, Okinawa. Acta Pathol. Jpn. 20:327-337.

Hoover, R. N., and P. H. Strasser. 1980. Editorial: Saccharin: A bitter after-taste? N. Engl. J. Med. 302:573-575.

Hormozdiari, H., N. E. Day, B. Aramesh, and E. Mahboubi. 1975. Dietary factors and esophageal cancer in the Caspian littoral of Iran. Cancer Res. 35:3493-3498.

Howe, G. R., J. D. Burch, A. B. Miller, B. Morrison, P. Gordon, L. Weldon, L. W. Chambers, G. Fodor, and G. M. Winsor. 1977. Artificial sweeteners and human bladder cancer. Lancet 2:578-581.

Howe, G. R., J. D. Burch, A. B. Miller, G. M. Cook, J. Esteve, B. Morrison, P. Gordon, L. W. Chambers, G. Fodor, and G. M. Winsor. 1980. Tobacco use, occupation, coffee, various nutrients, and bladder cancer. J. Natl. Cancer Inst. 64:701-713.

Howell, M. A. 1974. Factor analysis of international cancer mortality data and per capita food consumption. Br. J. Cancer 29:328-336.

Howell, M. A. 1975. Diet as an etiological factor in the development of cancers of the colon and rectum. J. Chronic Dis. 28:67-80.

Imai, T., T. Kubo, and H. Watanabe. 1971. Chronic gastritis in Japanese with reference to high incidence of gastric carcinoma. J. Natl. Cancer Inst. 47:179-195.

Irving, D., and B. S. Drasar. 1973. Fibre and cancer of the colon. Br. J. Cancer 28:462-463.

Ishii, K., K. Nakamura, H. Ozaki, N. Yamada, and T. Takeuchi. 1968. [In Japanese.] [Epidemiological problems of pancreas cancer.] Jpn. J. Clin. Med. 26:1839-1842.

Jain, M., G. M. Cook, F. G. Davis, M. G. Grace, G. R. Howe, and A. B. Miller. 1980. A case-control study of diet and colo-rectal cancer. Int. J. Cancer 26:757-768.

Jansson, B., M. M. Jacobs, and A. C. Griffin. 1978. Gastrointestinal cancer: Epidemiology and experimental studies. Adv. Exp. Med. Biol. 91:305-322.

Jensen, O. M. 1979. Cancer morbidity and causes of death among Danish brewery workers. Int. J. Cancer 23:454-463.

Jick, H., A. M. Walter, and K. J. Rothman. 1980. The epidemic of endometrial cancer: A commentary. Am. J. Public Health 70:264-267.

Joint Iran-International Agency for Research on Cancer Study Group. 1977. Esophageal cancer studies in the Caspian littoral of Iran: Results of population studies--a prodrome. J. Natl. Cancer Inst. 59:1127-1138.

Joossens, J. V., and J. Geboers. 1981. Nutrition and gastric cancer. Proc. Nutr. Soc. 40:37-46.

Kato, H., J. Tillotson, M. Z. Nichaman, G. C. Rhoads, and H. B. Hamilton. 1973. Epidemiologic studies of coronary heart disease and stroke in Japanese men living in Japan, Hawaii and California: Serum lipids and diet. Am. J. Epidemiol. 97:372-385.

Keen, P., and P. Martin. 1971. Is aflatoxin carcinogenic in man? The evidence in Swaziland. Trop. Geogr. Med. 23:44-53.

Keller, A. Z. 1980. The epidemiology of esophageal cancer in the west. Prev. Med. 9:607-612.

Kessler, I. I. 1970. Cancer mortality among diabetics. J. Natl. Cancer Inst. 44:673-686.

Kipling, M. D., and J. A. H. Waterhouse. 1967. Letter to the Editor: Cadmium and prostatic carcinoma. Lancet 1:730-731.

Knox, E. G. 1977. Foods and diseases. Br. J. Prev. Soc. Med. 31:71-80.

Kolonel, L. N. 1976. Association of cadmium with renal cancer. Cancer 37:1782-1787.

Kolonel, L. N. 1980. Cancer patterns of four ethnic groups in Hawaii. J. Natl. Cancer Inst. 65:1127-1139.

Kolonel, L. N., and W. Winkelstein, Jr. 1977. Letter to the Editor: Cadmium and prostatic carcinoma. Lancet 2:566-567.

Kolonel, L. N., M. W. Hinds, and J. H. Hankin. 1980. Cancer patterns among migrant and native-born Japanese in Hawaii in relation to smoking, drinking, and dietary habits. Pp. 327-340 in H. V. Gelboin, M. MacMahon, T. Matsushima, T. Sugimura, S. Takayama, and H. Takebe, eds. Genetic and Environmental Factors in Experimental and Human Cancer. Japan Scientific Societies Press, Tokyo.

Kolonel, L. N., J. H. Hankin, J. Lee, S. Y. Chu, A. M. Y. Nomura, and M. W. Hinds. 1981. Nutrient intakes in relation to cancer incidence in Hawaii. Br. J. Cancer 44:332-339.

Kriebel, D., and D. Jowett. 1979. Stomach cancer mortality in the north central states: High risk is not limited to the foreign-born. Nutr. Cancer 1(2):8-12.

Lea, A. J. 1967. Neoplasms and environmental factors. Ann. R. Coll. Surg. Engl. 41:432-438.

Lee, F. I. 1966. Cirrhosis and hepatoma in alcoholics. Gut 7:77-85.

Lee, J. A. H. 1976. Recent trends of large bowel cancer in Japan compared to United States and England and Wales. Int. J. Epidemiol. 5:187-194.

Lemen, R. A., J. S. Lee, J. K. Wagoner, and H. P. Blejer. 1976. Cancer mortality among cadmium production workers. Ann. N. Y. Acad. Sci. 271:273-279.

Lilienfeld, A. M. 1981. The Humean fog: Cancer and cholesterol. Am. J. Epidemiol. 114:1-4.

Lin, R. S., and I. I. Kessler. 1981. A multifactorial model for pancreatic cancer in man: Epidemiologic evidence. J. Am. Med. Assoc. 245: 147-152.

Lingeman, C. H. 1974. Etiology of cancer of the human ovary: A review. J. Natl. Cancer Inst. 53:1603-1618.

Linsell, C. A., and F. G. Peers. 1977. Aflatoxin and liver cell cancer. Trans. R. Soc. Trop. Med. Hyg. 71:471-473.

Lipworth, L. L., and C. A. Rice. 1979. Correlations in mortality data involving cancers of the colorectum esophagus. Cancer 43:1927-1933.

Lubin, J. H., W. J. Blot, and P. E. Burns. 1981. Breast cancer following high dietary fat and protein consumption. Am. J. Epidemiol. 114:422. Abstract.

Lui, K., D. Moss, V. Persky, J. Stamler, D. Garside, and I. Soltero. 1979. Dietary cholesterol, fat, and fibre, and colon-cancer mortality. An analysis of international data. Lancet 2:782-785.

Lynch, H. T., H. Guirgis, J. Lynch, F. D. Brodkey, and H. Magee. 1975. Cancer of the colon: Socioeconomic variables in a community. Am. J. Epidemiol. 102:119-127.

Lyon, J. L., and A. W. Sorenson. 1978. Colon cancer in a low-risk population. Am. J. Clin. Nutr. 31:S227-S230.

Lyon, J. L., M. R. Klauber, J. W. Gardner, and C. R. Smart. 1976. Cancer incidence in Mormons and non-Mormons in Utah, 1966-1970. N. Engl. J. Med. 294:129-133.

Lyon, J. L., J. W. Gardner, and D. W. West. 1980a. Cancer risk and lifestyle: Cancer among Mormons (1967-1975). Pp. 273-290 in H. V. Gelboin, B. MacMahon, T. Matsushima, T. Sugimura, S. Takayama, and H. Takebe, eds. Genetic and Environmental Factors in Experimental and Human Cancer. Japan Scientific Societies Press, Tokyo.

Lyon, J. L., J. W. Gardner, and D. W. West. 1980b. Cancer risk and life-style: Cancer among Mormons from 1967-1975. Pp. 3-28 in J. Cairns, J. L. Lyon, and M. Skolnick, eds. Cancer Incidence in Defined

Populations. Banbury Report 4. Cold Spring Harbor Laboratory, Cold Spring Harbor, N.Y.

MacLennan, R., J. Da Costa, N. E. Day, C. H. Law, Y. K. Ng, and K. Shanmugaratnam. 1977. Risk factors for lung cancer in Singapore Chinese, a population with high female incidence rates. Int. J. Cancer 20:854-860.

MacLennan, R., O. M. Jensen, J. Mosbech, and H. Vuori. 1978. Diet, transit time, stool weight, and colon cancer in two Scandinavian populations. Am. J. Clin. Nutr. 31:S239-S242.

MacMahon, B., P. Cole, and J. Brown. 1973. Etiology of human breast cancer: A review. J. Natl. Cancer Inst. 50:21-42.

MacMahon, B., S. Yen, D. Trichopoulos, K. Warren, and G. Nardi. 1981. Coffee and cancer of the pancreas. N. Engl. J. Med. 304:630-633.

Malhotra, S. L. 1977. Dietary factors in a study of cancer colon from cancer registry, with special reference to the role of saliva, milk and fermented milk products and vegetable fibre. Med. Hypotheses 3:122-126.

Marasas, W. F. O., S. J. van Rensburg, and C. J. Mirocha. 1979. Incidence of Fusarium species and the mycotoxins, deoxynivalenol and zearalenone, in corn produced in esophageal cancer areas in Transkei. J. Agric. Food Chem. 27:1108-1112.

Martínez, I. 1969. Factors associated with cancer of the esophagus, mouth and pharynx in Puerto Rico. J. Natl. Cancer Inst. 42:1069-1094.

Martínez, I., R. Torres, Z. Frías, J. R. Colón, and M. Fernández. 1979. Factors associated with adenocarcinomas of the large bowel in Puerto Rico. Pp. 45-52 in J. M. Birch, ed. Advances in Medical Oncology, Research and Education. Volume 3: Epidemiology. Pergamon Press, Oxford, New York, Toronto, Sydney, Paris, and Frankfurt.

Mason, T. J., F. W. McKay, R. Hoover, W. J. Blot, and J. F. Fraumeni, Jr. 1975. Atlas of Cancer Mortality for U.S. Counties: 1950-1969. DHEW Publication No. (NIH) 75-780. U.S. Department of Health, Education, and Welfare, Washington, D.C. 102 pp.

McMichael, A. J., J. D. Potter, and B. S. Hetzel. 1979. Time trends in colo-rectal cancer mortality in relation to food and alcohol consumption: United States, United Kingdom, Australia and New Zealand. Int. J. Epidemiol. 8:295-303.

Meinsma, L. 1964. [In Dutch; English Summary.] Nutrition and Cancer. Voeding 25:357-365.

Mettlin, C., and S. Graham. 1979. Dietary risk factors in human bladder cancer. Am. J. Epidemiol. 110:255-263.

Mettlin, C., S. Graham, and M. Swanson. 1979. Vitamin A and lung cancer. J. Natl. Cancer Inst. 62:1435-1438.

Mettlin, C., S. Graham, R. Priore, J. Marshall, and M. Swanson. 1980. Diet and cancer of the esophagus. Nutr. Cancer 2:143-147.

Miller, A. B. 1978. An overview of hormone-associated cancers. Cancer Res. 38:3985-3990.

Miller, A. B. 1980. Epidemiology and etiology of lung cancer. Pp. 9-26 in H. H. Hansen and M. Rørth, eds. Lung Cancer, 1980. Excerpta Medica, Amsterdam, Oxford, and Princeton.

Miller, A. B. 1981. Epidemiology of gastrointestinal cancer. Compr. Therapy 7(8):53-58.

Miller, A. B., and R. D. Bulbrook. 1980. The epidemiology and etiology of breast cancer. N. Engl. J. Med. 303:1246-1248.

Miller, A. B., A. Kelly, N. W. Choi, V. Matthews, R. W. Morgan, L. Munan, J. D. Burch, J. Feather, G. R. Howe, and M. Jain. 1978. A study of diet and breast cancer. Am. J. Epidemiol. 107:499-509.

Miller, C. T., C. I. Neutel, R. C. Nair, L. D. Marrett, J. M. Last, and W. E. Collins. 1978. Relative importance of risk factors in bladder carcinogenesis. J. Chronic Dis. 31:51-56.

Modan, B., F. Lubin, V. Barrell, R. A. Greenberg, M. Modan, and S. Graham. 1974. The role of starches in the etiology of gastric cancer. Cancer 34:2087-2092.

Modan, B., V. Barrell, F. Lubin, M. Modan, R. A. Greenberg, and S. Graham. 1975. Low-fiber intake as an etiologic factor in cancer of the colon. J. Natl. Cancer Inst. 55:15-18.

Monson, R. R., and J. L. Lyon. 1975. Proportional mortality among alcoholics. Cancer 36:1077-1079.

Moolgavkar, S. H., N. E. Day, and R. G. Stevens. 1980. Two-stage model for carcinogenesis: Epidemiology of breast cancer in females. J. Natl. Cancer Inst. 65:559-569.

Nomura, A., B. E. Henderson, and J. Lee. 1978. Breast cancer and diet among the Japanese in Hawaii. Am. J. Clin. Nutr. 31:2020-2025.

Oettle, A. G. 1965. The aetiology of primary carcinoma of the liver in in Africa: A critical appraisal of previous ideas with an outline of the mycotoxin hypothesis. S. Afr. Med. J. 39:817-825.

Okamura, T., and F. Matsuhisa. 1965. [In Japanese; English Summary.] Fluorine and other related components of Japanese foods. V. Fluorine and salt contents of miso and other foods rich in salt, and their geographical correlation with mortality from gastric cancer. Eiyo To Shokuryo 18(4):253-257.

Peers, F. G., and C. A. Linsell. 1973. Dietary aflatoxins and liver cancer--a population based study in Kenya. Br. J. Cancer 27:473-484.

Peers, F. G., G. A. Gilman, and C. A. Linsell. 1976. Dietary aflatoxins and human liver cancer. A study in Swaziland. Int. J. Cancer 17:167-176.

Pernu, J. 1960. An epidemiological study on cancer of the digestive organs and respiratory system. A study based on 7078 cases. Ann. Med. Intern. Fenn. Suppl. 33:1-137.

Phillips, R. L. 1975. Role of life-style and dietary habits in risk of cancer among Seventh-Day Adventists. Cancer Res. 35:3513-3522.

Phillips, R. L., J. W. Kuzma, and T. M. Lotz. 1980a. Cancer mortality among comparable members versus nonmembers of the Seventh-Day Adventist Church. Pp. 93-102 in J. Cairns, J. L. Lyon and M. Skolnick, eds. Cancer Incidence in Defined Populations. Banbury Report 4. Cold Spring Harbor Laboratory, Cold Spring Harbor, N.Y.

Phillips, R. L., J. W. Kuzma, W. L. Beeson, and T. Lotz. 1980b. Influence of selection versus lifestyle on risk of fatal cancer and cardiovascular disease among Seventh-Day Adventists. Am. J. Epidemiol. 112:296-314.

Pottern, L. M., L. E. Morris, W. J. Blot, R. G. Ziegler, and J. F. Fraumeni, Jr. 1981. Esophageal cancer among black men in Washington, D.C. I. Alcohol, tobacco, and other risk factors. J. Natl. Cancer Inst. 67:777-783.

Potts, C. L. 1965. Cadium proteinuria--The health of battery workers workers exposed to cadmium oxide dust. Ann. Occup. Hyg. 8:55-59.

Purtilo, D. T., and L. S. Gottlieb. 1973. Cirrhosis and hepatoma occurring at Boston City Hospital (1917-1968). Cancer 32:458-462.

Radomski, J. L., D. Greenwald, W. L. Hearn, N. L. Block, and F. M. Woods. 1978. Nitrosamine formation in bladder infections and its role in the etiology of bladder cancer. J. Urol. 120:48-50.

Reddy, B. S., A. R. Hedges, K. Laakso, and E. L. Wynder. 1978. Metabolic epidemiology of large bowel cancer. Fecal bulk and constituents of high-risk North American and low-risk Finnish population. Cancer 42:2832-2838.

Reddy, B. S., C. Sharma, L. Darby, K. Laakso, and E. L. Wynder. 1980. Metabolic epidemiology of large bowel cancer. Fecal mutagens in high- and low-risk population for colon cancer. A preliminary report. Mutat. Res. 72:511-522.

Reimer, R. R., R. Hoover, J. F. Fraumeni, Jr., and R. C. Young. 1978. Second primary neoplasms following ovarian cancer. J. Natl. Cancer Inst. 61:1195-1197.

Rose, G., H. Blackburn, A. Keys, H. L. Taylor, W. B. Kannel, O. Paul, D. D. Reid, and J. Stamler. 1974. Colon cancer and blood-cholesterol. Lancet 1:181-183.

Rothman, K., and A. Keller. 1972. The effect of joint exposure to alcohol and tobacco on risk of cancer of the mouth and pharynx. J. Chronic Dis. 25:711-716.

Rotkin, I. D. 1977. Studies in the epidemiology of prostatic cancer: Expanded sampling. Cancer Treat. Rep. 61:173-180.

Ruddell, W. S. J., E. S. Bone, M. J. Hill, and C. L. Walters. 1978. Pathogenesis of gastric cancer in pernicious anaemia. Lancet 1:521-523.

Sakula, A. 1976. Letter to the Editor: Vitamin A and lung cancer. Br. Med. J. 2:298.

Schmidt, W., and R. E. Popham. 1981. The role of drinking and smoking in mortality from cancer and other causes in male alcoholics. Cancer 47:1031-1041.

Schoenberg, B. S., J. C. Bailar III, and J. F. Fraumeni, Jr. 1971. Certain mortality patterns of esophageal cancer in the United States, 1930-67. J. Natl. Cancer Inst. 46:63-73.

Schrauzer, G. N., D. A. White, and C. J. Schneider. 1977a. Cancer mortality correlation studies.--III. Statistical associations with dietary selenium intakes. Bioinorg. Chem. 7:23-34.

Schrauzer, G. N., D. A. White, and C. J. Schneider. 1977b. Cancer mortality correlation studies.--IV. Associations with dietary intakes and blood levels of certain trace elements, notably Se-antagonists. Bioinorg. Chem. 7:35-56.

Schuman, L. M., J. S. Mandel, A. Radke, U. Seal, and F. Halberg. 1982. Some selected features of the epidemiology of prostatic cancer: Minneapolis-St. Paul, Minnesota case control study, 1976-1979. Pp. 345-354 in K. Magnus, ed. Trends in Cancer Incidence: Causes and Practical Implications. Hemisphere Publishing Corp., Washington, New York, and London.

Segi, M. 1975. Tea-gruel as a possible factor for cancer of the esophagus. Gann 66:199-202.

Shank, R. C., J. E. Gordon, G. N. Wogan, A. Nondasuta, and B. Subhamani. 1972a. Dietary aflatoxins and human liver cancer. III. Field survey of rural Thai families for ingested aflatoxins. Food Cosmet. Toxicol. 10:71-84.

Shank, R. C., N. Bhamarapravati, J. E. Gordon, and G. N. Wogan. 1972b. Dietary aflatoxins and human liver cancer. IV. Incidence of primary liver cancer in two municipal populations of Thailand. Food Cosmet. Toxicol. 10:171-179.

Shekelle, R. B., M. Lepper, S. Liu, C. Maliza, W. J. Raynor, Jr., A. H. Rossof, O. Paul, A. M. Shryock, and J. Stamler. 1981. Dietary vitamin A and risk of cancer in the Western Electric study. Lancet 2:1185-1190.

Shennan, D. H. 1973. Letter to the Editor: Renal carcinoma and coffee consumption in 16 countries. Br. J. Cancer 28:473-474.

Simon, D., S. Yen, and P. Cole. 1975. Coffee drinking and cancer of the lower urinary tract. J. Natl. Cancer Inst. 54:587-591.

Smith, P. G., and H. Jick. 1978. Cancers among users of preparations containing vitamin A. Cancer 42:808-811.

Stemmermann, G. N., M. Mandel, and H. F. Mower. 1979. Colon cancer: Its precursors and companions in Hawaii Japanese. Natl. Cancer Inst. Monogr. 53:175-179.

Stocks, P. 1957. Cancer incidence in North Wales and Liverpool region in relation to habits and environment. British Empire Cancer Campaign, Thirty Fifth Annual Report, Supplement to Part II. Cancer Research Campaign, London. 156 pp.

Stocks, P. 1970. Cancer mortality in relation to national consumption of cigarettes, solid fuel, tea and coffee. Br. J. Cancer 24:215-225.

Stukonis, M. K. 1978. Cancer Incidence Cumulative Rates--International Comparison Based on Data from "Cancer Incidence in Five Continents". IARC Technical Report No. 78/002. International Agency for Research on Cancer, Lyon, France. 54 pp.

Surgeon General. 1979. Smoking and Health. A Report of the Surgeon General. ·U.S. Department of Health, Education, and Welfare, Washington, D.C. 1222 pp.

Surgeon General. 1980. The Health Consequences of Smoking for Women. A Report of the Surgeon General. U.S. Department of Health, Education and Welfare, Washington, D.C. 359 pp.

Tannenbaum, S. R., D. Moran, W. Rand, C. Cuello, and P. Correa. 1979. Gastric cancer in Colombia. IV. Nitrite and other ions in gastric contents of residents from a high-risk region. J. Natl. Cancer Inst. 62:9-12.

Teppo, L., E. Pukkala, M. Hakama, T. Hakulinen, A. Herva, and E. Saxén. 1980. Way of life and cancer incidence in Finland. A municipality-based ecological analysis. Scand. J. Soc. Med. Suppl. 19:1-84.

Tung, T. C., and K. H. Ling. 1968. Study on aflatoxin of foodstuffs in Taiwan. J. Vitaminol. 14 (Suppl.):48-52.

Tuyns, A. J., G. Péquinot, and O. M. Jensen. 1977. [In French; English Summary.] Oesophageal cancer in Ille-et-Vilaine in relation to levels of alcohol and tobacco consumption: Multiplicative risks. Bull. Cancer 64:45-60.

Tuyns, A. J., G. Péquignot, and J. S. Abbatucci. 1979. Oesophageal cancer and alcohol consumption: Importance of type of beverage. Int. J. Cancer 23:443-447.

van Rensburg, S. J. 1981. Epidemiologic and dietary evidence for a specific nutritional predisposition to esophageal cancer. J. Natl. Cancer Inst. 67:243-251.

van Rensburg, S. J., J. J. van der Watt, I. F. H. Purchase, L. P. Coutinho, and R. Markham. 1974. Primary liver cancer rate and aflatoxin intake in a high cancer area. S. Afr. Med. J. 48:2508a-2508d.

Vitale, J. J., and L. S. Gottlieb. 1975. Alcohol and alcohol-related deficiencies as carcinogens. Cancer Res. 35:3336-3338.

Vitale, J. J., S. A. Broitman, and L. S. Gottlieb. 1981. Alcohol and carcinogenesis. Pp. 291-301 in G. R. Newell and N. M. Ellison, eds. Nutrition and Cancer: Etiology and Treatment. Raven Press, New York.

Warwick, G. P., and J. S. Harington. 1973. Some aspects of the epidemiology and etiology of esophageal cancer with particular emphasis on the Transkei, South Africa. Adv. Cancer Res. 17:81-229.

Waterhouse, J., C. Muir, P. Correa, and J. Powell, eds. 1976. Cancer Incidence in Five Continents, Volume III. IARC Scientific Publications No. 15. International Agency for Research on Cancer, Lyon, France. 584 pp.

Weisburger, J. H., and R. Raineri. 1975. Dietary factors and the etiology of gastric cancer. Cancer Res. 35:3469-3474.

Weisburger, J. H., B. S. Reddy, E. S. Fiala, Y. Y. Wang, L. L. Vuolo, E. L. Wynder, and N. E. Spingarn. 1981. Dietary factors in the causation and prevention of neoplasia. Pp. 595-612 in J. Burchenal and H. Oettgen, eds. Cancer: Achievements, Challenges, and Prospects for the 1980s, Volume 1. Grune and Stratton, New York, London, Toronto, Sydney, and San Francisco.

Williams, R. R., and J. W. Horm. 1977. Association of cancer sites with tobacco and alcohol consumption and socioeconomic status of patients: Interview study from the Third National Cancer Survey. J. Natl. Cancer Inst. 58:525-547.

Wogan, G. N. 1975. Dietary factors and special epidemiological situations of liver cancer in Thailand and Africa. Cancer Res. 35:3499-3502.

Wynder, E. L. 1975. The epidemiology of large bowel cancer. Cancer Res. 35:3388-3394.

Wynder, E. L., and I. J. Bross. 1961. A study of etiological factors in cancer of the esophagus. Cancer 14:389-413.

Wynder, E. L., and R. Goldsmith. 1977. The epidemiology of bladder cancer. A second look. Cancer 40:1246-1268.

Wynder, E. L., and T. Shigematsu. 1967. Environmental factors of cancer of the colon and rectum. Cancer 20:1520-1561.

Wynder, E. L., and S. D. Stellman. 1977. Comparative epidemiology of tobacco-related cancers. Cancer Res. 37:4608-4622.

Wynder, E. L., J. Kmet, N. Dungal, and M. Segi. 1963. An epidemiological investigation of gastric cancer. Cancer 16:1461-1496.

Wynder, E. L., G. C. Escher, and N. Mantel. 1966. An epidemiological investigation of cancer of the endometrium. Cancer 19:489-520.

Wynder, E. L., K. Mabuchi, and W. F. Whitmore, Jr. 1971. Epidemiology of cancer of the prostate. Cancer 28:344-360.

Wynder, E. L., K. Mabuchi, N. Maruchi, and J. G. Fortner. 1973. Epidemiology of cancer of the pancreas. J. Natl. Cancer Inst. 50:645-667.

Wynder, E. L., K. Mabuchi, and W. F. Whitmore, Jr. 1974. Epidemiology of adenocarcinoma of the kidney. J. Natl. Cancer Inst. 53:1619-1634.

Yang, C. S. 1980. Research on esophageal cancer in China: A review. Cancer Res. 40:2633-2644.

Zaldívar, R. 1977. Nitrate fertilizers as environmental pollutants: Positive correlations between nitrates ($NaNO_3$ and KNO_3) used per unit area and stomach cancer mortality rates. Experientia 33:264-265.

Ziegler, R. G., L. E. Morris, W. J. Blot, L. M. Pottern, R. Hoover, and J. F. Fraumeni, Jr. 1981. Esophageal cancer among black men in Washington, D.C. II. Role of nutrition. J. Natl. Cancer Inst. 67:1199-1206.

18 Assessment of Risk to Human Health

The literature on risk assessment has expanded rapidly in recent years. Some of the most comprehensive reports have been prepared by committees of the National Academy of Sciences (1977, 1980a,b). This chapter is only intended to supplement that literature with primary reference to risk analysis of the effects of diet, particularly nutrients, on the process of carcinogenesis. In this context, risk is defined as the probability that an individual will develop cancer within a given time. Such risk can be estimated by examining retrospective data.

To determine dietary and nutritional effects on cancer, it is useful to relate risk analysis to the basic concepts of carcinogenesis. That is, chemically induced carcinogenesis may include (a) an initiation phase, when chemicals or other agents possessing genotoxic activity interact with the genome of somatic cells, and (b) a modification phase, when a variety of events modify that process either simultaneously with, or subsequent to, the initiation phase.

Initiators of carcinogenesis are generally mutagenic in one or more systems (McCann et al., 1975; Purchase et al., 1978; Sugimura et al., 1976) and form covalent adducts with DNA and other cellular macromolecules, usually after enzymatic metabolism (Boyland and Levi, 1935) to chemically reactive metabolites (Magee et al., 1975; Miller, 1970). If such adducts or other interactions between DNA sites are not removed or repaired, and if the cell, through replication, transmits this molecular aberration to future cell generations, then the initiating event is considered to be irreversible.

In contrast to compounds that act as initiators, many other compounds may modify either the initiating events per se, or the subsequent multi-staged events responsible for the progression of the initiated cell to the fully developed neoplastic cell (Slaga, 1980). A wide variety of chemicals can modify later stages of carcinogenesis. Many of them act exclusively as modifiers; others are also initiators (complete carcinogens).

The process of carcinogenesis may be modified through a great many diverse mechanisms, which can involve the intervention of several physiological/biochemical systems, including changes in the function of the enzymes, hormones, immune response, membrane transport and communication activities, etc. Some modifiers have positive effects (i.e., they are promoters or cocarcinogens), whereas others have negative effects (i.e., they are inhibitors of initiation, antipromoters, or anticocarcinogens) on the progression of the initiated cell to the tumorigenic state. In contrast to initiation, the progress of positive modification (promotion) appears to be more reversible (Doll and Hill, 1964; Roe and Clack, 1963).

This distinction between initiation and modification is necessary for an understanding of the literature on risk analysis. Most such literature assumes that carcinogenic substances act as initiators. Models developed for initiation, e.g., those for threshold response, additivity vs. nonadditivity of toxic response, dose-response kinetics, and extent of exposure ("hitness"), do not necessarily apply to assessment of risk due to tumor modifiers. For example, one of the most straightforward differences is the direct correlation between dose and tumor response for initiators versus the inverse correlation between the tumor response and the dose of certain modifiers such as several nutrients and certain antioxidants.

Food may contain both initiators and modifiers of carcinogenesis (see Chapters 12 and 14). The great diversity of initiators to which humans are exposed is suggested by the wide variety of mutagens with a broad range of potencies present in the food we eat and the excreta produced (Bruce et al., 1977; Sugimura, 1979). There will always be an ample supply of modifiers in food, including a variety of nonnutritive substances and most, if not all, nutrients (when consumed in amounts that either exceed or are less than those required for optimum nutrition). These modifiers may affect carcinogenesis by influencing hormone status (Alberti, 1980), immune response (Axelrod, 1980; Gross and Newberne, 1980), and the activity of carcinogen-metabolizing enzymes (Campbell, 1979; Conney, 1967).

INITIATORS OF CARCINOGENESIS

In general, two procedures may be used to estimate acceptable levels of risk for toxic compounds. One method estimates the acceptable daily intake (ADI); the second is the "risk estimate" approach (National Academy of Sciences, 1980a).

The ADI is an arbitrary estimate that "is not an estimate of risk nor a guarantee of absolute safety" (National Academy of Sciences, 1980a). It has been widely used for noncarcinogenic toxic chemicals and is based on empirical data pertaining to acute toxicity. This procedure was modified by the Safe Drinking Water Committee to estimate acceptable daily intake for contaminants in drinking water because of the paucity of data for these compounds (National Academy of Sciences, 1977). To establish an ADI, the highest experimental dose that produces no observable effects is decreased by an "uncertainty factor" or "safety factor" (ranging from

10 to 5,000) in order to minimize the probability of harm to the more sensitive members of the general population. A commonly used safety factor for chronic toxicity tests is 100, which assumes a factor of 10 to allow for variability of individual responses within the test species and a second factor of 10 for the assumed differences in response between the test species and humans (Lehman and Fitzhugh, 1954). Although the 100-fold safety factor has been widely used to evaluate food additives and other chemicals (World Health Organization, 1958, 1972), there are no empirical data to support this specific factor. In general, the greater the uncertainty in the experimental data, the larger the safety factor (National Academy of Sciences, 1977). The ADI method is unacceptable for estimating risk for initiators because there is a great variation among species in susceptibility to carcinogens, and because of the serious consequences for regulatory action if the estimates are misleading (National Academy of Sciences, 1980a).

The more appropriate approach for estimating risk for initiators of carcinogenesis is to estimate the response of humans to low doses based on data derived from exposure of laboratory animals to high doses. This approach is comprised of two quantitative estimations: first, interpolation from responses obtained at high doses to estimate the response at low doses within the test species and, second, extrapolation of the data from the test species to estimate the response in humans.

Several mathematical models have been proposed to interpolate from high to low doses within the test species (Scientific Committee of the Food Safety Council, 1978; National Academy of Sciences, 1980a). The greatest uncertainty in these models is whether or not the kinetic characteristics of the responses at high doses are similar to those at low doses. This is a particularly important consideration when determining whether there is a threshold. For example, is the risk directly proportional to dosage level or is there a threshold dose below which the response is negligible? Even though mechanistic arguments may be developed in favor of a threshold effect (Gehring and Blau, 1977; see dose-response curves in the report of Scientific Committee of the Food Safety Council, 1978), most mathematical models that have been used in the regulatory process assume the nonexistence of a threshold for the general population (National Academy of Sciences, 1980a). At the very least, were thresholds to exist for individuals, there would undoubtedly be a distribution of threshold values for which population parameters would need to be estimated. That is considered impractical.

Assuming thresholds to be either nonexistent or unmeasurable, the simplest mathematical model for high dose to low dose interpolation is the linear dose-response model, wherein the response is directly proportional to the dose at low levels of exposure. Mathematical models using dose-response curves other than linear include the log-linear, log-normal, and log-logistic models. Models based on "target theory," which are used for radiation-induced carcinogenesis, assume that the site of action has a finite number of target sites that require some finite number of "hits" to elicit a response (see review by Turner, 1975). A more recent extension of this model was proposed by Cornfield (1977). According to the Scientific Committee of the Food Safety Council (1978), this model, in which multiple hits are assumed and which has the strongest biological foundation, provides a better description of dose-response data than the single-hit model. This "gamma hit model" was found to fit dose-response data for various types of toxic responses better than did some of the simpler models (Scientific Committee of the Food Safety Council, 1978).

There is little support for and use of other models that mathematically describe a tolerance distribution, because they do not take into consideration the multistep nature of chemical carcinogenesis (Finney, 1952). Some models (Druckrey, 1967; Peto et al., 1972; Pike, 1966) include additional parameters such as the time from initiation of exposure to the development of tumor or, where there is no response, the total period of observation. This period of observation would include the time during which chemical modifiers would be expected to exert their effects.

As mentioned earlier, the greatest difficulty with all of these models is the interpolation of the response to low doses. Traditional bioassays in animals are limited to the use of levels high enough to produce an observable response. Virtually none of the data resulting from such bioassays can be used to determine the most appropriate model for interpolation to low doses. For example, even though similar risk estimates were obtained from three common dose-response models (the lognormal, log-logistic, and single-hit models) over a 256-fold experimental dose range at relatively high doses, the projected risks at lower doses were increasingly divergent (Food and Drug Administration Committee on Protocols for Safety Evaluation, 1971). At a dose of 0.01%, which gave a 50% response, the single-hit model yielded a risk estimate 70,000 times higher than that obtained with the log-normal model.

Seriously compounding this uncertainty even further is the selection of the most appropriate basis for expressing the dose. When more meaningful comparative pharmacokinetic data are unavailable, it becomes necessary to select a common unit to express the dose received by various small, short-lived rodent species in order to compare that dose to the dose received by humans. There is no unanimous agreement on whether to express the dose as quantity per unit of body weight, body surface area, or over a lifetime. To calculate the risk to humans from saccharin, the Committee for a Study on Saccharin and Food Safety Policy (National Academy of Sciences, 1978) compared results from four models for high dose to low dose interpolation (the single-hit, multistage, multihit, and probit models) and expressed them as dose received from all three base units (body surface area, body weight, and lifetime). The estimate of risk derived from a Canadian study (Arnold et al., 1980) ranged from 0.001×10^{-6} lifetime cases to $5,200 \times 10^{-6}$ lifetime cases for exposed individuals, a range of 6 orders of magnitude. Most of this variance was attributable to the differing risks predicted by linear and probit models.

The Office of Technology Assessment (OTA) of the U.S. Congress recently issued a report on the assessment of technologies for determining cancer risks from the environment (Office of Technology Assessment, 1981). Although this group accepted the nonthreshold extrapolation from high dose measurements in animals to low dose estimates for humans, it acknowledged that there can be as much as a fortyfold variation in the risk estimate for low doses in humans, depending upon the scaling factor used for determining the relationships between laboratory animals and humans with respect to body size and rate of metabolism. Generally, toxicologists adjust exposures for the differences in scale between species on the basis of milligram per unit of body weight. This provides the lowest estimate of risk to humans. When the experimental dose is measured in parts per million (e.g., mg/kg diet, mg/cm^3 air, or mg/liter water) and humans are exposed through ingestion, the dose of the chemical can be expressed as parts per million. This method is generally used by the Food and Drug Administration (FDA) and, in some cases by the Environmental Protection Agency (EPA), but it produces an estimate of risk in humans 6 times greater than that estimated by the former method if the mouse is the laboratory animal or 3 times greater if the rat is used. Another method used by EPA takes the scale differences between species into account and adjusts exposure on the basis of the relative body surface areas of the test animal and humans. This gives a projected risk for humans 6 to 14 times higher than that of the first method. The fourth approach is to adjust exposures on the basis of relative body weight over a lifetime. This gives a projected risk for humans 40 times higher than that of the first method.

An additional factor to be considered is the shape of the dose-response curve. In general, linear interpolation provides the most conservative estimate. This approach is used by most regulatory agencies and is supported in the OTA report (Office of Technology Assessment, 1981).

The ultimate choice of a model for high to low dose interpolation is, therefore, arbitrary. Not only is there great uncertainty in the mathematical modeling procedures, but also there is no sound biological basis for any of them (Scientific Committee of the Food Safety Council, 1978). The Safe Drinking Water Committee concluded that the most suitable model may be the multistage model because of the multistep nature of carcinogenesis and because of the model's relatively conservative estimate of risk (National Academy of Sciences, 1980a). The committee sees no reason to modify that conclusion except to suggest that it should be reserved for initiators of carcinogenesis and that there should be awareness of the large variability among the heterogeneous human population.

MODIFIERS OF CARCINOGENESIS

For modifiers of carcinogenesis a different approach may have to be considered. There have been few systematic attempts to assess the risk for such compounds. However, the models discussed above may provide some leads to potentially useful approaches, such as time to tumor response, originally defined as the latent period by Armitage and Doll (1961). For example, experiments using doses of the initiator producing a high tumor response would be useful in studying dose-dependent effects of negative modifiers; conversely, experiments that produce barely perceptible responses could be used to examine dose-dependent responses of enhancers of carcinogenesis. Although more data are needed to develop this concept, several investigators have proposed specific mathematical models that incorporate time to tumor response (Druckrey, 1967; Peto et al., 1972; Pike, 1966). Moreover, continuous exposure to a "carcinogen" is considered in some models and time to tumor response has been incorporated as a function of dose in order to yield the age-specific incidence rate (Armitage and Doll, 1961; Crump, 1978; Hartley and Sielken, 1977). Although the time to tumor response may have considerable hypothetical and experimental utility for modifiers of carcinogenesis, such models are severely limited for use in population-based studies because of the unknown contribution and variable distribution of initiators.

Furthermore, withdrawal of an initiator may intercept progression of carcinogenesis (Boutwell 1964; Sivak, 1979; Teebor and Becker, 1971). Halving the dose-dependent progression of carcinogenesis should decrease the final response by that amount, regardless of when such interception occurred (Peto et al., 1981).

The Safe Drinking Water Committee concluded that conventional risk extrapolation methodology accompanied by sufficient data and reasonable models would predict risk to humans from studies in animals using low doses with a precision varying from 1 to 2 orders of magnitude (National Academy of Sciences, 1980a). Because of the differences in individual susceptibility, the precision may, in fact, be much less.

USE OF MUTAGENICITY TESTS

As discussed in Chapter 3, the estimation of risk to humans from exposure to mutagens is beset with uncertainties. First, it is difficult to determine the dose of such substances in the diet. For example, the general population may eat small or very small amounts of some extremely strong mutagens (e.g., aflatoxin B_1) and large quantities of certain weak mutagens (e.g., flavonoids in vegetables), and the capability of our biological defense mechanisms to protect us from either of these is not well understood. Presumably, the effects of such exposure will be a function of potency and dose, both of which extend over a very wide range. To translate the product of potency and dose for a specific mutagen into an estimate of absolute risk for a human population, it is necessary to know how to convert the values of mutagenicity obtained in simple test systems into estimates of carcinogenicity. Unfortunately, no way has been found to predict the carcinogenicity of any specific mutagen. One of the major difficulties in attempting such a determination is the known interspecies variation in susceptibility to the effect of carcinogens and mutagens. Until the variables that control susceptibility are better understood, it is impossible to extrapolate from tests for mutagenicity to obtain estimates of carcinogenicity in humans. Therefore, mutagenicity tests, which usually detect initiators, can be used only as qualitative indicators of possible carcinogenicity. In the absence of evidence derived from epidemiological studies, it is not possible to estimate the likelihood that such substances will affect the occurrence of cancer in humans.

USE OF EPIDEMIOLOGICAL STUDIES

Chapter 3 describes the approach used in epidemiological studies to assess the importance of exposures to carcinogens or risk factors such as diet or dietary components. The risk that disease will occur in humans during a given time period is measured by the incidence of that disease. Incidence can be accumulated over a lifetime in a population to measure cumulative incidence, which is approximately equivalent to the lifetime risk of disease (Day, 1976).

In cohort studies, the incidence of disease is measured directly: the ratio of incidence in exposed and unexposed cohorts provides a measure of the relative risk. The difference in incidence of disease between exposed and unexposed groups provides a second measure of risk--the attributable risk, which is simply the proportion of disease that can be attributed to the exposure to that particular variable, if it is causal. Such measurements of risk are valid only if the two populations compared differ only by the exposure (variable) being studied and if other factors influencing the risk of disease are controlled in the analysis. The derivation of the attributable risk is dependent on the reasonable assumption that the exposed group would have had an incidence similar to that of the unexposed group if it had not been exposed.

In case-control studies, estimates of the relative risk can be derived. A large body of statistical and epidemiological literature has accumulated to confirm that the odds ratios derived from case-control studies are approximately equivalent to the relative risk determined in cohort studies. Indeed, the same terminology is normally used in both types of studies. Estimates of population-attributable risk can also be derived from case-control studies. Such estimates are equivalent to those expected in the general population, provided that the cases and the controls are representative of their respective target populations so that estimates of exposure in the population can be derived from the control series.

These estimates of risk do not take into account the extent to which risk may vary with age. Almost invariably there is a latent period between first exposure and the expression of a risk. For many diseases, risk may appear to remain constant with age, but risk may decrease in older groups because the population may have lost most persons susceptible to the effect, especially if a risk factor or constellation of risk factors is responsible for more than one disease and if these diseases are relatively common in a population or because of a birth cohort effect that is increasing. An additional complexity is that risk may vary in populations because the extent of exposures to various risk factors may vary with time. This may lead to different expectations of lifetime incidence for different birth cohorts. In this respect, incidence among different age groups during the same time period may not accurately reflect the expected lifetime incidence in a population. For example, there has been a decline in risk for tuberculosis in successive cohorts in the United States. The risk for this disease in the present generation is largely restricted to elderly males. Another example is the risk for lung cancer, which has been increasing with successive cohorts, especially among males, so that cross-sectional incidence curves show maximum risk at middle ages and declining risk at older ages. For cervical cancer, there have been complex birth cohort effects. For example, those who were in their twenties during the depression years show a low incidence of cervical cancer, whereas others, particularly those who are now in their twenties, appear to have a higher incidence. Thus, it is difficult to interpret trends in incidence. However, for most of the cancers believed to be influenced by diet and nutrition, the incidence has been relatively stable for many years. Therefore, estimates of the proportion of these cancers attributable to dietary factors are not likely to be severely in error because of differences in risk encountered by different birth cohorts.

Because the causation of cancer is often multifactorial, the summation of estimates of the percentage of cancers attributable to individual factors often exceeds 100%. However, this does not invalidate the concept. Rather, it indicates that it may be possible to adopt different approaches to preventing a number of cancers.

DIET-RELATED CARCINOGENESIS

Given the limitations of traditional methods of risk assessment using data from experimental and epidemiological studies, what factors would be the most appropriate to consider in analysis of risk for diet-related carcinogenesis?

Because food contains both initiators and modifiers of carcinogenesis, there is a need for two very different kinds of risk analysis. For the initiators (mostly nonnutritive components of food), the Safe Drinking Water Committee's conclusion that a multistage mathematical model would be most appropriate (National Academy of Sciences, 1980a) is still considered to be valid. For the modifiers in food (including nutrients and nonnutritive substances), a mathematical model that includes time to tumor response may be preferable. For enhancers, an experimental titration of a dose of the modifier, which has a potency for increasing a near-zero tumorigenic response, may be an acceptable approach. Conversely, for inhibitors, titration of the dose of the modifier with the potency for eliminating nearly 100% of the response may be preferable. Any experiment to determine the carcinogenic response to a dose of a nutrient will be specific for the initiator, species, diet, and other experimental variables used in the test.

Caution will have to be exercised when extrapolating the resultant data to humans. In general, such extrapolation should initially be limited to qualitative rather than to quantitative conclusions. Greater confidence in the initial results may be gained by testing more initiators, species, and diets. The necessity for testing additional diets arises from the knowledge that there is an extremely broad array of nutrient-nutrient interactions. Thus, these reactions must be considered when selecting the new diets to be tested.

As new data become available, it may become possible to do more quantitative extrapolation from the test species to humans with respect to the risk from nutrient intake. The specific dose-response relationship for the effects of nutrients on carcinogenesis will necessarily be limited by the requirement for nutrients for metabolic functions. This suggests, therefore, that "risk" from nutrient intake should be defined in terms of the Recommended Dietary Allowances (RDA) (National Academy of Sciences, 1980c).

Beginning with the RDA's as the point of reference, the "risk" for a nutrient could be defined in terms of RDA multiples (or fractions thereof). This approach would introduce a broader perspective into the interpretation of the "carcinogenic" effects of nutrients. It would acknowledge that nutrients are essential and admit the existence of some level of risk, even if that risk were negligible. The dose-response slope constants will undoubtedly differ for various nutrients, and acceptable upper limits of intake, however arbitrary, will vary broadly as functions of the RDA's for different nutrients. Analogous phenomena for noncarcinogenic toxicity of nutrients have been evaluated elsewhere (Campbell et al., 1980; National Nutrition Consortium, 1978).

The Food and Nutrition Board's most recent edition of the Recommended Dietary Allowances (National Academy of Sciences, 1980c) provides ranges of intake for three vitamins and six minerals, the upper limits being defined as "safe" on the basis of available information. But, it is clear that epidemiological studies will be needed to confirm or deny whatever risk estimates for nutrient intake may be obtained from experiments in animals.

Doll and Peto (1981) suggest that laboratory data may be used for setting priorities for regulation. However, they point out that even tests in animals are unreliable, suffering not only from random errors, but also probably from large systematic errors of unknown direction and magnitude. Since there are thousands of chemicals that affect carcinogenesis to some extent or other, in one laboratory test or another, it is difficult to determine what, if any, practicable regulations should be enacted on the basis of laboratory tests. Nevertheless, they suggest that an appropriate use of results from laboratory tests might be to estimate risk for humans by multiplying the potency of each chemical studied by estimates, however crude, of the degree to which humans are exposed to that chemical. This would yield an index of risk for humans. Resultant estimates might provide a basis from which priorities for regulatory action could be determined.

There is one major difficulty with this approach. Although experimental or epidemiological studies may have identified risk factors as either potentially hazardous or protective for humans, it is difficult to label many of them as carcinogens or modifiers of carcinogenesis. Furthermore, even if such assessments were possible, the feasibility of modifying the diet of humans would have to be considered.

It is impossible to enact regulations pertaining to diet, except for those few substances that clearly qualify as food additives, which are currently regulated according to the provisions in the Delaney Clause (see Section B). Thus, it may not be appropriate to assess priorities for regulatory action at this time, especially since changes in the economy and in the sources of our food supply may well combine to impose dietary changes upon us. The dietary changes now under way appear to be reducing our dependence on foods from animal sources. It is likely that there will be continued reduction in fats from animal sources and an increasing dependence on vegetable and other plant products for protein supplies. Hence, diets may contain increasing amounts of vegetable products, some of which may be protective against cancer. However, if it is decided that changes have to be instigated, we should consider reducing exposure of the population to total dietary fat and increasing exposure to protective substances such as those found in fruits and vegetables, while ensuring the maintenance of an ideal body weight for height and well-balanced but varied nutrition.

CONTRIBUTION OF DIET TO OVERALL RISK OF CANCER

Higginson and Muir (1979) estimated the proportion of cancers related to various aspects of the environment. They believed that precise proportions of cancer incidence could not be attributed to diet, but they did include dietary factors among the general heading "Lifestyle." They estimated that possibly 30% of cancers in men and 60% in women in the

Birmingham and West Midland regions of England and Wales could be attributed to lifestyle. Wynder and Gori (1977) were more specific. On the basis of international and intranational comparisons of cancer incidence, the differences between U.S. mortality rates and the lowest reported worldwide mortality rates for each site, and results of specific case-control studies, they concluded that a little more than 40% of cancers in men and almost 60% of cancers in women in the United States could be attributed to dietary factors.

Using a similar approach, Doll and Peto (1981) were somewhat more cautious. They agreed that a substantial proportion of cancers in both sexes in the United States was likely to be attributable to dietary factors, but, by surveying the literature, they provided a rather wide range of estimates (i.e., 10% to 70%) for the proportion of deaths from cancer that could be reduced by practical dietary means. They stated that it might not be possible to achieve a large reduction in the near future, but that dietary modifications might eventually result in a 35% reduction of deaths from cancer in the United States. This reduction was estimated to include a 90% reduction in deaths from cancers of the stomach and large bowel; a 50% reduction in deaths from cancers of the endometrium, gallbladder, pancreas, and breast; a 20% reduction in deaths from cancers of the lung, larynx, bladder, cervix, mouth, pharynx, and esophagus; and a 10% reduction in deaths from other sites. These investigators placed a greater degree of confidence in the projected 35% reduction in overall mortality than in the estimated contribution from specific groups of cancer sites.

Only two case-control studies of dietary factors and cancer provided estimates of the proportion of cancers at specific sites that are attributable to dietary factors. On the basis of a case-control study of breast cancer in Canada, Miller (1978) estimated that 27% of the risk of breast cancer for women was attributable to total dietary fat intake. For colorectal cancer, Jain et al. (1980) estimated that 41% of the risk for males and 44% of the risk for females was attributable to saturated fat intake. Both of these estimates are probably too low, because artifacts in the diet tend to lead to low estimates of relative risk (Marshall et al., 1981). This is particularly true for breast cancer, since estimated effects of dietary factors based on current intake are likely to be substantially below the true effect for a factor that is operational earlier in life, possibly during adolescence.

The evidence reviewed by the committee suggests that cancers of most major sites are influenced by dietary patterns. However, the committee concluded that the data are not sufficient to quantitate the contribution of diet to the overall cancer risk or to determine the percent reduction in risk that might be achieved by dietary modifications.

REFERENCES

Alberti, K. G. M. M. 1980. Metabolic pathways--Hormone-metabolite interrelations. Pp. 5-19 in S. J. Karran and K. G. M. M. Alberti, eds. Practical Nutritional Support. Pitman Medical Publishing Co., Tunbridge Wells, Kent, England.

Armitage, P., and R. Doll. 1961. Stochastic models for carcinogenesis. Pp. 19-38 in Proceedings of the Fourth Berkeley Symposium on Mathematical Statistics and Probability. Volume 4, Contributions to Biology and Problems of Medicine. University of California Press, Berkeley and Los Angeles.

Arnold, D. L., C. A. Moodie, H. C. Grice, S. M. Charbonneau, B. Stavric, B. T. Collins, P. F. McGuire, Z. Z. Zawidzka, and I. C. Munro. 1980. Long-term toxicity of ortho-toluenesulfonamide and sodium saccharin in the rat. Toxicol. Appl. Pharmacol. 52:113-152.

Axelrod, A. E. 1980. Nutrition in relation to immunity. Pp. 578-591 in R. S. Goodhart and M. E. Shils, eds. Modern Nutrition in Health and Disease. Lea and Febiger, Philadelphia.

Boutwell, R. K. 1964. Some biological aspects of skin carcinogenesis. Prog. Exp. Tumor Res. 4:207-250.

Boyland, E., and A. A. Levi. 1935. Metabolism of polycyclic compounds. I. Production of dihydroxydihydroanthracene from anthracene. Biochem. J. 29:2679-2683.

Bruce, W. R., A. J. Varghese, R. Furrer, and P. C. Land. 1977. A mutagen in the feces of normal humans. Pp. 1641-1646 in H. H. Hiatt, J. E. Watson, and J. D. Winsten, eds. Origins of Human Cancer, Book C. Human Risk Assessment. Cold Spring Harbor Laboratory, Cold Spring Harbor, N.Y.

Campbell, T. C. 1979. Influence of nutrition on metabolism of carcinogens. Adv. Nutr. Res. 2:29-55.

Campbell, T. C., R. G. Allison, and C. J. Carr. 1980. Feasibility of Identifying Adverse Health Effects of Vitamins and Essential Minerals in Man. Prepared for Bureau of Foods, Food and Drug Administration, Washington, D. C. under Contract Number FDA 223-75-2090. Life Sciences Research Office, Federation of American Societies for Experimental Biology, Bethesda, Md. 76 pp.

Conney, A. H. 1967. Pharmacological implications of microsomal enzyme induction. Pharmacol. Rev. 19:317-366.

Cornfield, J. 1977. Carcinogenic risk assessment. Science 198:693-699.

Crump, K. S. 1978. Low dose extrapolation of animal carcinogenicity data. Biometrics 34:155. Abstract 2568.

Day, N. E. 1976. A new measure of age standardized incidence, the cumulative rate. Pp. 443-445 in J. Waterhouse, C. Muir, P. Correa, and J. Powell, eds. Cancer Incidence in Five Continents, Volume 3. IARC Scientific Publications No. 15, International Agency for Research on Cancer, Lyon, France.

Doll, R., and A. B. Hill. 1964. Mortality in relation to smoking: Ten years' observations of British doctors. Br. Med. J. 1:1399-1410; 1460-1467.

Doll, R., and R. Peto. 1981. The causes of cancer: Quantitative estimates of avoidable risks of cancer in the United States today. J. Natl. Cancer Inst. 66:1192-1308.

Druckrey, H. F. 1967. Quantitative aspects in chemical carcinogenesis. Pp. 60-77 in R. Truhaut, ed. Potential Carcinogenic Hazards from Drugs: Evaluation of Risks. UICC Monograph Series, Volume 7, Springer-Verlag, Berlin, Heidelberg, and New York.

Finney, D. J. 1952. Probit Analysis. 2nd Edition. Cambridge University Press, London and New York. 318 pp.

Food and Drug Administration Committee on Protocols for Safety Evaluation. 1971. Panel on Carcinogenesis Report on Cancer Testing in the Safety Evaluation of Food Additives and Pesticides. Toxicol. Appl. Pharmacol. 20:419-438.

Gehring, P. J., and G. E. Blau. 1977. Mechanisms of carcinogenesis: Dose response. J. Environ. Pathol. Toxicol. 1(1):163-179.

Gross, R. L., and P. M. Newberne. 1980. Role of nutrition in immunologic function. Physiol. Rev. 60:188-302.

Hartley, H. O., and R. L. Sielken, Jr. 1977. Estimation of "safe doses" in carcinogenic experiments. Biometrics 33:1-30.

Higginson, J., and C. S. Muir. 1979. Environmental carcinogenesis: Misconceptions and limitations to cancer control. J. Natl. Cancer Inst. 63:1291-1298.

Jain, M., G. M. Cook, F. G. Davis, M. G. Grace, G. R. Howe, and A. B. Miller. 1980. A case-control study of diet and colo-rectal cancer. Int. J. Cancer 26:757-768.

Lehman, A. J., and O. G. Fitzhugh. 1954. 100-fold margin of safety. Q. Bull. Assoc. Food Drug Off. U. S. 18:33-35.

Magee, P. N., A. E. Pegg, and P. F. Swann. 1975. Molecular mechanisms of chemical carcinogenesis. Pp. 329-419 in E. Grundmann, ed. Handbuch der Allgemeinen Pathologie, Bd. 6, T. 6., Geschwülste-Tumors II. Springer-Verlag, Berlin, Heidelberg, and New York.

Marshall, J. R., R. Priore, S. Graham, and J. Brasure. 1981. On the distortion of risk estimates in multiple exposure level case-control studies. Am. J. Epidemiol. 113:464-473.

McCann, J., E. Choi, E. Yamasaki, and B. N. Ames. 1975. Detection of carcinogens as mutagens in the Salmonella/microsome test: Assay of 300 chemicals. Proc. Natl. Acad. Sci. U.S.A. 72:5135-5139.

Miller, A. B. 1978. An overview of hormone-associated cancers. Cancer Res. 38:3985-3990.

Miller, J. A. 1970. Carcinogenesis by chemicals: An overview--G. H. A. Clowes memorial lecture. Cancer Res. 30:559-576.

National Academy of Sciences. 1977. Chemical contaminants: Safety and risk assessment. Pp. 19-62 in Drinking Water and Health. A report prepared by the Safe Drinking Water Committee. National Academy of Sciences, Washington, D.C.

National Academy of Sciences. 1978. Saccharin: Technical Assessment of Risks and Benefits. Part 1 of a 2-part study of the Committee for a Study on Saccharin and Food Safety Policy. National Academy of Sciences, Washington, D.C. [240] pp.

National Academy of Sciences. 1980a. Problems of risk estimation. Pp. 25-65 in Drinking Water and Health. Volume 3. A report of the Safe Drinking Water Committee. National Academy Press, Washington, D.C.

National Academy of Sciences. 1980b. Regulating Pesticides. A report prepared by the Committee on Prototype Explicit Analyses for Pesticides. National Academy of Sciences, Washington, D.C. 288 pp.

National Academy of Sciences. 1980c. Recommended Dietary Allowances, 9th edition. A report of the Committee on Dietary Allowances, Food and Nutrition Board. National Academy of Sciences, Washington, D.C. 187 pp.

National Nutrition Consortium. 1978. Vitamin-Mineral Safety, Toxicity, and Misuse. Report of the Committee on Safety, Toxicity, and Misuse of Vitamins and Trace Minerals. American Dietetic Association, Chicago, Ill. 36 pp.

Office of Technology Assessment. 1981. Assessment of Technologies for Determining Cancer Risks from the Environment. Office of Technology Assessment, Congress of the United States, Washington, D.C. 242 pp.

Peto, R., P. N. Lee, and W. S. Paige. 1972. Statistical analysis of the bioassay of continuous carcinogens. Br. J. Cancer 26:258-261.

Peto, R., R. Doll, J. D. Buckley, and M. B. Sporn. 1981. Can dietary beta-carotene materially reduce human cancer rates? Nature 290:201-208.

Pike, M. C. 1966. A method of analysis of a certain class of experiments in carcinogenesis. Biometrics 22:142-161.

Purchase, I. F. H., E. Longstaff, J. Ashby, J. A. Styles, D. Anderson, P. A. Lefevre, and F. R. Westwood. 1978. An evaluation of 6 short-term tests for detecting organic chemical carcinogens. Br. J. Cancer 37:873-959.

Roe, F. J. C., and J. Clack. 1963. Two-stage carcinogenesis: Effect of length of promoting treatment on the yield of benign and malignant tumours. Br. J. Cancer 17:596-604.

Scientific Committee, Food Safety Council. 1978. Proposed system for food safety assessment. Food Cosmet. Toxicol. 16(Suppl. 2):1-136.

Sivak, A. 1979. Cocarcinogenesis. Biochim. Biophys. Acta 560:67-89.

Slaga, T. J. 1980. Cancer: Etiology, mechanisms, and prevention--A summary. Pp. 243-262 in T. J. Slaga, ed. Carcinogenesis--A Comprehensive Survey. Volume 5: Modifiers of Chemical Carcinogenesis. Raven Press, New York.

Sugimura, T., S. Sato, M. Nagao, T. Yahagi, T. Matsushima, Y. Seino, M. Takeuchi, and T. Kawachi. 1976. Overlapping of carcinogens and mutagens. Pp. 191-213 in P. N. Magee, S. Takayama, T. Sugimura, and T. Matsushima, eds. Fundamentals in Cancer Prevention. University Park Press, Baltimore, London, and Tokyo.

Teebor, G. W., and F. F. Becker. 1971. Regression and persistence of hyperplastic hepatic nodules induced by N-2-fluorenylacetamide and their relationship to hepatocarcinogenesis. Cancer Res. 31:1-3.

Turner, M. E., Jr. 1975. Some classes of hit-theory models. Math. Bioscience 23:219-235.

World Health Organization. 1958. Procedures for the Testing of Intentional Food Additives to Establish Their Safety for Use. Second Report of the Joint FAO/WHO Expert Committee on Food Additives. W.H.O. Tech. Rep. Ser. 144:1-19.

World Health Organization. 1972. Evaluation of Certain Food Additives and the Contaminants Mercury, Lead, and Cadmium. Sixteenth Report of the Joint FAO/WHO Expert Committee on Food Additives. W.H.O. Tech. Rep. Ser. 505:1-32.

Wynder, E. L., and G. B. Gori. 1977. Contribution of the environment to cancer incidence: An epidemiologic exercise. J. Natl. Cancer Inst. 58:825-832.

Glossary

Acceptable daily intake (ADI): The daily dosage of a drug or a chemical residue that appears to present no appreciable risk to health during the entire lifetime of a human being.

Age-adjusted cancer incidence or mortality: The incidence or mortality rate for cancer, adjusted for differences in the age distribution of the populations being compared, i.e., the study population and a standard reference population.

Anticarcinogen: A substance that inhibits or eliminates the activity of a carcinogen.

Antimutagen: A substance that inhibits or eliminates the activity of a mutagen.

Antioxidant: A substance that retards oxidation. Examples include vitamin C, vitamin E, and butylated hydroxyanisole (BHA).

Benign tumor: A tumor that is confined to the territory in which it arises, i.e., it does not invade surrounding tissue or metastasize to distant organs. These tumors can usually be excised by local surgery.

Bioassay: A test in which living organisms are used.

Cancer: Any of the various types of malignant neoplasms. See malignant tumor, neoplasm.

Carcinogen: A chemical, physical, or biological agent that increases the incidence of cancer.

Carcinoma: Cancer in an epithelial tissue, including external epithelia (mainly skin and linings of the gastrointestinal tract, lungs, and cervix) and internal epithelia (which line glands such as the breast, pancreas, and thyroid).

Cocarcinogenesis: A general term that refers to augmentation of tumor induction.

Cohort: 1. A group of people with a defined history of exposure who are studied for a specific length of time to determine cancer incidence or mortality. 2. A group of individuals born within the same time period (usually within 5 or sometimes 10 years of each

447

other). Such groups are called "birth cohorts." The diseases among individuals in one birth cohort followed throughout their lifetimes may be different from those in another, implying differences in exposures to factors causing disease.

Complete carcinogen: An agent that can act as both initiator and promoter.

Comutagen: A nonmutagenic substance that enhances the activity of a mutagen or imparts mutagenic activity to another nonmutagenic substance.

Contaminant: A substance that is present in foods or feed but is not intentionally added.

Delaney Clause: Legislation passed by the U.S. Congress in 1958 that forbids the addition to food any additives shown to be carcinogenic in any species of animal or in humans.

Diet: The total composition of ingested food, including nutrients, naturally occurring contaminants, and additives.

Dietary factors: Substances that are present in or characteristics that are associated with the diet; for example, the amount of total fat, dietary fiber, the ratio of saturated versus unsaturated fat, and the method of cooking.

Environment: Anything external to humans, i.e., lifestyle factors and anything to which humans are exposed, including all forms of radiation and substances eaten, drunk, and inhaled. See lifestyle factors.

Epidemiology: The study of the distribution of diseases and their determinants in human populations.

Epigenetic: As used in reference to cancer, an effect that does not directly involve a change in the sequence of bases in DNA.

Dietary fiber: Generic name for plant materials that are resistant to the action of normal digestive enzymes.

Food additive: Any substance that is added to food, either directly or indirectly.

Food disappearance data or per capita intake. Crude estimates of food or nutrients available for consumption by a specified population; based on food production, imports, exports, etc. They do not reflect the amount consumed since approximately 20% of the food is probably discarded, wasted, or spoiled. In the absence of data on actual food consumption, however, it may be the closest approximation of the per capita dietary intake of that population.

Genotoxicity: The quality of being damaging to genetic material.

Hyperplasia: An increase in the number of cells in a tissue or organ.

Incidence: The number of new cases of a disease expressed as a rate, i.e., the number of new cases of a disease occurring in a given population during a specific period, divided by the total number of persons at risk of developing the disease during that same period.

Initiator: An external stimulus or agent that produces a cell that can become malignant under certain conditions. Initiation events may be mutational changes in a cell's genetic material, where the change is initially unexpressed and causes no detectable alteration in the cell's growth pattern. The change is considered to be irreversible.

Latency or latent period: The interval between the first exposure to a carcinogenic stimulus and the appearance of a clinically diagnosable tumor. For a disease like cancer, which usually involves a sequence of steps over a long period, the term "latent period" may be ambiguous.

Leukemia: Cancers of the blood-forming organs, characterized by abnormal proliferation and development of leukocytes (white blood cells) and their precursors in the blood, lymph, bone marrow, and lymph glands.

Lifestyle factors: Identifiable and quantifiable parameters of living (e.g., diet, smoking, drinking, hobbies) that are useful in distinguishing population groups for epidemiological studies.

Lymphoma: A cancer of cells of the immune system (e.g., lymphocytes), where the tumor is confined to lymph glands and related tissues, such as the spleen.

Malignant tumor: A tumor with the potential for invading neighboring tissue and/or metastasizing to distant body sites, or one that has already done so.

Melanoma: Malignant melanoma is a cancer of the cells that produce the pigment melanin.

Menarche: The age at which menstruation begins.

Metaplasia: The abnormal transformation of an adult (mature), fully differentiated tissue of one kind into differentiated tissue of another kind.

Metastasis: The spread of a malignancy to distant body sites by cancer cells transported in blood or lymph circulation.

Modifier: A substance that can alter the course of carcinogenesis.

Morbidity: The condition of being diseased, or the incidence or prevalence of some particular disease. The morbidity rate is equivalent to the incidence rate.

Mortality: The number of overall deaths, or deaths from a specific disease, usually expressed as a rate, i.e., the number of deaths from a disease in a given population during a specified period, divided by the average number of people exposed to the disease and at risk of dying from the disease during that time.

Mutagen: A chemical or physical agent that interacts with DNA to cause a permanent, transmissible change in the genetic material of a cell.

Multiple myeloma: A malignant neoplasm of plasma cells usually arising in the bone marrow. Also called myelomatosis.

Neoplasm: A new growth of tissue with the potential for uncontrolled and progressive growth. A neoplasm may be benign or malignant.

Nutrient: A component of food (e.g., protein, fat, carbohydrates, vitamins, minerals) that provides nourishment for growth and maintenance of the organism.

Nutrition: The sum of the processes by which an organism utilizes the chemical components of food (which may or may not be synthesized in vivo) through metabolism to maintain the structural and biochemical integrity of its cells, thereby ensuring its viability and reproductive potential.

Papilloma: A benign epithelial neoplasm.

Per capita intake: See food disappearance data.

Permissible residue: The quantity of a residue (e.g., a pesticide residue in or on a food crop) permitted when the product is first made available for consumption. The value may be calculated from the ADI (See acceptable daily intake).

Precancerous lesion: A lesion or visible abnormality that has a significant probability of later developing into cancer.

Prevalence (point prevalence): The number of existing cases of a disease, usually expressed as a proportion, i.e., number of cases of a disease in a given population at a specified time, divided by the estimated number of eligible persons in the population at that same time.

Promoter: An agent that causes an initiated cell to produce a tumor after prolonged exposure. Promotion events or, more generally, late events can occur only in "initiated" cells and are somewhat reversible. Discontinuation of exposure to a promoter before tumor development may prevent the appearance of a tumor.

Pyrolysis: The decomposition of a substance by heat.

Recommended Dietary Allowance (RDA): The level of intake of essential nutrients that is adequate to meet the nutritional needs of practically all healthy persons, as judged by the Committee on Dietary Allowances of the Food and Nutrition Board, National Research Council.

Risk: As used in epidemiological sections of this report, risk refers to the probability of occurrence of a disease (cancer) in a given population.

Relative risk: An estimate obtained by dividing the incidence of cancer in the exposed group by the incidence in the corresponding unexposed or control group.

Sarcoma: Cancers of various supporting tissues of the body (e.g., bone cells, blood vessels, fibrous tissue cells, muscle).

Synergism: When two or more substances enhance each other's effects, achieving more than the sum of their individual effects.

Threshold dose: A non-zero dose below which exposure is safe and not associated with risk.

Tolerance level: The maximum level or concentration of a drug or chemical that is permitted in or on food at a specified time during slaughter (or harvesting), processing, storage, and marketing up to the time of consumption by an animal or human being.

Transformed cell: A cell that has undergone both initiation and promotion and has the potential for leading to the develement of a neoplasm.

Tumor: An uncontrolled and progressive growth of tissue. A neoplasm. It encompasses both benign and malignant neoplasms, but occasionally may refer merely to a swelling of tissue.

Unintentional residue or contaminant: The residue of a compound in feed or food resulting from circumstances not intended to protect the feed or food against attack by infectious or parasitic diseases. The residue may be acquired during any phase in the growth, production, processing, or storage of feed or food.

Appendix A Committee on Diet, Nutrition, and Cancer— Affiliations and Major Research Interests

CHAIRMAN:

Clifford Grobstein
Professor of Biological Sciences
  and Public Policy
University of California
San Diego, Calif.
Major interests: Developmental
  biology and biomedical tech-
  nology assessment

VICE CHAIRMAN:

John Cairns
Professor
Department of Microbiology
Harvard School of Public
  Health
Boston, Mass.
Major interest: Molecular biology

MEMBERS:

Robert J. Berliner
Dean
Yale University
School of Medicine
New Haven, Conn.
Major interests: Physiology of
  the kidney, particulary with
  respect to fluid and electrolyte
  transport

Selwyn A. Broitman
Assistant Dean and Professor of
  Microbiology and Nutritional
  Sciences
Department of Microbiology
Boston University School of
  Medicine
Boston, Mass.
Major interests: Intestinal
  microflora and experimental
  gastroenterology

MEMBERS (CONTINUED)

T. Colin Campbell
Professor of Nutritional
  Biochemistry and
Director of Nutrition and
  Cancer Program Project
Division of Nutritional
  Sciences
Cornell University
Ithaca, N.Y.
Major interests: Mechanisms
  of nutrient effects on
  chemical carcinogenesis, afla-
  toxin-induced hepatocarcino-
  genesis, and carcinogen metabolism

Joan Dye Gussow
Chair
Department of Nutrition Education
Teachers College
Columbia University
New York, N.Y.
Major interests: Social and
  technological changes affecting
  the human food chain

Laurence N. Kolonel
Director
Epidemiology Program,
  Cancer Center of Hawaii and
Professor of Public Health
University of Hawaii
Honolulu, Hawaii
Major interest: Cancer epidemiology

David Kritchevsky
Associate Director
Wistar Institute
Philadelphia, Pa.
Major interests: Lipid metabolism
  and atherosclerosis

453

A-1

MEMBERS (CONTINUED):

Walter Mertz
Director
Human Nutrition Research Center
Agricultural Research Service
U.S. Department of Agriculture
Beltsville, Md.
Major interests: Nutrition and
    trace elements

Anthony Bernard Miller
Director
National Cancer Institute of Canada
    Epidemiology Unit and
Professor
Preventive Medicine and Biostatis-
    tics
Division of Community Health
University of Toronto
Toronto, Canada
Major interest: Cancer epidemiology

Michael J. Prival
Research Microbiologist
Genetic Toxicology Branch
U.S. Food and Drug Administration
Washington, D.C.
Major interest: Mutagenicity testing
    using bacteria

Thomas Joseph Slaga
Senior Staff Member
Biology Division
Oak Ridge National
    Laboratory
Oak Ridge, Tenn.
Major interests: Chemical
    carcinogenesis, pharma-
    cology, biochemical endo-
    crinology, and gene
    regulations

MEMBERS (CONTINUED):

Lee W. Wattenberg
Professor
Department of Laboratory
    Medicine and Pathology
University of Minnesota
    Medical School
Minneapolis, Minn.
Major interests: Chemical
    carcinogenesis and chemo-
    prevention

ADVISOR:

Takashi Sugimura
Director
National Cancer Center
    Research Institute, Tokyo, and
Professor, Institute of Medical
    Sciences
Tokyo University
Tokyo, Japan
Major interests: Chemical
    carcinogenesis and bio-
    chemistry

NATIONAL RESEARCH COUNCIL STAFF:

Sushma Palmer
Project Director
Assembly of Life Sciences and
Adjunct Assistant Professor
    of Pediatrics
Georgetown University
    School of Medicine
Washington, D.C.
Major interests: Nutrition,
    growth and development,
    and nutrition and immune
    response

NRC STAFF (CONTINUED):

Kulbir Bakshi
Staff Scientist
Assembly of Life Sciences and
Adjunct Graduate Assistant Professor
Howard University
Washington, D.C.
Major interest: Chemical
  mutagenesis

Robert Hilton
Research Associate
Assembly of Life Sciences
Washington, D.C.
Major interest: General biology

Frances Peter
Editor
Assembly of Life Sciences
Washington, D.C.
Major interest: Scientific
  communication

Index

A

AαC (2-amino-9H-pyrido
  [2,3-b]indole),
  280-284 *passim**
absinthe, 202
Acceptable Daily Intake
  (ADI), 321, 324,
  431-432
achlorhydria, 172, 393
acrylonitrile, 13, 315,
  332; *see also*
  food additives
additives, food, *see*
  food additives
adriamycin, 292
aflatoxins, 12, 26, 42,
  87, 112-115
  passim, 142, 151,
  204, 234-240, 257,
  291, 392, 401, 402,
  435; *see also*
  mycotoxins
agar, 133
Agaricus bisporus
  (mushroom), 240,
  242, 257
agaritine, 240
age, and cancer, 376-377
air, 1, 23, 24, 162,
  253, 279
alcohol consumption
  alimentary tract
    cancer and, 205
  and cancer, 11, 16,
    108, 202-208, 383
  carcinogens and,
    206-208 *passim*
  cigarette smoking and,
    11, 16, 205-206,
    207, 208, 391
  colon cancer and,
    203, 400
  colorectal cancer
    and, 11, 202-203,
    208, 400
  epidemiological
    evidence on, 202-206

esophageal cancer
    and, 11, 140, 144,
    202-208 *passim*,
    391-393, 402
  experimental evidence
    on, 206-208
  gastrointestinal
    cancer and, 16, 202
  head and neck cancer
    and, 206
  intestinal cancer
    and, 108, 400
  kidney cancer and,
    202
  laryngeal cancer and,
    11, 139, 145, 202,
    204, 208, 383, 391
  liver cancer and, 11,
    204, 208, 401-402
  lung cancer and, 202,
    204
  malnutrition and, 206
  mechanisms for cancer
    induction, 205,
    206-208
  microsomal enzymes
    and, 207
  Mormons and, 381
  nutritional status
    and, 206
  oral cavity cancer
    and, 11, 202-208
    passim, 383, 391
  pancreatic cancer
    and, 202, 403
  pharyngeal cancer
    and, 202, 204
  Plummer-Vinson
    syndrome and, 206
  prostate cancer and,
    202
  rectal cancer and,
    202, 203, 208, 400,
    401
  renal cancer and, 406
  respiratory tract
    cancer and, 11, 16,
    205, 206, 208

stomach cancer and,
    202
  urinary bladder
    cancer and, 406
  vinyl chloride and,
    313
  *see also specific
    alcoholic beverages*
alcoholic beverages, *see*
  alcohol consumption
  *and specific
  alcoholic beverages*
aldicarb, 319, 323, 324
aldrin, 319
alfalfa, 133, 245, 364
alimentary tract cancer
  alcohol consumption
    and, 205
  cigarette smoking
    and, 205
  iron and, 173
alkyl derivatives, 285
alkylating agents, 39,
  277
allylic benzene deriva-
  tives, 243-244
almonds, 235
American Cancer Society,
  381
Ames test, 39, 185, 207
  243-251 *passim*,
  257, 278, 307, 311,
  314, 315, 317, 328,
  330, 331; *see also*
  mutagenicity tests;
  *Salmonella
  typhimurium*
amides, 145, 252, 396
amines, 144, 145, 247,
  252, 253, 254, 285,
  396
amino acids
  deficiency, 109-112
  hydrolysate, 89
  leukemia and, 110
  mutagens from, 279-284
  protein and, 42-43,
    109-112, 114

---

*Subject mentioned at intervals throughout page range cited.

W

X